Evaluating Research in Health and Social Care

EDITED BY
Roger Gomm, Gill Needham and Anne Bullman

The Open
University

in association with

SAGE Publications
London • Thousand Oaks • New Delhi

SAGE Publications Ltd
6 Bonhill Street
London EC2A 4PU

SAGE Publications Inc
2455 Teller Road
Thousand Oaks, California 91320

SAGE Publications India Pvt Ltd
32, M-Block Market
Greater Kailash – I
New Delhi 110 048

British Library Cataloguing in Publication data

A catalogue record for this book is
available from the British Library

ISBN 0 7619 6490 8
ISBN 0 7619 6491 6 (pbk)

Library of Congress catalog card record available

Typeset by Photoprint, Torquay, Devon
Printed in Great Britain by The Cromwell Press Ltd,
Trowbridge, Wiltshire

CONTENTS

Resource Chapters

PART 2 SURVEY RESEARCH

Exemplar Chapters

Resource Chapters

PART 3   QUALITATIVE RESEARCH
Exemplar Chapters

Resource Chapter

PART 4   RESEARCH APPRAISAL QUESTIONS

ACKNOWLEDGEMENTS

The majority of resource materials that illustrate this book have been abbreviated as appropriate to the overall theme and purpose of this collection.

The editors and publishers are grateful to both the authors and original publishers and wish to thank the following for permission to use copyright material.

Chapter 1: EMAP for I. Wilkinson, S. Buttfield, S. Cooper and E. Young (1997) 'Trial of two bandaging systems for chronic venous leg ulcers', *Journal of Wound Care*, 6 (7): 339–40.

Chapter 2: The Lancet Ltd for M. Marshall, A. Lockwood and D. Gath (1995) 'Social Services case-management for long-term mental disorders: a randomised controlled trial', *The Lancet*, 345 (8947): 409–12.

Chapter 3: BMJ Publishing Group for S. Shepperd, D. Harwood, A. Gray, M. Vessey and P. Morgan (1998) 'Randomised controlled trial comparing hospital at home care with inpatient hospital care. II: cost minimisation analysis', *British Medical Journal*, 316: 1791–6.

Chapter 4: BMJ Publishing Group for I. Roberts, M.S. Kramer and S. Suissa (1996) 'Does home visiting prevent childhood injury? A systematic review of randomised controlled trials', *British Medical Journal*, 312: 29–33.

Chapter 8: BMJ Publishing Group for G. Cohen, J. Forbes and M. Garraway (1996) 'Can different patient satisfaction survey methods yield consistent results? Comparison of three surveys', *British Medical Journal*, 313: 841–4.

Chapter 9: BMJ Publishing Group for N. Payne and C. Saul (1997) 'Variations in use of cardiology services in a health authority: comparison of artery revascularisation rates with prevalence of angina and coronary mortality', *British Medical Journal*, 314: 257–61.

Chapter 12: Routledge for M. Blaxter (1993) 'Why do the victims blame themselves?' from *Worlds of Illness: Biographical and Cultural Perspectives on Health and Disease* edited by Alan Radley, Chapter 7. pp. 124–42.

Chapter 13: Blackwell Publishers Ltd/Editorial Board for I. Bowler (1993) ' "They're not the same as us": midwives' stereotypes of South Asian descent maternity patients', *Sociology of Health & Illness*, 15 (2): 157–78.

Chapter 15: Triangle Journals Ltd for C. Winter (1996) 'Creating quality care for children in the family centre', *Educational Action Research*, 4 (1): 49–57.

INTRODUCTION

WHAT THIS BOOK IS FOR, AND HOW TO USE IT

The problem

> Pooled odds ratios were then calculated as an inverse variance weighted average of the study specific odds ratios.
>
> Roberts et al., 1996: 30 (see Chapter 4 in this volume)

The demand that practice should be 'evidence based' requires practitioners in health and social care to be able to interpret, evaluate and apply published research findings in their work. Unfortunately, much research is written by researchers, for researchers and in a language which is opaque to outsiders, as the quotation above will illustrate for most readers. Researchers could certainly make their publications more accessible to practitioners. Some do try to do so with bullet point summaries of 'Practice implications'. But researchers publish under very severe constraints. Usually publication space is not available for researchers both to report on the research and to bring lay readers up to speed on the techniques they used to do it. And were they to try to do this, the substance of the research would get overwhelmed by including huge swathes of textbook material on, say, the theory of sampling or the difference between parametric and non-parametric statistics.

Thus, if practitioners and their clients are to benefit from published research studies, practitioners will have to learn to interpret research publications more or less as they are. In fact many of the obscurities in research publications do not matter a great deal to the practitioner reader. But the problem is that such readers do not always know which ones matter and which ones don't. The quotation which heads this section is a case in point: coming across a sentence like this when reading an article is likely to stop readers in their tracks. 'What does it mean?' 'What implications does it have for the interpretation of the research as a whole?' 'Without understanding this, can the remainder be understood?' In this case, as you can discover elsewhere in the book, all the practitioner needs to know here is the kind of thing that is going on and why, without necessarily understanding it more thoroughly.

This book is pitched at the level of 'understanding the kind of thing which is going on'. It is certainly not a textbook on research methods in the ordinary sense of the term. There are many excellent textbooks on research methods. Some of them are recommended as 'further reading' in this book. But these still leave a gap between reading the textbook and reading the research. This book gets into that gap by presenting you with 9 pieces of published research, of moderate difficulty, reprinted almost exactly as they were originally, and helping you to interpret them. What we hope is that in using the book you will get some feeling for which technicalities you can safely skip over, and which you really need to understand thoroughly.

This book is not about practitioners doing research. A good case can be made for practitioners doing some first hand research, but in practical terms the amount of time a busy practitioner can afford for this is very limited. Since there are so many matters on which research might focus, a practitioner could only hope to address a few topics in a lifetime. Moreover, there are many topics which simply cannot be investigated by someone in a practitioner role. For evidence based practice, most research evidence will always have to be derived from reading research publications.

The structure of the book and how to use it

This book makes a traditional distinction between experimental approaches (Part 1), surveys (Part 2) and qualitative research (Part 3). Each of these parts contains two kinds of chapter. In each part the *first* chapters are 'Exemplar Studies'. Except in one case, these are pieces of previously published research, reprinted almost exactly as in the original. We have chosen exemplars as being fairly typical for the kind of research they represent, and as being moderately difficult to understand for the non-researcher. They represent what published research is really like. Each exemplar starts with an editorial introduction and a checklist of matters you would need to understand in order to understand the research study. This checklist cross-refers to the second kind of chapter in each part, 'Resource Chapters'. These are much more like the chapters of a research methodology textbook. Although they could be read from beginning to end, they have been written to be dipped into, as and when you need information in order to understand points in one of the exemplars. The resource chapters also contain advice on further reading.

We have presented the exemplars first, and the resources to understand them second. This is to suggest that you use them in this order, or rather, use them in parallel, trying to see how much sense you can make of an exemplar before looking for further guidance. At the end of each exemplar chapter there are some suggestions for activities you could do in order to further what you have learned from reading it.

Part 4 of the book contains a series of checklists of 'critical appraisal questions' with titles such as 'Questions to Ask about Experiments', or 'Questions to Ask about Surveys'. Most of these pose two kinds of question. One kind is about the internal validity of a piece of research: is it believable in its own terms? The other kind of question concerns matters of generalisability, transferability or applicability of the research in practice: for example, could what happened in the experiment be made to happen in practice, and would it be a good idea to try to do so? Where appropriate, the questions are cross-referenced to the resource chapters, so that you can appreciate why asking a particular question is important, and understand the implications of different answers.

These questions can be applied to the exemplar studies to carry out a more thorough-going appraisal of them than can be accomplished on first reading. However, they can also be used with other pieces of research of the same kind, so that you can transfer what you have learned from reading an exemplar to reading other research of a similar kind. The Appendix to the volume contains advice on how to find published research relevant to your own practice.

EXPERIMENTAL APPROACHES

CHAPTER I

EXPERIMENTAL METHODS AND SIMPLE INTERVENTIONS: BANDAGES FOR LEG ULCERS

Wilkinson, I., Buttfield, S., Cooper, S. and Young, E. (1997) 'Trial of two bandaging systems for chronic venous leg ulcers', *Journal of Wound Care*, 6 (7): 339–40

EXEMPLAR

What you need to understand in order to understand the exemplar
The basics of experimental design. *See Chapter 5, throughout but particularly sections 1 to 5, 9 and 12*
The table of results in the exemplar, how the data in it were tested for statistical significance and what this means. *See Chapter 7, sections 1 and 2*
The importance of blinding subjects and researchers to the treatments received and the problems of not doing so. *See Chapter 5, section 5*
The implications of randomising ulcers to treatments rather than individuals to treatments. *See Chapter 5, section 4*
Reporting by intention to treat. *See Chapter 5, section 8*
Odds ratios and confidence intervals. *See Chapter 7, section 10.4; see also sections 4 and 5*

Introduction

The treatment of leg ulcers is one of the largest single costs of medical and nursing care for older people. Even a small reduction in the cost of treatment, or a small increase in the rate of healing, would have a considerable impact on NHS costs when multiplied by the large number of people who suffer from the condition. This is to say nothing of the pain, inconvenience and restriction caused to those who have ulcerated legs. The exemplar study for this chapter investigates the relative effectiveness of two compression bandaging systems. One of these is more expensive than the other. Thus, if they proved equally effective, and equally acceptable to patients, the way would be clear for deciding to use the cheaper system. The experiment is a randomised controlled trial (RCT), without blinding, and the topic is particularly suitable for investigation using the RCT design (see Chapter 5, sections 9, 11 and 12). There are unambiguous measures of success and the treatments are simple and easy to standardise. The key process is a physiological one, and it seems likely that what would facilitate wound healing under experimental conditions, would also do so in routine practice. However, there is other research which shows that rates of leg ulcer healing can be influenced by patients' beliefs and practitioners' faith in particular treatments. Hence the failure to blind subjects or practitioners is a design weakness, even though such blinding would have been impracticable (Chapter 5, section 5). Random allocation of ulcers to treatments probably ensured that practitioner/ researcher bias could not influence who got which treatment.

As the authors themselves note, the sample for this trial was a little too small for confidence as to whether the two bandaging systems are indeed equally effective. The results are good enough, however, to be sure that if one treatment were more effective than the other the difference would not be very great. The experiment compared two treatments. Thus the finding that the treatments were 'equally effective' might mean that they were equally effective in promoting healing, or that they were equally ineffective in doing so. Healing might have occurred whether compression bandages were used or not. But this seems very unlikely since the research follows on from other published research comparing compression bandaging with other treatments and with no treatment at all, showing that compression bandages do increase healing rates. None the less, only some of the healing will be attributable to the use of compression bandages. Evidence from other research quoted in the text suggests that roughly 25 per cent of the ulcers would have healed had they been subjected to treatments other than compression bandaging.

TRIAL OF TWO BANDAGING SYSTEMS FOR CHRONIC VENOUS LEG ULCERS

I. Wilkinson, MFPHM, S. Buttfield, RGN, DNCert,
S. Cooper, MRCGP, E. Young, FRCP

Summary

A four-layer bandaging system developed at Charing Cross Hospital has been found to be effective in healing chronic venous ulcers but is not available on the *Drug Tariff*. An alternative system was devised from bandages available on the *Drug Tariff* and a community-based randomised controlled trial was undertaken to compare the two systems. Twenty-nine patients with a total of 35 ulcerated legs were recruited.

Equal numbers of ulcerated legs healed using the two compression systems. Nineteen ulcerated legs did not heal, of which six were withdrawn from the trial – two in the trial system and four in the Charing Cross system. Of the 13 remaining ulcerated legs, for which treatment was completed, the mean reduction in ulcer area was 34% with the trial system and 39% with the Charing Cross system. The change in ulcer area was not statistically significant. However, a much larger trial is required in order to demonstrate definitively that the two bandaging systems are equivalent.

Introduction

Compression bandages have been advocated for the healing of leg ulcers since 1805.[1] Their two main functions are to control oedema and counteract the effects of venous hypertension. Physiological studies have shown that graduated compression (compression decreasing from the ankle to the knee) is most effective.[2] It has also been shown that compression bandages vary greatly in their characteristics,[3,4] with some losing 60% of the sub-bandage pressure exerted within four hours.

The four-layer bandaging system developed at Charing Cross Hospital[5] is widely used for applying compression.[6,7] It has the advantage of requiring changing only once a week as the bandages maintain the required degree of compression. In the Charing Cross study, healing rates of up to 69% were obtained at 12 weeks,[8] but the bandaging system has not previously been tested against a high-compression bandage in a randomised controlled trial. Other researchers have failed to reach these levels of healing, obtaining rates of 40%–50% at 12 weeks.[7,9] These are, nevertheless, a marked improvement on the 25% healing rate achieved with traditional treatments.[10]

However, as three of the component bandages for the Charing Cross system are not available on the *Drug Tariff*, they cannot be used in the community. We were uncertain whether other bandages available on the *Drug Tariff* could be used in a combination that would be as effective as the Charing Cross system. Such a treatment would then be available for use by nurses working in primary care.

Method

A four-layer bandaging system using bandages available on the *Durg Tariff* was designed to give a degree of compression (30–40 mmHg at the ankle) similar to that of the Charing Cross system. The system comprised a lightweight elasticated tubular bandage (Tubifast) over the dressing, lint applied in separate strips horizontally around the leg to absorb exudate and pad bony prominences, a high-compression bandage (Setopress) and a lightweight elasticated tubular bandage (Tubifast) to hold the high-compression bandage in position and prevent it from 'rucking up'.

The Charing Cross system was used as supplied in the package (Profore). This consists of orthopaedic wool (Soffban), a crêpe bandage, a light compression crêpe bandage (Litepress) and a cohesive bandage (Coplus). A knitted viscose primary dressing (Tricotex) was used under both systems and the cleansing solutions and emollients used were standardised.

Patients with an uncomplicated chronic venous ulcer on the lower leg who were being treated by a district or practice nurse were recruited with their GPs' permission. Exclusion criteria included a resting ankle brachial pressure index (ABPI) of <0.8, a known contact allergy to latex, evidence of cellulitis or an ankle circumference of <18 cm or >25 cm. Details of each patient's medical history and medications were noted.

When patients were considered suitable to enter the trial, informed consent was obtained and the patients' ulcerated legs allocated to one of two groups using numbers generated by random number tables. If there was more than one ulcer on a leg then the largest (<10 cm^2 and $\geq$10 cm^2) was included in the trial. Ulcer area is a strong predictor for healing. Ulcer size was calculated by multiplying the maximum length and width of the ulcer. All patients were reviewed by a dermatologist within two weeks of starting treatment to confirm that they had uncomplicated venous ulcers.

Nurses were taught to apply the bandages by the research nurse who continued to attend the surgery until agreement on competency was met. Measurements of sub-bandage pressure were not made under either regimen.

Patients were reviewed weekly when the bandages were changed. The ulcers were measured at four, eight and 12 weeks. The main outcome measure was healing of the ulcer, defined as a continuous layer of epithelial cells across the ulcer surface. This was assessed by the community nurse, who was not 'blind' to the bandaging system. When ulcers healed, the patients were supplied with Class 2 compression stockings.

Results

Twenty-nine patients with a total of 35 ulcerated legs were recruited. Recruitment was slow as fewer suitable patients than anticipated were willing to enter the trial. There were no significant differences between the groups in age, sex, duration or size of current ulcer, number of smokers or other medical conditions. Initial ulcer area was not significantly different – trial system mean 8.6 cm^2 (range 0.25–45 cm^2), Charing Cross system 11.2 cm^2 (0.25–49.6 cm^2).

The outcome of treatment for all ulcers is shown in Table 1. The odds ratio for healing with the Charing Cross system compared with the trial system is 1.11 (95%

Table 1   Outcome of treatment at 12 weeks

Bandaging system	Healed	Not healed	Withdrawn
Charing Cross ($n = 17$)	8 (47%)	5 (29%)	4 (24%)
Trial system ($n = 18$)	8 (44%)	8 (44%)	2 (12%)

$\chi^2 = 1.3$; df = 2; p = 0.51

Table 2   Reasons for withdrawal from treatment

Bandaging system	No. of ulcerated legs	Reasons for withdrawal
Charing Cross	1	Developed cellulitis
	1	Bandage uncomfortable/slipped
	1	?Allergic to bandage
	1	Bandage too painful
Trial system	1	Leg painful, possibly infected
	1	Bandage too painful

confidence interval 0.24–5.19). Nineteen ulcers did not heal. Of the 13 ulcers that completed the trial without healing, the mean reduction in area was 34% with the trial system and 39% with the Charing Cross system. This difference is not significant (*t*-test 1.4, df 5, $p = 0.89$). Six ulcers were withdrawn from the trial – four in the Charing Cross group and two in the trial group (Table 2). No patients were lost to follow-up. The results were analysed on the basis of intention to treat.

Discussion

The healing rates obtained with both systems at 12 weeks are similar to other published rates using four-layer bandaging. This suggests that the bandaging technique is correct.

The trial system was better tolerated by patients than the Charing Cross system as shown by the smaller number of withdrawals from the trial group, but with the small numbers involved this may be due to chance.

There is no significant difference in the number of ulcers healed by the two systems but the 95% confidence interval for the odds ratio is very wide (0.24–5.19) because of the small number of participants. A much larger trial is needed to demonstrate definitively that the two bandaging systems are equivalent. This study has, however, highlighted the difficulty in recruiting a large number of patients with suitable ulcers into a trial.

The majority of patients with leg ulcers are managed in primary care. It is therefore important to have effective treatments that can be used without referral to hospital. Nurses applying the bandages must receive adequate training in the assessment of leg ulcers, including measurement of ABPI, and in applying compression bandages. Inappropriate application or excessive compression can cause considerable damage to the underlying skin.

The results of this trial show that the benefits of compression bandaging in the treatment of chronic venous leg ulcers can be available to all patients in the community as the bandages used are available on prescription.

References

1 The Inquirer. What are the comparative advantages of the different modes proposed for the treatment of ulcerated legs? *Edin Med & Surg J* 1805; 1: 187–193.

2 Ruckley, C.V. Treatment of venous ulceration: compression therapy. *Phlebology* 1992; (Suppl 1), 22–26.

3 Barbenel, J.C., Sockalingham, S., Queen, D. *In vivo* and laboratory evaluation of elastic bandages. *Care Sci & Pract* 1990; 8: 2, 72–74.

4 Tennant, W.G., Park, K.G.M., Ruckley, C.V. Testing compression bandages. *Phlebology* 1988; 3: 55–61.

5 Moffatt, C.J., Dickson, D. The Charing Cross high compression four-layer bandage system. *J Wound Care* 1993; 2: 2, 91–94.

6 Simon, D.A., Freak, L. Kinsella, A. et al. Community leg ulcer clinics: a comparative study in two health authorities. *Br Med J* 1996; 312: 1648–1651.

7 Thompson, B., Hooper, P., Powel, R., Wann, A.P. Four-layer bandaging and healing rates of venous leg ulcers. *J Wound Care* 1996; 5: 5, 213–216.

8 Moffatt, C.J., Franks, P.J., Oldroyd. M. et al. Community clinics for leg ulcers and impact on healing. *Br Med J* 1992; 305: 1389–1392.

9 Duby, T., Hofman, D., Cameron. J. et al. A randomised trial in the treatment of venous leg ulcers comparing short stretch bandages, four layer bandage system, and a long stretch-paste bandage system. *Wounds: Compend Clin Res & Pract* 1993; 5: 276–279.

10 Cullum, N. *Leg Ulcers: An evidence-based approach.* Harrow: Scutari Press, 1995.

What you might do now

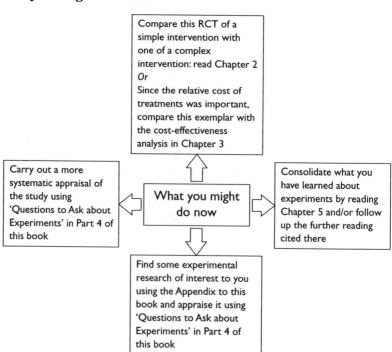

Compare this RCT of a simple intervention with one of a complex intervention: read Chapter 2
Or
Since the relative cost of treatments was important, compare this exemplar with the cost-effectiveness analysis in Chapter 3

Carry out a more systematic appraisal of the study using 'Questions to Ask about Experiments' in Part 4 of this book

What you might do now

Consolidate what you have learned about experiments by reading Chapter 5 and/or follow up the further reading cited there

Find some experimental research of interest to you using the Appendix to this book and appraise it using 'Questions to Ask about Experiments' in Part 4 of this book

EXPERIMENTAL METHODS AND COMPLEX INTERVENTIONS: CASE MANAGEMENT IN MENTAL HEALTH CARE

Marshall, M., Lockwood, A. and Gath, D. (1995) 'Social Services case-management for long-term mental disorders: a randomised controlled trial', *The Lancet*, 345: 409–12

EXEMPLAR

What you need to understand in order to understand the exemplar
The basics of experimental design. *See Chapter 5, throughout but particularly sections 1 to 3, 5 to 9 and 12*
'the data were first evaluated to ensure normality of sampling distributions, linearity and homogeneity of variance' *See Chapter 7, section 6*
The table of results (Table 3). *See Chapter 7, section 10.1*
Why the researchers used 'off-the-peg' instruments rather than inventing their own. *See Chapter 6, section 1*
The problems caused by subjects dropping out of experiments. *See Chapter 5, section 8*
That given the extreme scores of all subjects on entry, some of the improvement shown may be due to regression to the mean. *See Chapter 5, section 6*
The difficulties arising from non-standardised treatment of subjects within arms of an experiment. *See Chapter 5, section 7; Chapter 7, section 7*
The problem of conducting experiments about complex interventions. *See Introduction to this Chapter; Chapter 5, section 9*

> The way most of the instruments used generated interval
> level data or better, which is analysed with parametric
> statistics (ANCOVA, *F*-test) though measures in days were
> treated as ordinal data and analysed with the non-parametric
> Mann-Whitney *U* test.
> *See Chapter 6, sections 3 and 4; Chapter 7, section 6*

> You do *not* need to understand how to do the statistical
> calculations in this research but you do need to understand
> the meaning of statistical significance and the interpretation
> of confidence intervals.
> *See Chapter 7, sections 1, 2 and 4*

Introduction

The exemplar for this chapter is a study of case (or care) management
in social work for people living in the community and diagnosed as
suffering from severe mental illness. The idea of case management
for mental health emanated in the USA, and in the UK became a
constituent of community care for mentally ill people with the introduction of the 'Care Programme Approach', first in England and Wales
from 1990 and later in Scotland. But neither in the USA, nor in the
UK was there much sound evidence from research to show that case
management for people with severe mental health problems would
have better outcomes than alternative ways of organising care in the
community.

The study takes a randomised controlled trial format, without
blinding (see Chapter 5). Blinding practitioners would have been
impracticable in this situation and the fact that practitioners knew
what treatment subjects were receiving creates room for practitioner
bias to influence the results (Chapter 5, section 5). However, such bias,
if it occurred, would be most likely to create differences in outcomes,
while the result of this trial was of similar outcomes for subjects dealt
with differently.

There is a case for saying that the topic of case management is at or
beyond the limits of what can be investigated using randomised
controlled trials, or other experimental structures, at least with the
kinds of sample size they usually have. This is because of the complex-
ity of the interventions concerned (Chapter 5, section 9). Community
mental health care is supposed to involve practitioners customising
the care to the particular needs of individual clients and there is no
reason to suppose that practitioners involved in this trial did otherwise. Thus while the researchers behave as if they were conducting a
trial with two arms – treatment and control – it can be suggested that

in reality this was a trial with a large but undetermined number of arms; many different modalities of treatment; many different modalities of alternatives (see Chapter 7, section 7). In this trial there are also likely to be differences *within* arms of the trial between practitioners; their levels of skill, their congeniality to particular clients, and so on. These comments would be more important if this experiment had shown significant differences in improvement in mental health between the two groups, because failures to create and maintain similar groups and failures to standardise treatments within arms of a trial are more likely to produce outcome differences than outcome similarities. In fact, the trial showed little difference in mental health outcomes for two groups on most of a number of different measures.

There is no reason not to accept the researchers' conclusion that *in this case*, with the exception of deviant behaviour measurement, there were no significant differences in the outcomes measured between the group subjected to case management and the group dealt with otherwise. The authors, quite rightly, do not claim that either treatment actually caused the improvements made. These might have been due to the fact that those selected for the experiment were in a severe condition, and for that reason were more likely to get better than worse (see Chapter 5, section 6) in both arms of the experiment. Or it may be that those least likely to improve were those most likely to drop out of either arm of the experiment. A weakness of this study is that at the end there are no data for 24 per cent of the subjects who were entered into the experiment at the beginning (Chapter 5, section 8).

There are problems in this experiment about the extent to which its results can be generalised (Chapter 5, section 12). The generalisability question is 'how far can the results of this study serve as a confident judgement on "case management" elsewhere?'. The research report gives very little information as to what case management meant in the experiment. Nor does it describe the way in which the controls were treated. Readers have no way of judging how different these two interventions were from each other, or how similar the case management of one client was to the case management of another (Chapter 5, section 7). To add to this difficulty, the term 'case management' has no fixed meaning, and what is called case management in one place may be very different from what is called case management in another, particularly in terms of face-to-face relations between client and practitioner. Thus readers do not really know what was done, and do not know how it compares to what happens in their own practice. This makes it extremely difficult to base generalisations on this study. However, most other studies in the same field give similar results. This suggests that even though there is a wide variety of practices going under the name of case management, none of them has much effect, and the result of this study strengthens this conclusion.

The analysis of experimental and quasi-experimental research tends to concentrate on differences *between* arms of a trial. Restricting comparisons to those between means (averages) for groups leads prematurely to the conclusion that had the case managed and the control groups been reversed, then the outcomes would have been much the same, not only group score on group score, but individual by individual. This may be a cogent assumption where interventions are simple and standardised and the important mechanisms are physiological, but it seems unlikely where relationships and interpretations are the important mechanisms for change. Almost certainly there will be some people who made more improvement under the alternative treatment, who would have made less if case managed, and some people who made less improvement under case management and who would have made more under the alternative regime. The bald question 'does case management work?' around which this study is framed is less interesting than the questions 'is case management the best option for anyone, and if so, for whom and under what circumstances and why?' This is a question which is amenable to experimental research but would require a very large sample indeed in order to pursue it; large enough to distinguish distinctive sub-groups within arms of the trial and to analyse the factors associated with more improvement under one regime than another (see Chapter 7, section 7).

SOCIAL SERVICES CASE-MANAGEMENT FOR LONG-TERM MENTAL DISORDERS: A RANDOMISED CONTROLLED TRIAL

M. Marshall, A. Lockwood, D. Gath

Summary

Case-management arose in the USA as a solution to the difficulties of providing community care to people with severe mental disorders. The basic principle of the approach is that a case-manager takes responsibility for a client; arranges an assessment of need, a comprehensive service plan, delivery of suitable services, and monitoring and assessment of services delivered. The case-management approach has been widely accepted, to the extent that recent legislation has made case-management the cornerstone of community care in the UK.

We did a randomised controlled trial to evaluate a social services case-management team for people with long-term mental disorders. Subjects were referred from hostels for the homeless, night shelters, a general practitioner clinic for the homeless, the Oxford City Council homelessness unit, and local voluntary-sector group homes. Of 103 subjects referred, 80 consented to be randomised to treatment or control groups. At 14-month follow-up, as assessed by standardised interviews, there were no significant differences between groups in number of needs, quality of life, employment status, quality of accommodation, social behaviour, or severity of psychiatric symptoms. In the case-management group there was a significant reduction in deviant behaviour on a standardised behaviour rating scale (REHAB) (mean = 0.79; 95% confidence interval (CI) 0.26–1.32).

It is unfortunate, in view of the limited effectiveness we have shown, that social services case-management was not evaluated in randomised controlled trials before its implementation in the UK.

Introduction

People with long-term mental disorders have many social and psychiatric needs.[1] Since the closure of psychiatric hospitals in the UK, services required to meet these needs have become dispersed among different sites and providing authorities,[2] with the consequence that many people with mental disorders are unable to obtain the care they need.[3] In the USA, case-management arose as a solution to this problem of dispersion; this approach has been widely accepted[4,5] and recently became the cornerstone of community care in the UK.

In the UK, as elsewhere, the practice, composition, and organisation of case-management teams vary. Some UK teams work entirely within social services departments; others are jointly managed by social services and mental health services, or by mental health services alone.[6] Nevertheless, teams share basic principles of the case-management approach: a case-manager, who takes responsibility for a client, arranges an assessment of need, a comprehensive service plan, delivery of suitable services, monitoring and assessment of services delivered, and also evaluates results.[2,7] The expectation was that, by working alongside existing services, case-management teams would improve the quality and efficiency of care for patients with long-term mental disorders.[8]

The case-management approach has been described as 'intuitively appealing',[9] but there is little evidence that it is efficacious. The only randomised trial of an approach comparable to that practised by UK case-management teams was carried out in the USA and showed that the case-management group received more services than the control group and were more often admitted to mental hospitals, but showed no improvements in quality of life.[9] We report the findings of a randomised controlled trial of the effectiveness of a social services case-management team set up by Oxford Social Services in September 1991.

Subjects and methods

The study was a randomised controlled trial. Subjects were assessed before allocation to treatment or control groups and at 7 and 14 months after entering the study.

Entry and randomisation

Before the study, researchers and the case-management team approached two local night shelters, three hostels for the homeless (two of which also provided sheltered accommodation), a general practice clinic for the homeless, the city council homelessness unit, housing associations providing sheltered care, a local voluntary organisation providing group homes, and a health authority employment rehabilitation service in contact with people living in poor-quality bedsits. These organisations were asked to refer subjects to the study over a 6-month recruitment period.

Subjects were considered for inclusion if they were judged by the referrer to have a severe, persistent, psychiatric disorder; were homeless (roofless, or living in a night shelter or hostel for the homeless); at risk of homelessness (i.e., facing a threat of eviction, or having a recent history of homelessness, or frequent changes of accommodation); living in accommodation which was temporary, or supported (such as a group home), or of poor quality; were coping badly, experiencing social isolation, or causing disturbances; and were not clients of another case-management service.

Subjects who had a well-documented psychiatric history were assessed either by a trained research nurse or a research psychiatrist; others were assessed by a research psychiatrist. One of the authors (M.M.) then allocated an ICD-10 diagnosis.

After initial assessment, subjects were randomly allocated to case-management or control groups. Randomisation was by sealed envelop. Random permuted blocks were used to keep the numbers of subjects balanced in both groups. Once a subject had been allocated to the case-management team, the senior case-manager was notified of the subject's name, address and principal carer.

Case-management

Case-managers chose how much time to offer each subject. As a minimum, each was offered an assessment of need from a case-manager, a discussion of the findings of this assessment with the subject's carer, intervention from the case-manager to meet needs that were identified, monitoring of the subject's progress by the case-manager, and further assistance should needs arise. In addition, case-managers were free to choose how far they would personally assist the subject with transport, counselling, organisation of activity programmes, assistance with completion of forms, crisis intervention, help with finding accommodation, assistance with benefits, finding work or places on training courses, and help with obtaining furnishings and domestic appliances. The extent to which case-managers should act as advocates was likewise an individual choice.

Control

Subjects continued to receive any assistance that they had been receiving before the study. Staff working with subjects were at liberty to obtain any further care they saw fit. However, no control subjects were taken on by the study case-management team, or by any other case-management team.

Rating scales

The needs of subjects for psychiatric and social care were assessed with a modified version of the MRC Needs for Care Schedule,[10] as described elsewhere.[11,12] Ratings of need were made by a psychiatrist and a psychiatric nurse, both experienced in psychiatric rehabilitation. Quality of life was assessed in terms of accommodation, employment status, and subjects' own ratings of their quality of life on the Quality of Life Interview.[13]

Social behaviour was measured by observer ratings and subjects' own ratings. The observer rating of social behaviour was made with a standardised behaviour scale (REHAB), which rates the frequency of items of embarrassing or disruptive behaviour, such as violence, self harm, shouting and swearing, and sexual offensiveness (deviant behaviour); and lack of general skills (general behaviour).[14] REHAB ratings were made by an observer trained by the researchers (e.g., a member of staff in a hostel, a voluntary worker, or a primary-care worker). The subject's perception of his or her own social behaviour was rated with the Social Integration Questionnaire.[15] Severity of psychiatric symptoms was assessed with the Manchester Scale.[16]

Analysis

The data were first evaluated to ensure normality of sampling distributions, linearity and homogeneity of variance. One-way repeated measures analyses of variance were used to compare scores at the start, and at 7 and 14 months. Two by two repeated measures analyses of covariance (incorporating experimental grouping as a between-subjects factor) were used to examine differences between groups in ratings of psychopathology, social functioning, quality of life and numbers of needs. In each of these analyses the scores on the dependent variable at baseline were used as the covariates.

Changes in the accommodation status of the subjects were analysed with non-parametric statistics. Control and treatment groups were compared in terms of the number of days in accommodation better than their baseline accommodation, days in accommodation worse than baseline, and days in hospital. Employment status was compared with non-parametric statistics, after adjustment for baseline differences between the groups. Comparisons were made of total days in employment, and of weighted days (paid employment receiving greater weight than voluntary work). (Details available from authors.)

Results

During the 6-month recruitment period, 103 subjects were referred to the study, of whom 14 declined to participate and 4 were unable to give informed consent. Mean age of these 18 subjects was 53.2 years; 2 were female. Case-notes indicated that 11 (61%) had a previous diagnosis of schizophrenia or a related disorder. Five subjects were excluded from the study before randomisation because they were involved with another case-management service. Eighty subjects entered the study.

After baseline assessment, they were randomly allocated to case-management (40) or control groups (40).

Baseline characteristics

There were no significant differences between the groups in terms of age, sex, housing status, previous psychiatric history, diagnosis (Table 1), or psychiatric symptoms (Table 2). At baseline, mean REHAB general behaviour score of the 80 subjects was high (43.5; SD 24.3; 95% CI 38.6–48.9). 36 (45.6%) were mildly socially disabled; 27 (34.2%) were moderately disabled; and 16 (20.3%) were severely disabled. The sample had high measures of deviant behaviour (mean 1.25; 0.89–1.61). At baseline, subjects had a mean of 1.0 psychiatric/medical needs, and 2.6 social needs (total 3.6 needs, SD 2.2).

Table 1   Characteristics of subjects

	Contol group (n = 40)		Case-management (n = 40)	
	No.	%	No.	%
Age grouping				
20–29	4	10.0	4	10.0
30–39	6	15.4	11	28.2
40–49	16	40.0	6	15.4
50–59	5	12.5	9	22.5
60+	9	22.5	9	22.5
Sex				
Male	34	85.0	34	85.0
Female	6	15.0	6	15.0
History				
Illness > 1 year	40	100	40	100
Previous psychiatric admission	34	85.0	34	85.0
In contact with psychiatric services	25	62.5	21	52.5
ICD 10 diagnosis				
Schizophrenia and related disorders	32	80.0	27	67.5
Mood disorders	3	7.5	6	15.0
Personality disorder	2	5.0	3	7.5
Neurotic disorders	1	2.5	3	7.5
Organic disorders	2	5.0	1	2.5
Housing status				
Hostels for the homeless	18	45.0	20	50.0
Staffed group homes	7	17.5	4	10.0
Unstaffed group home	5	12.5	5	12.5
Night shelter or sleeping rough	4	10.0	3	7.5
Supported flat	3	7.5	3	7.5
Own flat	2	5.0	3	7.5
Poor quality bedsit	0	0.0	2	5.0
With family	1	2.5	0	0.0

Table 2 Symptoms among study subjects

Subjects	Symptoms no. (%)				
	Psychotic*	Mood[†]	Negative[§]	Any	None
Control	21 (52.5)	21 (52.5)	14 (35)	32 (80)	8 (20.0)
Case-management	19 (47.5)	18 (45)	11 (27.5)	31 (77.5)	9 (22.5)
All	40 (50)	39 (48.8)	25 (31.3)	63 (78.8)	17 (22.2)

* Rating of two or more points on any of the following Manchester scale items: hallucinations, delusions, or incoherence of thought. [†] Rating of two or more points on any of the following Manchester scale items: depression, anxiety. [§] Rating of two or more points on any of the following Manchester scale items: psychomotor retardation, blunting of affect, or poverty of speech.

Outcome

Of the 80 subjects assessed at baseline, 61 were reassessed at 7 and 14 months after entering the study, and 8 at 7 but not at 14 months. Of 11 who dropped out, 6 were in the case-management and 5 were in the control group. Reasons for drop out were: moved to another town (6); refused further contact (2); died (2); and moved locally without leaving contact address (1). The 2 who died were in the case-management group.

The sample as a whole showed significant improvements in social behaviour (REHAB general behaviour, $F = 5.01$, $p < 0.01$) and social integration ($F = 4.28$, $p < 0.05$) over 14 months. Table 3 shows the results of the repeated measures analyses of covariance, which were used to compare measures of quality of life, social behaviour, deviant behaviour, social integration, and mental state at 7 and 14 months. Outcome was better for the case-management group on three of the five variables (REHAB general and deviant behaviour and mental state), but only deviant behaviour differed significantly between the two groups. Subjects in the case-management group had a mean of 44.3 days in better accommodation as against a mean of 32.3 for the control group; and a mean of 15.1 days in worse accommodation as against a mean of 33.4 for the control group. These differences were not significant (days in better accommodation, Mann–Whitney $U = 470$; $p = 0.17$; days in worse accommodation, $U = 515$; $p = 0.67$). Subjects in the control group spent a mean of 21.8 (SD 62.3) days in hospital during the study whereas subjects in the case-management group spent a mean of 14.6 (30.5) days in hospital. There was no significant difference between the groups in terms of days in hospital, after adjustment for days in hospital during the baseline period (mean of observed days − expected days [control group] = 5.3; mean of observed days − expected days [case-management] = 5.6; $U = -1.6$; $p = 0.1$).

Subjects in the case-management group spent slightly more days in employment than expected, whereas subjects in the control group spent slightly fewer days than expected; this difference between the groups is not statistically significant either for days in any kind of employment ($U = 726$; $p = 0.40$) or for days in employment weighted in favour of paid employment or training ($U = 733$; $p = 0.45$). There were significant falls in the numbers of needs for psychiatric/medical care and social care in both groups ($F = 18.7$; $p < 0.001$), but there were no significant differences between the groups (Table 3).

Throughout the study, case-managers kept a record of the time spent working with, or for, each subject. 4 subjects received no input from the case-management

Table 3 Outcome of control and case-management groups

Measure	Group	Baseline scores (n)	Change at 7 mth (n)	Change at 14 mth (n)	Mean diff at 14 mth (95% CI)*	F	Clinically relevant difference†
REHAB GB	Control	44.7 (40)	4.3 (35)	4.9 (30)	4.3 (−4.9 to 13.4)	0.87	15
	Case-management	42.2 (40)	5.3 (34)	7.5 (31)			
REHAB DB	Control	1.56 (40)	0.15 (35)	0.19 (30)	0.3 (0.15 to 0.46)	8.42§	0.5
	Case-management	0.98 (40)	0.26 (34)	0.42 (31)			
Manchester scale	Control	6.73 (40)	0.1 (35)	−0.8 (30)	0.75 (−1.0 to 2.5)	0.26	2.0
	Case-management	6.88 (40)	0.1 (34)	0.1 (31)			
Quality of life	Control	3.54 (38)	0.0 (32)	0.2 (27)	0.0 (−0.42 to 0.42)	0.19	1.0
	Case-management	3.59 (40)	0.2 (33)	0.2 (31)			
Social interactions	Control	1.77 (40)	0.0 (35)	0.2 (29)	−0.07 (−0.27 to 0.13)	1.36	0.5
	Case-management	1.80 (40)	0.1 (34)	0.2 (31)			
Needs	Control	3.60 (40)	1.2 (35)	1.3 (30)	−0.07 (−0.97 to 0.84)	0.02	1.0
	Case-management	3.68 (40)	1.7 (34)	1.3 (31)			

*Mean difference between the groups at 14 months and the 95% CIs were calculated with a linear regression model in which baseline scores were the independent variable. A negative score indicates a difference in favour of the control group. † Estimate of the change in score that would represent a clinically recognisable improvement.
§ $p < 0.01$. GB = general behaviour, DB = deviant behaviour.

team; of these, 1 left Oxford within 2 days of being recruited, 2 refused to be seen, and 1 was admitted to hospital. Case-managers gave a mean of 21.6 h (SD 32.4) to the remaining 36 subjects.

Discussion

The aim of the study was to determine the effectiveness of social services case-management in addition to services already provided in the community. After 14 months of case-management, case-management subjects showed no significant differences from controls on measures of need, quality of life, quality of accommodation, employment status, social behaviour, or psychopathology; they showed significantly less deviant behaviour. This limited effectiveness is in keeping with other findings.[5,9]

Our findings cannot be generalised to all case-management teams in the UK; variability between teams means that an overall judgement on the effectiveness of case-management has to be based on the accumulated findings of several trials. However, our results challenge the orthodoxy that case-management is effective. The case-managers we studied may not have spent enough time with subjects to bring about improvement, although case-managers decided how much time to spend with a subject, as happens in everyday practice.

References

1 Brewin CR, Wing JK, Mangen SP, Brugha TS, MacCarthy B, Lesage A. Needs for care among the long-term mentally ill: a report from the Camberwell High Contact Survey. *Psychol Med* 1988; 18: 457–68.

2 Shepherd G. Case management. *Health Trends* 1990; 22: 59–61.

3 Audit Commission. Making a reality of community care. London: HM Stationery Office, 1986.

4 Thornicroft G. The concept of case management for long-term mental illness. *Int Rev Psychiatry* 1991; 3: 125–32.

5 Rossler W, Loffler W, Fatkenheuer B, Reicher-Rossler A. Does case management reduce the rehospitalization rate? *Acta Psychiatr Scand* 1992; 86: 445–49.

6 Ford R, Repper J, Cooke A, Norton P, Beadsmoore A, Clark C. Implementing case management. London: Research and Development for Psychiatry, 1993.

7 Holloway F, McLean EK, Robertson JA. Case management. *Br J Psychiatry* 1991; 159: 142–48.

8 Holloway F. Case management for the mentally ill: looking at the evidence. *Int J Soc Psychiatry* 1991; 37: 2–13.

9 Franklin J, Solovitz B, Mason M, Clemons J, Miller G. An evaluation of case management. *Am J Public Health* 1987; 77: 674–78.

10 Brewin C, Wing J, Mangen S, Brugha T, MacCarthy B. Principles and practice of measuring needs in the long-term mentally ill: the MRC Needs for Care Schedule. *Psychol Med* 1987; 17: 971–81.

11 Marshall M. How should we measure need? Concept and practice in the development of a standardised schedule. *Philosophy, Psychology, and Psychiatry* 1994; 1: 27–36.

12 Marshall M, Hogg L, Lockwood A, Gath D. The Cardinal Needs Schedule: a modified version of the MRC Needs for Care Schedule. *Psychol Med* 1994 (in press).

13 Lehman A. The well being of chronic mental patients: assessing their quality of life. *Arch Gen Psychiatry* 1983; 40: 369–73.

14 Baker R, Hall J. Users manual for Rehabilitation Evaluation Hall and Baker. Aberdeen: Vine, 1983.
15 Segal S, Aviram U. Community-based sheltered care: a study of community care and social integration. New York: Wiley-Interscience, 1977.
16 Krawiecka M, Goldberg D, Vaughn M. A standardized psychiatric assessment scale for rating chronic psychotic patients. *Acta Psychiatr Scand* 1977; 55: 299–308.

What you might do now

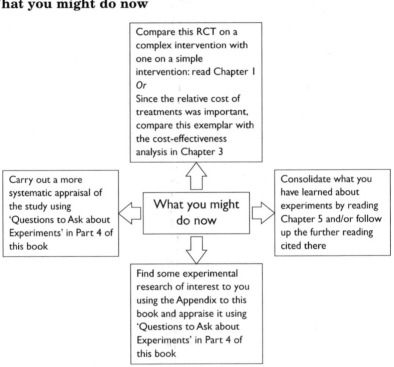

Compare this RCT on a complex intervention with one on a simple intervention: read Chapter 1
Or
Since the relative cost of treatments was important, compare this exemplar with the cost-effectiveness analysis in Chapter 3

Carry out a more systematic appraisal of the study using 'Questions to Ask about Experiments' in Part 4 of this book

What you might do now

Consolidate what you have learned about experiments by reading Chapter 5 and/or follow up the further reading cited there

Find some experimental research of interest to you using the Appendix to this book and appraise it using 'Questions to Ask about Experiments' in Part 4 of this book

CHAPTER 3

FROM EFFECTIVENESS TO COST-EFFECTIVENESS: A TRIAL OF A HOSPITAL AT HOME SCHEME

Shepperd, S., Harwood, D., Gray, A., Vessey, M. and Morgan, P. (1998) 'Randomised controlled trial comparing hospital at home care with inpatient hospital care. II: cost minimisation analysis', *British Medical Journal*, 316: 1791–6

EXEMPLAR

What you need to understand in order to understand the exemplar
You can accept that the RCT establishing the similar effectiveness of the two interventions was well-designed and well-conducted, but if you want to investigate experimental design for research on effectiveness, see the *Introduction to this chapter and Chapter 5*
'analysis was done on an intention to treat basis' *See Chapter 5, section 8*
'When appropriate, data with a non-normal distribution was log transformed before further parametric analysis was done.' (The use of the geometric mean is for the same reason.) *See Chapter 6, section 4 (data transformations); Chapter 7, section 6*
What the figures for standard deviation (SD) tell you. *See Chapter 7, section 9*
P values and how to interpret them (where no *p* values are cited the results are not statistically significant at the 0.05 (5%) level). *See Chapter 7, section 2 (especially Table 7.2)*
Confidence intervals and how to interpret them. *See Chapter 7, sections 4 and 5*
Sensitivity analysis. *See Chapter 7, section 12*
The problems of generalising from a cost-effectiveness study done in one locale to cost-effectiveness elsewhere. *See Chapter 5, section 12*

Introduction

During the 1990s in the UK many hospital at home schemes were established on the assumption that providing postoperative care in a patient's home would be cheaper than providing it on an inpatient basis. However, there was almost no research evidence to back up this assumption. The exemplar study for this chapter is one of a number investigating this towards the end of the 1990s. Often studies like this are called *cost-effectiveness analyses*, though more narrowly defined this one is *a cost-minimisation analysis*, where the object is to decide which of two equally effective interventions has the lowest costs. Cost-effectiveness analyses, narrowly defined, try to establish how much benefit is produced per unit cost. All such analyses have to include, or build on, research establishing the relative effectiveness of interventions, before their relative *cost*-effectiveness can be considered. The most convincing evidence about effectiveness comes from randomised controlled trials and the exemplar printed here is the second half of a study which began with an RCT (Figure 3.1).

The way that patients were recruited for the trial is shown in Figure 5.4 in Chapter 5. Table 3.1 below comes from the first half of the study. It refers only to the hip replacement patients. The trial included patients in other care groups as well, and these mainly show similar results. The results are produced from the use of COOP charts (Figure 6.1 in Chapter 6) and a clinical test for the Oxford hip score. The two groups were very similar at baseline. Their difference here was also tested for statistical significance separately. The standard deviation figures (SD) show that internally the two groups were not very different in diversity (Chapter 7, section 9). The outcome differences were calculated by subtracting one group's average (mean) change from baseline to 3 months from that of the other group (Chapter 7, section 10.1). A positive score would show more improvement for the hospital at home patients. Most of the 95% confidence intervals (Chapter 7, sections 4 and 5) give limits which span values that would

Figure 3.1   The main components of an analysis of cost-effectiveness

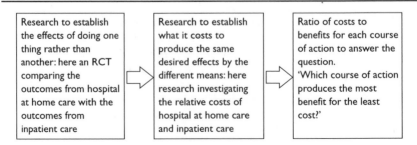

Table 3.1 Outcome measures reported by patients recovering from hip replacement who were allocated to hospital at home care (n = 37) or inpatient care (n = 49)

	Mean (SD) value at baseline		Mean change from baseline value at 3 month follow up		
	HaH (n = 36)	Hospital (n = 48)	HaH (n = 36)	Hospital (n = 45)	Difference (95% CI)
Dartmouth COOP charts[1]					
Physical fitness	4.58 (0.91)	4.73 (0.49)	0.42	0.51	−0.09 (−0.48 to 0.29)
Feelings	2.44 (1.08)	2.60 (1.16)	1.03	0.78	0.25 (−0.29 to 0.79)
Daily activities	3.17 (1.13)	3.40 (0.98)	1.00	0.93	0.07 (−0.39 to 0.53)
Social activities	2.92 (1.27)	3.10 (1.19)	1.43	1.02	0.41 (−0.15 to 0.97)
Pain	4.33 (0.76)	4.46 (0.68)	1.54	1.69	−0.15 (−0.78 to 0.49)
Change in health	2.44 (0.94)	2.44 (0.92)	0.74	0.13	0.61 (0.02 to 1.20)
Overall health	2.78 (0.76)	2.85 (1.01)	0.06	−0.04	0.10 (−0.35 to 0.55)
Social support	1.56 (0.84)	1.90 (1.34)	0.26	0.40	−0.14 (−0.57 to 0.28)
Quality of life	2.94 (0.83)	2.73 (0.74)	0.97	0.47	0.59 (0.13 to 0.88)
Oxford hip	(n = 34)	(n = 46)	(n = 43)	(n = 43)	
score[2]	25.56 (6.15)	27.34 (8.03)	4.77	3.13	1.64 (−1.23 to 4.50)

HaH, Hospital at home care.
[1] Scale 1–5 (low score = good quality of life).
[2] No data for some patients, scale 12–60 (high score = high level of impairment). Baseline score measured at 1 month.

Source: Shepperd, S., Harwood, D., Jenkinson, C., Gray, A., Vessey, M. and Morgan, P. (1998) 'Randomised controlled trial comparing hospital at home care with inpatient hospital care. I: three month follow up of health outcomes', *British Medical Journal*, 316: 1788

show more improvement for either group, thus suggesting no significant differences. All the outcome differences were tested for statistical significance (Chapter 7, sections 1 and 2). None in this table showed statistical significance at the 0.05 (5%) level, which is indicated by the authors not including any values for *p* (Table 7.2 in Chapter 7).

Overall then, the researchers could be confident that, in most respects, for most patient groups involved in the trial there was little difference in health outcomes associated with receiving inpatient care or hospital at home care. The exemplar study focuses on which of these two interventions 'cost' least.

In analyses like this it is important to note that:

1 'Costs' and 'benefits' are not restricted to monetary matters.
2 Combining monetary and non-monetary costs in the same analysis can lead to tricky problems: for example, how much should patient discomfort raise the cost of a treatment above its monetary cost? Or how much extra should service managers be willing to pay for an intervention which patients prefer, but which provides no additional health gain?

3   Cost–benefit ratios are always from someone's point of view. A cost
    for someone, may be a benefit to someone else.
4   For all these reasons and others, economic analysis entails making
    moral judgements about:
    - whose interests should be taken into consideration in deciding
      what to count as costs and benefits, and what to ignore;
    - whose interests should take highest priority when setting the
      costs for one party against benefits to another.

These are matters you might like to bear in mind when you read the
exemplar study.

You will see that the authors explain how they costed care, but do
not present a great deal of the data for this. This is common, since
such data would take a very large amount of space. However, the
authors offer to make it available if required. This is important if a
reader wants to compare unit costs in the study with unit costs in
their own practice area.

RANDOMISED CONTROLLED TRIAL COMPARING HOSPITAL AT HOME CARE WITH INPATIENT HOSPITAL CARE. II: COST MINIMISATION ANALYSIS

Sasha Shepperd, Diana Harwood, Alastair Gray, Martin Vessey,
Patrick Morgan

Abstract

Objectives: To examine the cost of providing hospital at home in place of some
forms of inpatient hospital care.

Design: Cost minimisation study within a randomised controlled trial.

Setting: District general hospital and catchment area of neighbouring community trust.

Subjects: Patients recovering from hip replacement ($n = 86$), knee replacement
($n = 86$) and hysterectomy ($n = 238$); elderly medical patients ($n = 96$); and patients
with chronic obstructive airways disease ($n = 32$).

Interventions: Hospital at home or inpatient hospital care.

Main outcome measures: Cost of hospital at home scheme to health service,
to general practitioners, and to patients and their families compared with hospital
care.

Results: No difference was detected in total health care costs between hospital at
home and hospital care for patients recovering from a hip or knee replacement, or

elderly medical patients. Hospital at home significantly increased health care costs for patients recovering from a hysterectomy (ratio of geometrical means 1.15, 95% confidence interval 1.04 to 1.29, $p = 0.009$) and for those with chronic obstructive airways disease (Mann–Whitney U test, $p = 0.01$). Hospital at home significantly increased general practitioners' costs for elderly medical patients (Mann–Whitney U test, $p < 0.01$) and for those with chronic obstructive airways disease ($p = 0.02$). Patient and carer expenditure made up a small proportion of total costs.

Conclusion: Hospital at home care did not reduce total health care costs for the conditions studied in this trial, and costs were significantly increased for patients recovering from a hysterectomy and those with chronic obstructive airways disease. There was some evidence that costs were shifted to primary care for elderly medical patients and those with chronic obstructive airways disease.

Introduction

There is little evidence to justify the widespread adoption of hospital at home on the basis of cost. A review of the subject identified only one randomised controlled trial that compared the cost of hospital at home with inpatient hospital care.[1] This trial, based in the United States, recruited patients with a terminal illness and found no difference in overall health care costs.[2] There is conflicting evidence from non-randomised studies.[3,4]

We report the results of a prospective economic evaluation, in the context of a randomised controlled trial, of the cost of providing hospital at home as a substitute for some forms of inpatient hospital care. The three questions addressed by the economic evaluation were

- Does substituting hospital at home care for hospital care result in a lower cost to the health service?
- Does hospital at home care, compared to hospital care, increase the cost to general practitioners?
- Does hospital at home care increase the cost borne by the patients and their families compared with hospital care?

Uses of health service resources that were recorded for cost minimisation analysis

Hospital care
- Number of inpatient days
- Number of inpatient days due to a hospital readmission related to the trial diagnosis
- Medication

Hospital at home care
- Number of hospital at home days
- Number of hospital at home visits (including duration of visit and grading of staff)
- Medication

Hospital transport
- Number of journeys made by ambulance or a health service car

General practitioner visits
- Number of visits to doctor's surgery
- Number of home visits

Methods

We describe patient recruitment and randomisation in our accompanying paper [not reprinted in this volume; see Introduction].[5] This economic evaluation took the form of a cost minimisation analysis, as the health outcomes of the two arms of the trial did not differ. Our primary interest was the cost to the health service, but we also examined the costs incurred by patients and families, as they could influence the acceptability of a hospital at home scheme.

We recruited five groups of patients: patients recovering from a hip replacement, a knee replacement, or a hysterectomy; patients with chronic obstructive airways disease; and elderly patients with a mix of medical conditions. All patients were aged 60 years or over, except those recovering from a hysterectomy, who were aged 20–70 years.

Data collection

The box lists the uses of health service resources on which data were collected. We obtained cost data for hospital care and hospital at home care from the respective trusts' finance departments for the financial year 1994–5, apportioned on the basis of activity for 1993–4. Details of the unit costs are available from the authors.

Hospital costs   The cost of hospital care included staffing costs, all non-staff running costs, and capital costs. Patient dependency scores were developed by hospital nursing and medical staff to reflect the marginal costs incurred during a patient's episode of hospital care (and hence the marginal savings of early discharge).[3,6] These scores were used to weight the costs for each day that a patient was in hospital. The costs of physiotherapy and occupational therapy were calculated according to the amount of time spent with a typical patient for each clinical group, and included a cost for non-contact time. Equipment costs (based on ward records), the cost of items not directly related to levels of patient care, and capital charges for land and buildings (based on valuation and including interest and depreciation) were divided by the number of ward bed days for the year 1994–5 to arrive at a charge per bed day. The cost of prescribed drugs was obtained from the hospital pharmacy department.

The time profile for costing hospital care differed for each clinical group. The costs for surgical patients excluded the costs of the operation, as these costs do not alter with different rehabilitative care. For patients having a hip or knee replacement, costs were calculated from the fourth postoperative day. For patients having a hysterectomy, costs were calculated from the first postoperative day. Cost data for medical patients were collected for the duration of their hospital stay.

Hospital at home costs   The cost of hospital at home care included all staffing and non-staff running costs. The costs of nurses, physiotherapists, and occupational therapists were based on the amount of time spent with patients, and included a cost for non-contact time. The following non-staff costs were included: central administration, travel, training, telephones and pagers, equipment, and office space. Medical supplies and equipment costs were depreciated over a 10 year period with a discount rate of 6%.[7] These costs were apportioned on an equal basis to each patient receiving hospital at home care, assuming costs were payable in advance at the start of the year. Administration and travel costs were apportioned according to the volume of patients. The cost of prescribed drugs was obtained from the hospital's pharmacy department.

General practitioner costs Research nurses visited each practice to record the number of general practitioners' home visits and number of patients' visits to the surgery. The community trust providing the hospital at home care reimbursed general practitioners visiting hospital at home patients at a rate of £100 per patient and £25 for each visit. General practitioner costs for the hospital care group were calculated with unit costs developed by the Personal Social Services Research Unit, Kent.[8]

Carer costs Carers were asked to record all expenditures related to the trial diagnosis (including equipment and adaptations, consumables, and travel) in a diary for one month, and any loss of earnings and days off work due to caring for their patient. Carers were also asked to record the number of hours a day they spent caring for the patient.

Statistical analysis

We describe the sample size calculations in our accompanying paper [not reprinted here].[5] Analysis was done on an intention to treat basis. When appropriate, data with non-normal distribution was log transformed before further parametric analysis was done. The Mann–Whitney U test was used for continuous variables that did not approximate a normal distribution after log transformation.

Sensitivity analyses were conducted for areas that could possibly restrict the generalisability of the trial results. These were the trial rate of reimbursing general practitioners, patients' duration of hospital at home care observed in the trial, and the use of average costs per inpatient day instead of dependency adjusted hospital costs.

Results

Results are presented by clinical condition for both arms of the trial. Inpatient hospital care and hospital at home care accounted for most of the health care costs. Tables 1, 2 and 3 show health service resources and costs for each patient group.

Early discharge of patients after elective surgery

Patients allocated to hospital at home care after a hip or knee replacement or a hysterectomy spent significantly fewer days in hospital (Tables 1 and 2). However, they received significantly more days of health care with the addition of hospital at home. For patients recovering from a hip or knee replacement, the total costs to the health service were not significantly different between the two groups. For patients recovering from a hysterectomy, total health service costs were significantly higher for those allocated to hospital at home care. Of the total numbers of patients undergoing these procedures during the study period, we recruited about 20% of all those having hip replacements, 25% of those having knee replacements, and 35% of those undergoing hysterectomy.

Table I   Health service resources and costs consumed at 3 months after hospital admission by patients allocated to hospital at home care or inpatient hospital care: orthopaedic patients recovering from hip or knee replacement

	Hospital at home	Hospital	Difference (95% CI)
Hip replacement:	(n = 36)*	(n = 49)	
Mean (SD) days in hospital care	8.11 (5.52)	11.87 (4.52)	−3.75 (−5.92 to −1.58)
Mean (SD) days in hospital at home care	6.58 (4.26)	—	—
Mean (SD) total days of care	14.69 (5.13)	11.87 (4.57)	2.84 (0.75 to 4.93)
Median (interquartile range) days of readmission	0 (0.00–0.00)	0 (0.00–0.00)	$p = 0.39$†
Mean (SD) hospital costs including readmission (£)	515.42 (473.20)	776.30 (364.53)	−260.87 (−441.56 to −80.19) $p < 0.01$
Mean (SD) hospital at home costs (£)	351.24 (240.58)	—	—
Median (interquartile range) GP costs: home and surgery visits (£)	42.84 (0.00–64.61)‡	15.49 (0.00–45.19)	$p = 0.06$†
Mean (SD) total health service costs (£)	911.39 (563.76)	815.70 (347.99)	Ratio of geometric mean 1.05 (0.87 to 1.27) $p = 0.59$
Knee replacement:	(n = 46)‡	(n = 39)	
Mean (SD) days in hospital care	10.28 (4.60)	13.31 (4.57)	−3.02 (−5.01 to −1.04)
Mean (SD) days in hospital at home care	5.72 (4.98)	—	—
Mean (SD) total days of care	16.00 (5.44)	13.31 (4.57)	2.69 (0.50 to 4.88)
Median (interquartile range) days of readmission	0 (0.00–0.00)	0 (0.00–0.00)	$p = 0.23$†
Mean (SD) hospital costs including readmission (£)	1092.24 (615.27)	1348.35 (625.94)	−256.11 (−524.61 to 12.38) $p = 0.06$
Mean (SD) hospital at home costs (£)	348.16 (275.25)	—	—
Median (interquartile range) GP costs: home and surgery visits (£)	15.49 (0.00–57.15)	15.49 (0.00–30.98)	$p = 0.22$†
Mean (SD) total health service costs (£)	1461.62 (666.61)	1375.36 (637.76)	Ratio of geometric mean 1.05 (0.88 to 1.26) $p = 0.55$

GP = general practitioner.
* No data available for 1 patient.
† Mann–Whitney U test.
‡ No data available for 1 patient.

Table 2 Health service resources and costs consumed at 3 months after hospital admission by patients allocated to hospital at home care or inpatient hospital care: patients recovering from hysterectomy

	Hospital at home (n = 111*)	Hospital (n = 123[†])	Difference (95% CI)
Mean (SD) days in hospital care	4.34 (1.86)	5.79 (2.98)	−1.44 (−2.09 to −0.79)
Mean (SD) days in hospital at home care	3.11 (2.64)	—	—
Mean (SD) total days of care	7.45 (2.59)	5.79 (2.98)	1.66 (0.94 to 2.39)
Median (interquartile range) days of readmission	0 (0.00–0.00)	0 (0.00–0.00)	$p = 0.21$[‡]
Mean (SD) hospital costs including readmission (£)	487.43 (350.20)	647.77 (496.27)	Ratio of geometric mean 0.76 (0.67 to 0.87) $p < 0.01$
Mean (SD) hospital at home costs (£)	250.18 (273.54)	—	—
Median (interquartile range) GP costs: home and surgery visits (£)	30.98 (15.49–61.96)	30.98 (15.49–61.96)	$p = 0.70$[‡]
Mean (SD) total health service costs (£)	771.78 (408.72)	679.39 (439.83)	Ratio of geometric mean 1.15 (1.04 to 1.29) $p < 0.01$

GP = general practitioner.
* No data available for 3 patients.
[†] No data available for 1 patient.
[‡] Mann–Whitney U test.

Table 3 Health service resources and costs consumed at 3 months after hospital admission by patients allocated to hospital at home care or inpatient hospital care: elderly medical patients and patients with chronic obstructive airways disease

	Hospital at home	Hospital	Difference (95% CI)
Elderly medical:	(n = 50)	(n = 44*)	
Mean (SD) days in hospital care	12.84 (14.69)	13.20 (14.19)	−0.36 (−6.30 to 5.57)
Mean (SD) days in hospital at home care	9.04 (7.79)	—	—
Mean (SD) total days of care	21.88 (18.30)	13.20 (14.19)	8.67 (1.90 to 15.45)
Median (interquartile range) days of readmission	0 (0.00–1.00)	0 (0.00–0.00)	$p = 0.08$†
Median (interquartile range) hospital costs including readmission (£)	913.76 (243.31–2045.68)	1366.16 (629.08–2033.50)	$p = 0.21$†
Mean (SD) hospital at home costs (£)	793.45 (811.36)	—	—
Median (interquartile range) GP costs: home and surgery visits (£)	67.84 (45.19–172.83)	45.19 (15.49–82.95)	$p < 0.01$†
Median (interquartile range) total health service costs (£)	1705.32 (913.83–3121.55)	1388.76 (645.06–2094.88)	$p = 0.09$†
Chronic obstructive airways disease:	(n = 15)	(n = 17)	
Mean (SD) days in hospital care	6.93 (3.39)	12.12 (7.49)	−5.18 (−9.48 to −0.89)
Mean (SD) days in hospital at home care	5.33 (3.94)	—	—
Mean (SD) total days of care	12.27 (3.69)	12.12 (7.49)	0.15 (−4.21 to 4.51)
Median (interquartile range) days of readmission	5.00 (0.00–10.0)	0.00 (0.00–3.00)	$p = 0.08$†
Median (interquartile range) hospital costs including readmission (£)	1389.53 (821.65–1993.97)	1198.53 (712.00–1508.24)	$p = 0.56$†
Mean (SD) hospital at home costs (£)	710.61 (526.50)	—	—
Median (interquartile range) GP costs: home and surgery visits (£)	115.38 (25.00–214.30)	15.49 (0.00–91.02)	$p = 0.02$†
Median (interquartile range) total health service costs (£)	2379.67 (1458.09–2759.05)	1247.64 (772.50–1619.19)	$p = 0.01$†

GP = general practitioner.
* No data available for 2 patients.
† Mann–Whitney U test.

Elderly medical patients and patients with chronic obstructive airways disease

No significant difference was detected between the two groups of elderly medical patients in the number of days spent in hospital, but, with the addition of hospital at home care, the total days of health care for the hospital at home group was significantly higher (Table 3). Patients with chronic obstructive airways disease in the hospital at home group spent significantly fewer days in hospital, but this reduction was offset by the time spent in hospital at home care so there was no significant difference between the two groups for the total days of health care (Table 3). For elderly medical patients, total costs to the health service were not significantly different between the two groups. Patients with chronic obstructive airways disease allocated to hospital at home care incurred significantly greater health care costs than did those receiving only hospital care. About 1% of all patients admitted for medical conditions during the study period were recruited to either the elderly medical or chronic obstructive airways disease groups. Nineteen of these patients were recruited by general practitioners, of whom nine were allocated to hospital care. However, only two of these patients received acute hospital care.

General practitioner costs

For patients discharged early after elective surgery, no significant differences in general practitioner costs were detected between the two groups. However, for elderly medical patients and those with chronic obstructive airways disease, the costs of general practitioner services were significantly higher for the patients allocated to hospital at home care compared with those in the hospital groups.

Costs to patients and carers

Patients' and carers' expenses made up a small proportion of total costs. There were no significant differences between the two groups for any of the categories of patients, and inclusion of these costs did not alter the results. The median cost for all patient groups was £0. The greatest expense was incurred by patients with chronic obstructive airways disease: median cost for the hospital at home group was £0 (interquartile range £0–£19.8) and for the hospital group was £0 (£0–£0). There were no significant differences between the two groups of carers in the time spent caring for the patient, although this was a substantial element in both groups. Few carers reported loss of earnings from caring for the patient, as most of the carers were retired. Further details of these costs will be published elsewhere.

Sensitivity analysis

Table 4 shows the results of the sensitivity analyses. Reducing length of stay in hospital at home care changed the difference in total health care costs for patients recovering from a hysterectomy and for those with chronic obstructive airways disease. A one day reduction eliminated the difference in cost for patients recovering from a hysterectomy, while a two day reduction altered the results so that hospital at home care became significantly less costly than hospital care for these patients. Costs remained significantly more expensive for patients with

Table 4 Sensitivity analysis: comparing costs of hospital care, dependency adjusted costs and average costs, with costs of hospital at home care after reducing lengths of stay by one or two days

	Hip replacement HaH (n = 36) v hospital (n = 49)	Knee replacement HaH (n = 46) v hospital (n = 39)	Hysterectomy HaH (n = 111) v hospital (n = 123)	Elderly medical HaH (n = 50) v hospital (n = 44)	Chronic obstructive airways disease HaH (n = 15) v hospital (n = 17)
Trial results: difference in total health care costs using dependency adjusted hospital costs					
Difference in cost (£)	Mean 95.68	Mean 86.26	Mean 92.40	Median 316.56	Median 1132.03
Ratio of geometric mean (95% CI)	1.05 (0.87 to 1.27)	1.05 (0.88 to 1.26)	1.15 (1.04 to 1.29)	—	—
p value	0.59	0.55	0.009	0.09	0.01
Sensitivity analysis: difference in total health care costs using average hospital costs					
Difference in cost (£)	Mean −36.80	Mean 35.23	Mean 60.85	Median 518.35	Median 741.36
Ratio of geometric mean (95% CI)	0.89 (0.73 to 1.09)	1.004 (0.82 to 1.22)	1.06 (0.98 to 1.23)	—	—
p value	0.27	0.96	0.10	0.05	0.02
Sensitivity analysis: length of stay in hospital at home care reduced by 1 day					
Difference in cost (£)	Mean 58.32	Mean −8.01	Mean −21.75	Median 227.25	Median 840.26
Ratio of geometric mean (95% CI)	1.02 (0.84 to 1.23)	1.002 (0.84 to 1.19)	0.99 (0.90 to 1.11)	—	—
p value	0.87	0.99	0.99	0.17	0.04
Sensitivity analysis: length of stay in hospital at home care reduced by 2 days					
Difference in cost (£)	Mean 10.61	Mean −49.10	Mean −80.48	Median 103.37	Median 757.23
Ratio of geometric mean (95% CI)	0.95 (0.78 to 1.15)	0.96 (0.81 to 1.15)	0.88 (0.78 to 0.99)	—	—
p value	0.59	0.68	0.03	0.38	0.06

HaH = hospital at home.

chronic obstructive airways disease when duration of hospital at home care was reduced by one day, but a reduction of two days resulted in a non-significant difference between the two groups.

Using average hospital costs instead of dependency adjusted costs reduced the difference in cost between hospital at home care and hospital care for all groups of patients except for the elderly medical patients. Using standard general practitioner costs[8] for both arms of the trial altered the results only for patients recovering from a hip replacement, and general practitioner costs for these patients became significantly more expensive (Mann–Whitney U test, $p = 0.03$).

Discussion

Many believe that hospital at home schemes will contain health care costs by reducing the demand for acute hospital beds. Our findings indicate that this is not the case. Instead, hospital at home care increased health service costs for some groups of patients, while for others there were no net differences in costs. This is perhaps not surprising, as patients who were discharged early to hospital at home care went home when their hospital care was least expensive. Once in hospital at home care some patients, particularly elderly patients with a medical condition, required 24 hour care. Furthermore, hospital at home increased the overall duration of an episode of health care. This pattern has been observed elsewhere.[4] It may be possible to decrease the amount of time patients spend in hospital at home, and thus reduce cost. However, this could have an adverse effect on patient outcomes. For elderly medical patients and those with chronic obstructive airways disease, hospital at home care increased general practitioner costs, providing evidence that some costs were shifted within the health service.

Perhaps surprisingly for a service that is intended to reduce the pressure on acute hospital beds, the proportion of patients eligible for hospital at home care was low. Other evaluations have also described a relatively low volume of eligible patients.[2,4,9–12] This contrasts with the numbers described by some service providers (Harrison V, Intermediate Care Conference, Anglia and Oxford NHS Executive, Milton Keynes, October, 1997). An increased volume of patients would not, however, alter the costs substantially as only a small proportion of hospital at home costs are fixed. It is possible that patients who would otherwise agree to use hospital at home are deterred by an evaluation. An alternative explanation may be that hospital at home provides extra care in the community but not necessarily care that would otherwise be carried out in a hospital setting.

Just as inappropriate admissions are a problem for acute hospitals, there is no reason to believe they do not pose a problem for services such as hospital at home. We found that some patients allocated to hospital care were never admitted to hospital and stayed at home with no extra services. This has been found elsewhere (A. Wilson, personal communication) and suggests that hospital at home schemes could potentially provide care to patients who would otherwise not be receiving health care services. Alternatively, hospital at home may be viewed as supplementing existing services, which may be an acceptable policy option for some groups of patients, particularly elderly medical patients who prefer this form of care.

The extent to which hospital at home care can substitute for hospital care in the United Kingdom is limited. This can partly be explained by the speed at which hospital at home schemes have been set up. Purchasers and providers have responded, quickly to initiatives, usually supported by 'ring fenced' monies, designed to ease the pressure on hospital beds. Schemes have usually been grafted onto primary care services, with minor alterations to the mix of skills already available. They may become out of date with changes in hospital practice. This is a particular problem for schemes admitting patients who are discharged early from hospital. As hospital lengths of stay decrease, the number of days that can be transferred into the community is correspondingly reduced.

Conclusions

The results of this trial suggest that simply shifting services from one location to another is unlikely to reduce health service costs. Patients discharged early after elective surgery go home at a time when they use least resources. When an inpatient stay involves relatively high nursing costs, as with elderly medical patients, early discharge to hospital at home is unlikely to be significantly cheaper than hospital based care as most of these nursing costs still have to be incurred. Hospital at home care may be cost effective for patients who are relatively independent but who require technical support, such as those receiving intravenous antimicrobial therapy. However, there is little evidence to support or refute this.[13] Service developments, as much as clinical interventions, need to be evidence based. Arguments for diverting resources away from hospital beds should be viewed in the light of the available evidence.

References

1 Shepperd S, Iliffe S. Hospital at home compared with in-patient hospital care [review]. In: Bero L., Grilli R., Grimshaw J., Oxman A., eds. *The Cochrane Library.* Cochrane Collaboration; Issue 1. Oxford: Update Software, 1998. (Updated quarterly.)
2 Hughes S.L., Cummings J., Weaver F., Manheim L., Braun B., Conrad K. A randomised trial of the cost effectiveness of VA hospital-based home care for the terminally ill. *Health Serv Res* 1992; 26: 801–17.
3 Hollingsworth W., Todd C., Parker M., Roberts J.A., Williams R. Cost analysis of early discharge after hip fracture. *BMJ* 1993; 307: 908–6.
4 Hensher M., Fulop N., Hood S., Ujah S. Does hospital at home make economic sense? Early discharge versus standard care for orthopaedic patients. *J R Soc Med* 1996; 89: 548–51.
5 Shepperd S., Harwood D., Jenkinson C., Gray A., Vessey M., Morgan P. Randomised controlled trial comparing hospital at home care with inpatient hospital care. I: three month follow up of health outcomes. *BMJ* 1998; 316: 1786–91.
6 Jonsson B., Lindren B. Five common fallacies in estimating the economic gains of early discharge. *Soc Sci Med* 1980; 14: 27–33.
7 Drummond M.F., O'Brien B., Stoddart G.L., Torrance G.W. *Methods for the Economic Evaluation of Health Care Programmes,* 2nd edn. Oxford: Oxford University Press, 1997.
8 Netten A., Dennett J. *Unit Costs of Health and Social Care 1996.* Canterbury: Personal Social Services Research Unit, 1996.
9 Adler M.W., Waller J.J., Creese A., Thorne S.C. Randomised controlled trial of early discharge for inguinal hernia and varicose veins. *J Epidemiol Community Health* 1978; 32: 136–42.
10 Ruckley C.V., Cuthbertson C., Fenwick N., Prescott R.J., Garraway W.M. Day care after operations for hernia or varicose veins: a controlled trial. *Br J Surg* 1978; 65: 456–9.

11 Martin F., Oyewole A., Moloney A. A randomised controlled trial of a high support hospital discharge team for elderly people. *Age Ageing* 1994; 12: 228–34.

12 Donald I.P., Baldwin R.N., Bannerjee M. Gloucester hospital at home: a randomised controlled trial. *Age Ageing* 1995; 24: 434–9.

13 Gilbert D.N., Dworkin R.J., Raber S.R., Leggett J.E. Outpatient parenteral antimicrobial drug therapy. *N Engl J Med* 1997; 337: 829–38.

What you might do now

This was a very elaborate economic analysis, partly because care was provided by various agencies and various practitioners. The exemplars in Chapters 1 and 2 also have economic implications. You might want to read them and consider whether they would have been more useful to practitioners if they had paid more attention to costing interventions

Carry out a more systematic appraisal of the study using 'Questions to Ask about Cost-effectiveness Studies' in Part 4 of this book

What you might do now

Consolidate what you have learned about experiments by reading Chapter 5, or about cost-effectiveness studies by using the further reading in that chapter

Find some cost-effectiveness research of interest to you using the Appendix to this book, and appraise it using 'Questions to Ask about Cost-effectiveness Studies' in Part 4 of this book

CHAPTER 4

COMPARING LIKE WITH LIKE: A SYSTEMATIC REVIEW AND META-ANALYSIS OF HOME VISITING SCHEMES AND CHILDHOOD INJURY

EXEMPLAR   Roberts, I., Kramer, M.S. and Suissa, S. (1996) 'Does home visting prevent childhood injury? A systematic review of randomised controlled trials', *British Medical Journal*, 312: 29–33

What you need to understand in order to understand the exemplar study
The idea of a systematic review. *See the introduction to this chapter.*
The importance of quality criteria for including studies in the review ('inclusion criteria'). *These are explained in the exemplar, but have a look at Figure 5.2 in Chapter 5 to see why these are the quality criteria adopted.*
'agreement on methodological criteria adopted evaluated with weighted κ' and the figures given for agreement relating to Table 1 *This refers to an inter-rater reliability test. See Chapter 6, section 6.*
The importance of publication bias and overcoming it. *Explained in the exemplar*
The idea of a meta-analysis. *See the introduction to this chapter.*
Odds ratios, their confidence intervals and how to read an odds ratio diagram from a meta-analysis. *See Chapter 7, section 5.*
You do not have to understand the details of the statistical methods used in the study. But many of the technicalities concern data transformations. *See Chapter 6, sections 3 and 4; Chapter 7, section 6.*

Introduction

Some studies suggest that home visiting schemes reduce rates of childhood injury, while others suggest that they do not. This diversity is hardly surprising since the studies were conducted at different times, in different places, for different kinds of visiting scheme, with regard to families at different degrees and kinds of risk, and using different measures of childhood injury. In addition, each study was relatively small for a 'complex' intervention such as home visiting (see Chapter 5, section 9) and concerning rare events such as childhood injury (see Chapter 7, section 7). And some studies were much better designed than others.

The term 'systematic review' refers to reviewing a number of pieces of research on approximately the same topic, using a stringent set of quality criteria, evaluating each in relation to each other in terms of its credibility, and discerning to where the combined evidence points, if anywhere, and identifying gaps in knowledge as priorities for further research. Systematic reviews should not be confused with other publications reviewing research. These are often propagandist, with the reviewer picking and choosing between bits of research and giving them a spin in order to support some case the author is making.

From a practitioner's point of view systematic reviews enormously reduce the amount of effort needed to keep up to date with research. The Appendix to this volume is particularly useful for accessing systematic reviews. The review will give a synopsis and expert comment on perhaps ten or more studies which otherwise would all have to be found, read and understood, sometimes in several languages. All this comes at a price, of course. Practitioners who rely on systematic reviews have to accept the quality standards adopted by systematic reviewers. These usually exclude all research except experimental research, and commonly all research except randomised controlled trials, as in the exemplar reading for this chapter. If the focus is on effectiveness there is a good case for doing this (see Chapter 5, Introduction and section 1). But such a narrowing is not to everyone's taste. It is certainly true that systematic reviews side-line all research other than experimental research. This does not just follow from judgements about quality, but also from the fact that experimental research tends to take similar formats which allows for point by point comparisons to be made between studies. This is rarely possible with other kinds of research, thereby raising puzzles as to whether differences in findings derive from real differences in what was studied, or merely from using different methods to study the same thing.

Some systematic reviews include a *meta-analysis*, as does the exemplar. Put simply, this involves pooling the results of several studies as if each were just part of a much larger study including them all. Meta-

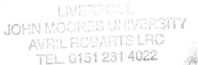

analysis can be controversial in three different ways. First, studies in the review are likely to have some differences, perhaps with different kinds of subjects entering the trial, somewhat different interventions, using different instruments and generating different kinds of baseline and outcome data. Hence like may not be being pooled with like. Second, different studies may have involved diverse kinds of statistical calculation to produce their results, hence there are good mathematical reservations about adding them together. When they are pooled this may involve complicated statistical manoeuvres to bring them all into the same scheme of measurement which may be controversial and often make it difficult to give a common-sense meaning to the results. In the exemplar Roberts et al. express the pooled results as the 'inverse variance weighted average of the study specific odds ratios'. This may be statistically appropriate, but it is difficult to understand in everyday terms (but see Chapter 7, section 6). Third, there is a possibility that a large, but badly conducted trial will over-influence the pooled results, despite reviewers' attempts to eliminate poorly conducted trials from the review using quality or 'inclusion' criteria.

While pooling may be problematic, doing something like it is unavoidable if conclusions are to be drawn from the quantitative data produced by a number of different pieces of research. It is probably appropriate to think of pooling as being quasi-mathematics rather than mathematics: rather more precise than saying 'most', but less precise than saying '73.24%'.

DOES HOME VISITING PREVENT CHILDHOOD INJURY? A SYSTEMATIC REVIEW OF RANDOMISED CONTROLLED TRIALS*

Ian Roberts, Michael S. Kramer, Samy Suissa

Abstract

Objective: To quantify the effectiveness of home visiting programmes in the prevention of child injury [...]

   Design: Systematic review of 11 randomised controlled trials of home visiting programmes. Pooled odds ratios were estimated as an inverse variance weighted average of the study specific odds ratios.

---

* Editorial note: The original publication also reviewed studies of the effect of home visiting on non-accidental injury rates. These sections have been edited out of the exemplar.

Setting: Randomised trials that were available by April 1995.

Subjects: The trials comprised 3433 participants.

Results: Eight trials examined the effectiveness of home visiting in the prevention of childhood injury. The pooled odds ratio for the eight trials was 0.74 (95% confidence interval 0.60 to 0.92). Four studies examined the effect of home visiting on injury in the first year of life. The pooled odds ratio was 0.98 (0.62 to 1.53).

Conclusions: Home visiting programmes have the potential to reduce significantly the rates of childhood injury.

Introduction

Home visiting programmes have long been advocated for improving the health of disadvantaged children. In Britain home visits by health visitors are considered to have a key role in accident prevention because of the advice given during the visits on child development and home safety.[1] In the United States home visiting has been promoted primarily for the prevention of child abuse and neglect.[2] In 1991 the United States Advisory Board on Child Abuse and Neglect called for the establishment of a universal programme of home visiting in an attempt to stem the increase in numbers of child abuse reports.[3]

Over the past two decades several randomised trials have examined the effect of home visiting programmes on the occurrence of child abuse and other child health outcomes. The results of these trials, however, have been conflicting. Although several published articles have reviewed the evidence from randomised trials,[4,5] none of these satisfies the methodological criteria that have been proposed for scientific overviews.[6] To quantify the effect of home visiting programmes on the occurrence of child injury and abuse we conducted a systematic review.

Methods

Inclusion criteria We included studies in the systematic review if they met all three of the following criteria: (*a*) the assignment of the study participants to the intervention or control group had to be random or quasi-random – for example, alternate record numbers; (*b*) the study intervention had to include one or more postnatal home visits; and (*c*) the study had to address the outcomes of child injury (unintentional).

Identification of relevant trials We identified trials by a computerised literature search of Medline (January 1966 to April 1995) and Embase (January 1975 to April 1995). We also searched the social sciences citation index for articles referencing randomised trials of home visiting. Key terms used for searching included social support, family support, home (and health) visitors, home (and health) visitation, child abuse and child neglect. We reviewed the references of all relevant papers found in the searches, as well as those of review articles and textbooks. Because home visiting is often encountered in the context of the prevention of child abuse, a hand search was conducted of the *Journal of Child Abuse and Neglect* (from 1977 1(1) through to 1995 19(3)). We contacted the authors of identified papers and experts in the field and asked about any published or unpublished work that they might be aware of. To access studies not formally published, such as research reports and abstracts, we searched relevant conference proceedings. If studies met the first two inclusion criteria but did not report outcomes of child injury or abuse we asked the authors to provide any unpublished data on child injury.

Data extraction and study appraisal We extracted the following data from each study: strategy for allocation concealment, number of randomised participants, duration of follow up, loss to follow up, blinding of outcome assessment, and the professional background of the home visitor (health or welfare professional or non-professional). We evaluated the quality of the trial using a modification of Prendiville's criteria.[7] With this approach trials are scored from 1 to 3 (1 = poorest score, 3 = best score) on three important aspects of study methodology: control of confounding at entry (adequacy of allocation concealment); control of selection bias (extent to which analyses are based on all randomised participants); and control of information bias in assessing outcome (blinding of observers). While the original criteria assigned a score of 3 for random assignment by telephone and 2 for using opaque sealed envelopes, we assigned a score of 3 for using either of these methods. Trials that assigned subjects to treatment by using methods intended to reduce the risk of foreknowledge of allocation but which were not as secure as random assignment by telephone or use of opaque sealed envelopes scored 2. Trials in which the authors did not report the method of allocation concealment (and were unable to provide further details or could not be contacted) and trials using alternate record numbers or other similar strategies scored 1. If a published report contained insufficient information for us to assess the quality of the trial, we asked the authors to provide further details. Two assessors performed the data extraction independently, with agreement on methodological criteria evaluated with weighted κ.[8] Each point of disagreement was settled by collaborative review.

Statistical methods The measure of association, the odds ratio, was calculated directly for studies in which injury was expressed in binary (yes/no) form, with the variance estimated by Wolf's method.[9] For studies in which injury occurrence was allowed to be multiple and expressed as an incidence density, the odds ratio was estimated on the assumption of a Poisson distribution, with the probability of a participant having at least one event being given by $1 - e - ^{ID}$, where ID is the incidence density. Pooled odds ratios were then calculated as an inverse variance weighted average of the study specific odds ratios.

Results

The combined search strategies identified 33 trials meeting the first two inclusion criteria (randomised trials of postnatal home visiting).[10–42] Eleven of these trials (with 3433 participants) reported outcome data on injury or abuse, or on both.[10–19,42] One of the eleven trials was published as an abstract only,[42] the author of this report was contacted, but the relevant outcome data were not available for inclusion in the review. Of the remaining 10 trials, one reported no differences in the occurrence of accidents,[13] and in another injury outcome data had been collected but not reported.[19] In both of these trials the authors gave us the relevant data. The authors of 13 of the 22 trials meeting the first two inclusion criteria but not reporting outcome data on injury or abuse responded to our request for information on unpublished injury outcomes. As a result of this process one further

Table I   Scores* for quality of methodology and study characteristics for
randomised trials of home visiting

Trial (year, country)	Allocation concealment	Analysed as randomised[†]	Blinding[†]	No. of participants randomised	Follow up (years)
IHDP (1995, USA)[43]	3	2	1	985	1
Marcenko et al. (1994, USA)[10]	2	2	1	225	0.8
Johnson et al. (1993, Republic of Ireland)[11]	3	2	1	262	1
Barth (1991, USA)[12]	1	2	1	313	3
Dawson et al. (1989, USA)[13]	1	1	1	145	1
Hardy et al. (1989, USA)[14]	1	2	2	290	1.9
Olds et al. (1986, USA)[15]	3	1	2	400	4
Lealman et al. (1983, England)[16]	3	2	3	312	1.5
Larson (1980, Canada)[17]	3	2	2	80	1.5
Siegel et al. (1980, USA)[18]	3	3	1	321	1
Gray et al. (1979, USA)[19]	3	2	1	100	1.4

IHDP = infant health and development program.
* On scale of 1 to 3 (1 = poorest score, 3 = best score).
[†] Judged for injury outcome measures whenever possible.

trial was identified that met all three inclusion criteria.[43] Eleven trials were therefore identified that had outcome data on injury or abuse, or both.

Table I shows the scores for the quality of methodology for the trials included in the systematic review. The weighted κ for agreement between the two assessors was 0.94 for adequacy of allocation concealment, 0.51 for the extent to which analyses were based on all randomised participants, and 0.78 for blinding. The mean scores for the unintentional injury outcomes were: adequacy of allocation concealment, 2.4; extent to which analyses were based on all randomised participants, 1.9; blinding, 1.5.

Table 2 shows the data for the eight trials that examined the effect of home visiting on the occurrence of childhood injury. Six of the eight trials reported a lower incidence of injury in the group that received home visits. One study reported three injury outcome measures, representing three different time periods of follow up. For this study, the overall injury rates and odds ratios were calculated for the entire (four year) follow up period (odds ratio 0.74 (95% confidence interval 0.55 to 0.99)). The pooled odds ratio for injury for the eight trials (figure) was 0.74 (0.60 to 0.92). Four studies examined the effect of home visiting on injury occurrence in the first year of life only. The pooled odds ratio was 0.98 (0.62 to 1.53).

Discussion

Although home visiting is unlikely to be associated with adverse effects, the widespread implementation or intensification of home visiting programmes may have important resource implications. Our meta-analysis of the results from eight randomised trials shows a significant preventive effect of home visiting on the occurrence of childhood injury.

Table 2   Home visiting and childhood injury

Trial (year, country)	Study population	Intervention	Outcome	Participants visited	Controls	Odds ratio (95% confidence interval)
IHDP (1995, USA)[43]	Parents of low birthweight premature infants	Postnatal, non-professional, emotional, social, practial, and informational support	'Non-hospitalised injuries by maternal report'	17/345	26/551	1.05 (0.56–1.96)
Johnson et al. (1993, Republic of Ireland)[11]	Disadvantaged first time mothers	Postnatal, non-professional support and encouragement in child rearing using the child development programme	'Suffered an accident'	3/127	8/105	0.29 (0.08–1.14)
Hardy et al. (1989, USA)[14]	Inner city mothers of poor infants	Postnatal, non-professional parenting and childcare education	'Outpatient diagnosis of closed head trauma'	8/131	15/132	0.51 (0.21–1.24)
Dawson et al. (1989, USA)[13]	Pregnant women attending for maternity care not selected for psychosocial risk	Antenatal and postnatal, non-professional emotional support; information and help in using community resources	'Accidents or ingestion requiring medical attention'	5/67	6/44	0.51 (0.15–1.79)
Olds et al. (1986, USA)[15]	Primiparas who were teenagers, unmarried, or of low socioeconomic status	Antenatal and postnatal parenting education in infant development from nurse; involvement of family members and friends in child care; linkage of family members with health and human services	'Emergency visit for accidents and poisoning (1st year of life)'	0.12*	0.06*	2.06 (0.83–5.15)
			'Emergency visit for accidents and poisoning (2nd year of life)'	0.15*	0.34*	0.40 (0.21–0.77)
			'Emergency department visits for injuries/ingestion (25 to 50 months)'	0.47*	0.61*	0.71 (0.49–1.04)
Lealman et al. (1983, England)[16]	Families predicted to be at risk of child abuse	Postnatal intervention and support from social worker	'Admissions with trauma'	1/103	4/209	0.50 (0.06–4.55)
Larson (1980, Canada)[17]	Working class families	Postnatal, non-professional emotional and informational support	'Significant falls, cuts, burns, poisonings or other injuries'	1.26**	1.55**	0.73 (0.46–1.16)
Gray et al. (1979, USA)[19]	Families most likely to exhibit abnormal parenting practices	Postnatal emotional support from physician/nurse/lay visitor	'Accidents by maternal report'	16/26	13/25	1.48 (0.49–4.5)
Pooled results						0.74 (0.60–0.92)

IHDP = infant health and development program.
* Adjusted mean.
** Cumulative accident rate per child.

Methodological issues

Publication bias is one of the most important potential threats to the validity of systematic reviews. Such bias may arise if certain outcome data are selectively omitted from published reports because the results fail to reach significance. To avoid this type of bias we wrote to the authors of all identified randomised trials of home visiting programmes, asking them to provide any unpublished outcome data on injury or abuse (one further trial was identified by this approach). The authors of nearly half of the studies meeting the first two inclusion criteria, however, could not be traced. These were predominantly small studies and so would make a comparatively minor impact on the overall result. Funnel plots can be used to estimate the extent of publication bias, but because their use is limited to meta-analyses that have enough trials to allow a funnel shape to be visualised, this approach is not helpful in this review.[44]

A recurring issue in the context of systematic reviews is the extent to which the interventions examined are sufficiently comparable for the results from the studies to be combined. The effectiveness of home visiting may depend on its timing, duration, and intensity. Nevertheless, for unintentional childhood injuries no clear heterogeneity was seen in the effect across studies.

Implications

Because most of the trials included in this review used non-professional home visitors, the question of the relative effectiveness of professional versus non-professional home visiting remains unanswered. The observed effect of home visiting on child injury is consistent with a generic effect of home based maternal support. In Britain a programme of home visiting is provided by health visitors. Current health visiting programmes, however, should not be assumed to achieve the

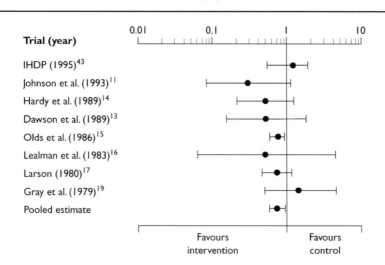

Odds ratio and 95% confidence intervals for effect of home visiting on child injury

effects on childhood injury that are implied by the results of this systematic review. Firstly, the experimental home visiting may have been more intense than that which is typically provided by health visitors. Secondly, in all but one of the trials the intervention was targeted at groups considered to be at increased risk for adverse child health outcomes. This may restrict the extent to which the results are generalisable to programmes of universal health visiting.

The Health of the Nation strategy established child accident prevention as a national priority. Few injury prevention interventions, however, have been shown to reduce injury rates in randomised controlled trials. Given the results of this systematic review, the effectiveness of home visiting by health visitors and non-professional support agencies in preventing childhood injury deserves further examination.

References

1 Avery J.G., Jackson R.H. *Children and their accidents*. Edward Arnold: London, 1933.
2 Kempe C.H. Approaches to preventing child abuse: the health visitor concept. *Am J Dis Child* 1976; 130: 941–2.
3 United States Advisory Board on Child Abuse and Neglect. *Child Abuse and Neglect: Critical First Steps in Response to a National Emergency*. Washington DC: US Government Printing Office, 1990. (Publication no 017–092–00104–5.)
4 Olds D.L., Kitzman H. Can home visitation improve the health of women and children at environmental risk? *Pediatrics* 1990; 86: 108–16.
5 Combs-Orme T., Reis J., Ward L.D. Effectiveness of home visits by public health nurses in maternal and child health: an empirical review. *Public Health Rep* 1985; 100: 490–9.
6 Oxman A.D., Cook D.J., Guyatt G.H. User's guides to the medical literature. VI. How to use an overview. *JAMA* 1994; 272: 1367–71.
7 Prendiville W., Elbourne D., Chalmers I. The effects of routine oxytocic administration in the management of the third stage of labor: an overview of the evidence from controlled trials. *Br J Obstet Gynaecol* 1988; 95: 3–16.
8 Cohen J.A. A coefficient of agreement for nominal scales. *Educational and Psychological Measurement* 1960; 20: 37–46.
9 Wolf B. On estimating the relation between blood group and disease. *Ann Hum Genet* 1965; 19: 251–3.
10 Marcenko M.O., Spence M. Home visitation services for at-risk pregnant and postpartum women: a randomised trial. *Am J Orthopsychiatry* 1994; 64: 468–78.
11 Johnson Z., Howell F., Molloy B. Community mother's programme: a randomised controlled trial of non-professional intervention in parenting. *BMJ* 1993; 306: 1449–52.
12 Barth R.P. An experimental evaluation of in-home child abuse prevention services. *Child Abuse Negl* 1991; 15: 363–75.
13 Dawson P., Van Doorninck W.J., Robinson J.L. Effects of home based, informal social support on child health. *J Dev Behav Pediatr* 1989; 10: 63–7.
14 Hardy J.B., Streett R. Family support and parenting education in the home: an effective extension of clinic-based preventive health care services for poor children. *J Pediatr* 1989; 115: 927–31.
15 Olds D.L., Henderson C.R., Chamberlin R., Tatelbaum R. Preventing child abuse and neglect: a randomised trial of nurse home visitation. *Pediatrics* 1986; 78: 65–78.
16 Lealman G., Haigh D., Philips J. Predicting and preventing child abuse – an empty hope? *Lancet* 1983; i: 1423–4.
17 Larson C.P. Efficacy of prenatal and postpartum home visits on child health and development. *Pediatrics* 1980; 66: 191–7.

18 Siegel E., Bauman K.E., Schaefer E.S., Saunders M.M., Ingram D.D. Hospital and home support in infancy: impact on maternal attachment, child abuse and neglect, and health care utilization. *Pediatrics* 1980; 66: 183–90.

19 Gray J.D., Cutler C.A., Dean J.G., Kempe C.H. Prediction and prevention of child abuse and neglect. *Journal of Social Issues* 1979; 35: 127–39.

20 Infante-Rivard C., Filion G., Baumgarten M., Labelle J., Messier M. A public health home intervention among families of low socioeconomic status. *Children's Health Care* 1989; 18: 102–7.

21 Casey P.H., Kelleher K.J., Bradley R.H., Kellogg U.W., Kirby R.S., Whiteside L. A multi-faceted intervention for infants with failure to thrive. *Arch Pediatr Adolesc Med* 1994; 148: 1071–7.

22 Greenberg R.A., Stretcher V.J., Bauman K.E., Boat B.W., Fowler M.G., Keyes L.L., et al. Evaluation of a home-based intervention program to reduce infant passive smoking and lower respiratory illness. *J Behav Med* 1994; 17: 273–90.

23 Currie A.L., Gehlbach S.H., Massion C., Thompson S. Newborn home visits. *J Fam Pract* 1983; 17: 635–8.

24 Thompson R.J., Cappleman M.W., Conrad H.H., Jordan W.B. Early intervention program for adolescent mothers and their infants. *J Dev Behav Pediatr* 1982; 3: 18–21.

25 Yanover M.J., Jones D., Miller M.D. Perinatal care of low-risk mothers and infants. *N Engl J Med* 1976; 294: 702–5.

26 Black M.M., Nair P., Kight C., Wachtel R., Roby P., Schler M. Parenting and early development among children of drug abusing mothers: effects of home intervention. *Pediatrics* 1994; 94: 440–8.

27 Hall L.A. Effect of teaching on primiparas' perceptions of their newborn. *Nursing Res* 1980; 29: 317–21.

28 Lowe M.L. Effectiveness of teaching as measured by compliance with medical recommendations. *Nursing Res* 1970; 19: 59–63.

29 Yauger R.A. Does family centered care make a difference? *Nursing Outlook* 1972; 20: 320–3.

30 Shyne A.W., LeMat A., Kogan L.S. Evaluating public health nursing service to the maternity patient and her family. *Nursing Outlook* 1963; 11: 56–8.

31 Stanwick R.S., Moffat M.E., Robitaille Y., Edmond A., Dok C. An evaluation of the routine public health nurse home visit. *Can J Public Health* 1982; 73: 200–5.

32 Field T.M., Widmayer S.M., Stringer S., Ignatoff E. Teenage, lower class, black mothers and their pre-term infants: an intervention and developmental follow-up. *Child Dev* 1980; 51: 426–36.

33 Powell C., Grantham-McGregor S. Home visiting of varying frequency and child development. *Pediatrics* 1989; 84: 157–64.

34 Beckwith L. Intervention with disadvantaged parents of sick pre-term infants. *Psychiatry* 1988; 51: 242–7.

35 Barnard K.E., Magyary D., Sumner G., Booth C.L., Mitchell S.K., Spieker S. Prevention of parenting alterations for women with low social support. *Psychiatry* 1988; 51: 248–53.

36 Scarr S., McCartney K. Far from home: an experimental evaluation of the mother-child home program in Bermuda. *Child Dev* 1988; 59: 531–43.

37 Madden J., O'Hara J., Levenstein P. Home again: effects of the mother–child home program on mother and child. *Child Dev* 1984; 55: 636–47.

38 Casiro O.G., McKenzie M.E., McFadyen L., Shapiro C., Seshia M.M., MacDonald N., et al. Earlier discharge with community base intervention for low birth weight infants: a randomised trial. *Pediatrics* 1993; 92: 128–34.

39 Vines S.W., Williams-Burgess C. Effects of a community health nursing parent-baby (ad)venture program on depression and other selected maternal child health outcomes. *Public Health Nursing* 1994; 11: 188–95.

40 Johnson D.L., Walker T. Primary prevention on behaviour problems in Mexican-American children. *Am J Community Psychol* 1987; 15: 375–85.

41 Nicol A.R., Stretch D.D., Davison I., Fundudis T. Controlled comparison of three interventions for mother and toddler problems: preliminary communication. *J R Soc Med* 1984; 77: 488–91.

42 Olds D.L., Kitzman H.J., Cole R.E. Effect of home visitation by nurses on caregiving and maternal life course. *Arch Pediatr Adolesc Med* 1995; 149: 76.

43 The Infant Health and Development Program. Enhancing the outcomes of low-birth-weight, premature infants. *JAMA* 1990; 263: 3035–42.

44 Dickersin K., Berlin J.A. Meta-analysis: state of the science. *Epidemiol Rev* 1992; 143: 154–76.

What you might do now

The main problems with this systematic review arose from the diversity of studies reviewed and the lack of information about the interventions concerned. These are the same problems as in the exemplar Chapter 2, but writ large. You might want to compare the two exemplars with this in mind

Carry out a more systematic appraisal of the systematic review using 'Questions to Ask about Systematic Reviews' in Part 4 of this book

What you might do now

Think some more about quality criteria for experimental research by reading Chapter 5 with this exemplar in mind

Find a systematic review of interest to you using the Appendix to this book and appraise it using 'Questions to Ask about Systematic Reviews' in Part 4 of this book

CHAPTER 5

THE BASICS OF EXPERIMENTAL DESIGN

Introduction — 1 Experiments as systems of safeguards — 2 Double-blinded, randomised controlled experiments or trials and other experimental designs — 3 Forming comparison groups — creating controls — 4 Sampling units — 5 Subject reactions, researcher bias and blinding — 6 Regression to the mean — 7 Replicability — 8 Intention to treat — 9 Simple and complex interventions — 10 Reliable and sensitive measurements — 11 The internal validity of experiments — 12 The external validity of experiments — 13 Single subject experiments — 14 Questions to ask about controlled experiments — 15 Further reading on controlled experiments in health and social care and cost-effectiveness studies – References and further reading

Introduction

Experiments are particularly important in health care research. It has been argued that they should be more important in social care research too (Oakley and Fullerton, 1996). Some people claim that experimental methods are the only methods capable of investigating causality. They are certainly superior to all other methods in this regard. It is not possible to decide whether some health or social care intervention is effective if it is not clear what causes what effects. Thus the most telling evidence about effective practice is evidence that comes from experimental work.

The major problem in investigating causality is that everything that happens has multiple causes. A controlled experiment is an artificial situation established so that the multiple causes of phenomena can be controlled, by excluding some influences, standardising others, while allowing others to vary. This is described as *controlling variables to prevent confounding*, where 'confounding' means muddling the picture so that it is difficult to discern what is causing what to happen. The principle is much the same as that used by an electrician in isolating a circuit in a complex electrical system and then running various charges between different points at known amplitudes and seeing what happens. This chapter describes the way in which experiments are designed. Chapter 6 looks at the instruments which are used for collecting data in experimental research and Chapter 7 at the more common ways in which the results of experiments are expressed.

In health and social care research the terms 'experiment' and 'trial' are often used interchangeably, though the use of the term 'trial' usually implies that what is being investigated is the effectiveness of a health or social care intervention.

1   Experiments as systems of safeguards

Experiments usually involve treating two or more groups differently. This is often expressed by saying that an experiment has 'arms', each arm consisting of a group of subjects who have been subjected to different treatments.

At the end of an experiment there will be some results which will show either that there is a difference in outcomes between the arms, or that there is not. Chapter 7 gives an account of some of the more usual ways in which the results of experiments are expressed. Any such difference may be statistically significant or not (see Chapter 7, sections 1 and 2). A *difference* in outcome between the arms of the experiment should show the effect of what was done differently and intentionally in different arms and nothing else except the effects of chance. Or *similarities* in outcomes should show that what was done differently and intentionally had much the same effect, and that except for the play of chance, there was nothing else creating this similarity. But unfortunately there are plenty of opportunities for the results of experiments to reflect matters other than the intended differences or similarities in treatment. Figure 5.1 shows the ways in which other factors may contaminate the results. Figure 5.2 tells the same story but identifies a number of safeguards which can be used to block off these routes of confusion.

2   Double-blinded, randomised controlled experiments or trials and other experimental designs

Figure 5.3 gives a picture of an RCT. The terms in it will be explained as the chapter proceeds. Figure 5.4 gives as an example the structure of the RCT that formed the basis for the economic analysis which is presented as the exemplar study in Chapter 3.

The randomised controlled experiment or trial (RCT), with double-blinding, is the experimental design which is regarded as the 'gold standard' in health research, particularly for testing the efficacy of drugs and other treatments. In terms of Figure 5.2, it contains the most stringent array of safeguards against confounding and against bias. Where it can be used, and used appropriately, it is certainly the design which produces the results that can be regarded with most confidence. Although it is often impracticable or unethical to use an RCT design, all other experimental designs can be regarded as

Figure 5.1 Routes of confusion in an experiment

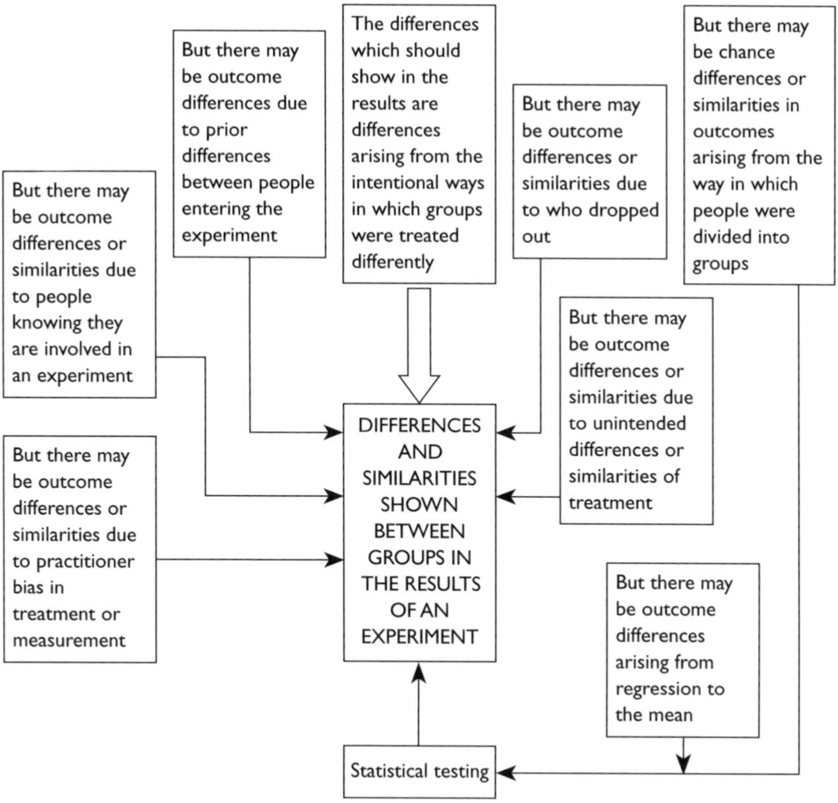

deficient versions of this format, lacking one or more of the characteristics which give the RCT its power to investigate causality. Other
experimental designs are often called 'quasi-experiments', the 'true'
experiment being the kind involving randomisation.

3 Forming comparison groups – creating controls

(See boxes 1 and 6 on Figure 5.2)
An RCT (Figures 5.3 and 5.4) starts with a sample of people drawn
from a wider population. How the sample is drawn, and whether it is
representative of a wider population, and what wider population it
is representative of, is important for the question of how far the
results can be generalised (see section 12 later). Matters other than
representativeness will also determine who enters the trial, such as
estimations of whether people would be harmed by participating, and
individual choice as to participate or not (see Figure 5.4). Once a pool
of subjects has been assembled they are divided *at random* into as

Figure 5.2   Safeguards against misleading results in a controlled experiment

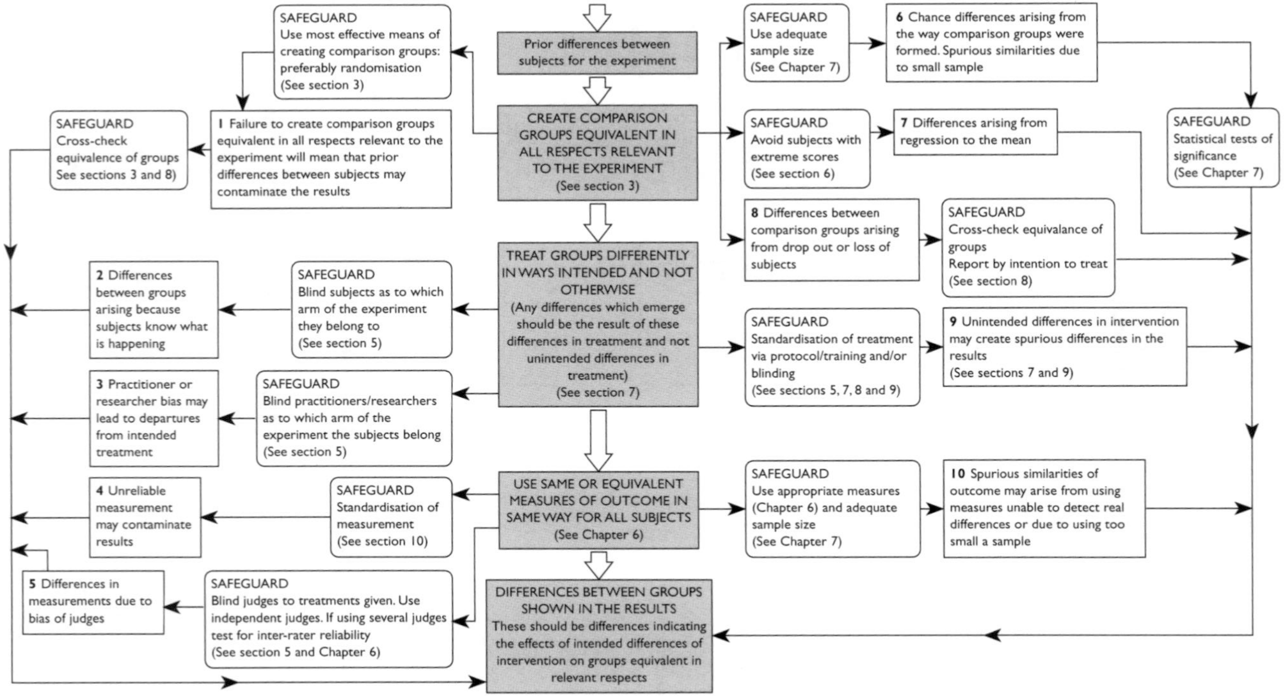

Figure 5.3 A basic randomised controlled trial

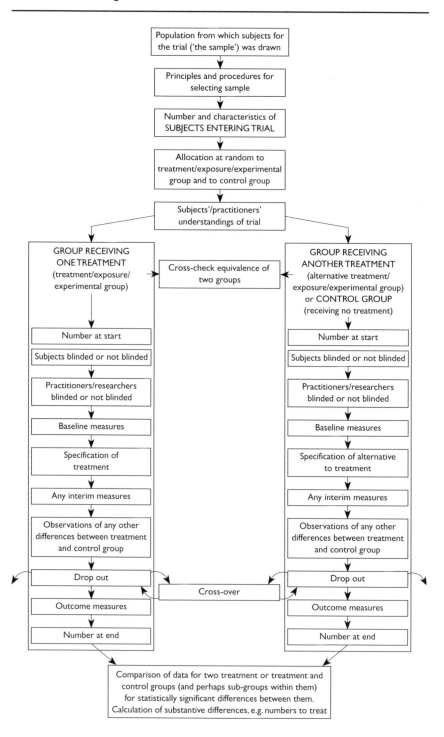

Evaluating Research in Health and Social Care

**Figure 5.4 Procedure for recruitment and randomisation of patients and data
collection in a randomised controlled trial comparing the relative effectiveness of a
hospital at home scheme with inpatient care (Shepperd et al., 1998: 1787)**

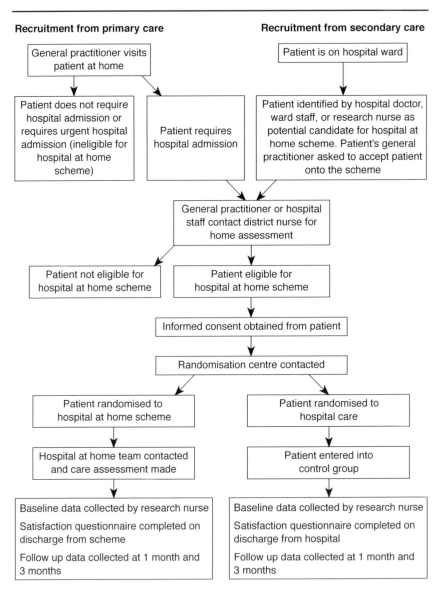

many groups as the trial has arms. The trials in Figures 5.3 and 5.4
have two arms. Random allocation might be done simply by tossing a
coin for each subject. Thus an RCT involves two (or more) random
samples, which together add up to 100 per cent of the subjects
involved.

Using randomisation to create comparison groups is the most effective way of creating groups that are similar. While groups can be created in other ways (see Box 5.1), most of the alternatives rely on dividing people according to known differences. So long as the sample is large enough, randomisation should also produce comparison groups that are similar with regard to unknown differences as well. Schultz and his colleagues (1995) suggest that failure to randomise properly can spuriously inflate outcome differences between arms of a trial by up to 40 per cent. Using methods for creating comparison groups other than randomisation may result in the entirety of any outcome differences between arms in an experiment being due to pre-existing differences between subjects, rather than due to the different ways subjects were treated.

Randomisation may need a helping hand to distribute the characteristics of subjects evenly across arms of the trial. For example, if age were an important variable a researcher might first divide the pool of subjects into age groups and then randomly allocate the members of each age group to arms of the trial, thus ensuring that each arm had a similar age profile (Bowling, 1997: 214–17).

Randomisation also excludes the possibility of subjects, practitioners or researchers influencing which treatment subjects are allocated to and hence biasing the results.

Cross-checks can be made to see whether randomisation has created similar groups in terms of known characteristics. For example, there should be nearly equal numbers of males and females in each group, or each group should have a similar age profile.

Box 5.1 gives a range of methods used for creating comparison groups.

4 Sampling units

In most experiments the sampling unit is an individual person and in an RCT it is usually individuals who are randomly allocated to different interventions. However, sometimes the units might be parts of people, clinics, or communities. The experiment reported in Chapter 1 compares the effects of two different bandaging systems on the healing of venous leg ulcers. In that experiment it was not individuals that were allocated to the two different bandaging systems, but ulcerated legs. Thus the same person might appear twice in the results, once for each leg. The sampling units for an experiment should be decided, and the experiment arranged, such that what happens to any one unit is independent of what happens to any other. Thus in an experiment concerning group therapy, what happens to one person in a therapy group will be influenced by and in turn influence what happens to others. There is a case for saying that a therapy group of ten

Box 5.1   Some ways of attempting to create comparison groups which are similar in all relevant respects*

Randomised controlled trials

Subjects already selected to be rather similar to each other are allocated at random to separate groups: to a control group and one or more experimental/treatment group(s) *or* to two or more groups receiving different interventions (see Figures 5.3 and 5.4). Randomisation may be *unrestricted* or *stratified*. The latter means that the initial pool of subjects is first divided into categories (age groups, genders, ethnic groups) and each subject in each of these groups is then is randomly allocated (Bowling, 1997: 214–17).

Cross-over designs

The same people feature as both experimental and control subjects. For example, the subjects for the experiment are divided into two groups. One group gets the placebo first (see section 5) and then the drug being tested and one group first gets the drug being tested, and then the placebo. Where this design is used it is often as an additional feature of an RCT, with random allocation to groups. And sometimes an RCT will use four groups (or more): *c* then *c*, *c* then *e*, *e* then *c* and *e* then *e* (*c* = control, *e* = experimental group). Where this is possible this is an extremely powerful design, but the opportunities for using it are limited to situations where the intervention received has no long-lasting effect (Roberts and Sibbald, 1998). N-of-1 experiments and single case evaluations are special versions of cross-over designs (see section 13).

Matched pairs designs

Subjects for the experiment are paired off to create pairs of people who are similar to each other in ways considered relevant to the experiment. One of each pair is allocated to one arm and the other to the other arm of the trial – usually at random (Bowling, 1997: 220–2); though this is usually described as 'quasi-randomisation'. Sometimes matched pairs designs are attempted retrospectively where 'control pairs' are found for subjects of an experiment which has already been done. This is one approach used in 'case control studies' (see Chapter 10).

Purposive sampling, sometimes called 'factorialisation'

Two groups are created which are as near identical in all respects except one – for example, a group of males and a group of females with similar age, social class and ethnic profiles. Then males and females are subjected to the same intervention and any outcome differences are attributed to differences of gender. Sometimes the same effect is created through a matched pairs design (Bowling, 1997: 219). Sometimes factorialisation is done to create sub-groups within an RCT.

Reference group/area designs

There is an experimental group who are subjected to some intervention. The results of this are compared with the 'before and after' characteristics of some other group deemed to be similar but who have not received the intervention, or have received a different one. For example, the smoking behaviour of children in a school in which there has been anti-smoking health education is compared with the smoking behaviour in a school where there has been no such health education campaign. Attempts are made to select areas/groups who are similar in at least their demographic characteristics: age, gender, deprivation, ethnicity, for example. However, the possibilities for confounding factors to muddy the results are many. This is the other major strategy used in 'case control studies' (see Chapter 10).

Pre- and post-test designs without controls

Subjects for the experiment are studied prior to intervention to provide some baseline measures. All are subject to the intervention, the outcomes are measured and compared with the baseline measures. In effect 'the controls' are these same people prior to intervention. However, there is rarely any way of deciding which of the differences between the pre- and post-test were due to the intervention, which were due to the characteristics of the people chosen (for example due to their propensity for spontaneous remission from a condition being treated), or to the elapsing of time, or which were due to the fact that they were subjects of an experiment, over and above the effects of the intervention itself. Where designs like this are used to investigate causality, including effectiveness, little confidence should be placed in the results.

* In this box 'intervention' is used as a shorthand to include treatments such as drug treatments or surgical operations, exposure to health education, exposure to pathogens (as in influenza research), or modes of care delivery (such as care management) and so on.

people is actually a sample of one and that the experimental 'subject' is the group as a whole. It is a moot point as to whether the healing of an ulcer on one leg is independent of the healing of an ulcer on the other leg of the same person. The experiment in Chapter 1 involved 35 ulcerated legs and 29 people. Was this a sample of 35 or of 29?

5 Subject reactions, researcher bias and blinding

(See boxes 2, 3 and 5 on Figure 5.2)
The understandings of subjects, practitioners and researchers will, of course, influence what happens in an experiment. That cannot be avoided. What can be avoided is such influences affecting one arm of

the trial more or differently from another. Preventing subjects, practitioners and researchers knowing which arm of the trial particular subjects are in standardises this influence across all arms of the trial. This is rather unfortunately known as 'blinding'.

There is a large, and long-established, research literature showing how the expectancies of subjects can influence research outcomes, and how the unwitting biases of practitioners and researchers can influence the results. Although the physiological processes of wound healing might seem immune to this influence, there is research showing that the expectations of practitioners can affect the speed at which leg ulcers heal (Schwartz et al., 1988). The 'double-blind randomised controlled trial' is one where neither the subjects themselves nor the practitioners/researchers know to which arm of the experiment subjects belong, group membership only being disclosed at the end of the trial or earlier if it has to be broken off prematurely for safety reasons. Random allocation helps with blinding, but blinding usually also involves secret codes, sealed envelopes and perhaps the use of an independent agency to allocate subjects to treatments. The 'randomisation centre' in Figure 5.4 blindly allocated patients to treatments, though it did not blind patients or practitioners to the mode of care patients received. Blinding may also involve making treatments look, taste or feel similar; for example two different drugs or a drug and a placebo (a dummy drug), made up into tablets of identical appearance.

It is impossible or unethical to blind practitioners/researchers and difficult to blind subjects where the intervention is surgery, or diet, a health education programme, or counselling, and in the study in Chapter 3 it was impossible to blind either as to whether patients were being cared for in hospital or at home. Where blinding is impossible, confidence in the results must be lower because there is always a possibility that any outcome differences came from knowledge of what the treatment was, rather than from the effects of the treatment itself. Schultz and colleagues suggest that the absence of double-blinding may create spurious outcome differences of up to 17 per cent (Schultz et al., 1995), but other research suggests even greater effects (Rosenthal and Rubin, 1978).

6   Regression to the mean

(See box 7 on Figure 5.2)
Regression to the mean is a particularly common cause of confounding in experimental research. Imagine that you threw six dice and gained a score of 9 – you threw all 1s and 2s. You know intuitively that if you were to throw the dice a second time you would be likely to get a higher score. This is simply because there are more other scores to score than 1s and 2s. The same regression effect would be true if on

the first throw you scored mainly 5s and 6s. Then the next throw would be more likely to result in a lower score. Similarly, if subjects for an experiment are chosen because they have extreme scores for some illness, or behaviour or social problem, chance alone is likely to mean that they will show improvement over time. In investigations without controls there is no way of knowing whether all improvement shown is due to this statistical artefact, that is, changes that are not due to the intervention at all. If one arm of an experiment started with subjects with more extreme scores than the other, more improvement shown for that arm may be due to the regression effect. Unfortunately usual tests for statistical significance (see Chapter 7) will not distinguish regression effects from real effects. More complicated statistical analysis is needed to do this (Senn, 1997). However, even without statistical analysis readers of research may have a reasonable suspicion that the results are affected by regression to the mean if the subjects in one arm of the trial have notably more extreme baseline scores than the subjects in the other arm *and* if those with the more extreme scores also show the greatest improvement.

7 Replicability

As the philosopher Daniel Dennett says, science is 'making mistakes for all to see, in the hopes of getting others to help with the corrections' (1995: 380). For experiments this means researchers specifying exactly what was done, so that, in principle at least, someone else can repeat the experiment. The possibility of replication is what makes experimental researchers so much more accountable to their readers than other kinds of researchers. RCTs in medicine are one of the fields of science where replication, or near replication, is widely practised. As Chapter 4 shows, practitioners may often be able to draw on evidence from several experiments of much the same kind. In applying research results to practice it is also important that what was done in the experiment was clearly specified. If it is not, it will be impossible for practitioners to know how to 'do the same', and hence difficult for them to achieve similar results. Achieving replicability may be difficult with complex interventions – see section 9 and Chapter 2).

8 Intention to treat

(See box 8 on Figure 5.2)
It is not essential that each arm of an experiment has equal numbers of subjects. But once under way, it is problematic if people drop out. This is because differences in outcomes between arms might then be due to the people dropping out from one arm of the experiment being different from those dropping out from another arm. Drop out may, or

may not, have to do with the treatments received. Prejudices on behalf of practitioners may influence the drop out. Sometimes, for therapeutic reasons, a subject will be swapped from an arm of the trial which receives a placebo treatment, to an arm which receives an active treatment; an unplanned cross-over. Sometimes subjects do not comply with their treatment, and do something which is very like what happens in a different arm of the trial. The way in which drop outs, unplanned cross-overs and non-compliance should be managed is to regard all subjects as still belonging to the groups to which they were originally allocated. This is called reporting the results in terms of *intention to treat*. Thus in a diet experiment where someone on a low fat diet cheats and eats a high fat diet, s/he will still be counted as a member of the low fat arm of the trial. There may, of course, be problems of researchers knowing about compliance and non-compliance.

At the end of the trial the subjects remaining should be analysed to see whether the characteristics of the groups have changed due to drop out, cross-over and so on, and whether this might have influenced the results.

9   Simple and complex interventions

In the blinded RCT, treatments should seem similar to subjects and practitioners, thus eliminating one possibility for confounding. And whether blinded or not, most medical RCTs conducted in academia put a premium on a standardised performance by practitioners, using written protocols and sometimes special training, specifying what should be done, how measurements should be taken and how judgements should be made. However, there has been considerable concern expressed about laxity in these regards concerning RCTs by drug companies, particularly those carried out in general practice (*British Medical Journal*, 1998; Boseley, 1999).

Standardisation is important if the experiment is to be replicable (see section 7 above and box 9 on Figure 5.2). Standardisation is more possible where treatments are simple to administer and it is justifiable to administer them in a standardised way. This is often not the case. Counselling, psychotherapy, most social work interventions and some nursing interventions are customised to the particularities of each individual client. If this happens in experimental research, then each arm of the trial will actually contain not the same, but diverse treatments. There may then be more similarities between some treatments in different arms of the experiment, than between some treatments in the same arm of the experiment. In fact, the overwhelming majority of experimental studies in social work and counselling show 'no difference' between 'different treatments' (Newman, 1994; Oakley and Fullerton, 1996). This is sometimes interpreted benignly through issuing the dodo bird verdict – 'everyone a winner', and sometimes adversely with the verdict that there is no evidence that social work or counselling are more effective than leaving people alone (Brugha and Glover, 1998). But it is equally likely to be due to the fact that these interventions are so variable in practice that, either they are not amenable to experimental research, or, if they are, they would need enormously large samples to accommodate the diversity *within* arms of the trial (Chapter 7, section 7) and a great effort to record the differences accurately.

Complex interventions then, make for difficulties in replication (section 7 above). Where interventions are complex it may be difficult for researchers to know which are the important ingredients of the intervention and hence which to record. Similarly, complex interventions will be more difficult for practitioners to emulate. The experiment which features in Chapter 2 exemplifies these problems.

10   Reliable and sensitive measurements

(See boxes 4, 5 and 10 on Figure 5.2)
It is crucial that the same assessments and measurements are made of all subjects, each in the same way, otherwise it will be unclear as to whether different baseline and outcome measures reflect real differences, or merely inconsistency in measurement. If practitioners are not blinded to the intervention subjects have received, it is common to involve an independent party who does not know this to do the assessments to avoid bias contaminating the measurements.

Chapter 6 discusses measurement instruments, but here it is worth noting that insensitive instruments may give results which are spuriously similar. For example, designating ulcers as merely 'healed' or 'not healed' may miss the fact that some 'not-healed' ulcers are more healed than others and perhaps making the superiority of one treatment over another invisible. Unfortunately, measurement instruments which discriminate finely also set up the ideal conditions for regression effects (section 6 above), since there are more positions on the scale for subjects to regress from. Consistency of judgement by practitioners and researchers is also important. Testing for this is dealt with in Chapter 6, section 6.

11   The internal validity of experiments

Roughly speaking, internal validity refers to whether what researchers claim to be true is indeed true for the subjects in the setting in which they did their research. Much of the critical appraisal of the internal validity of any experiment revolves around three kinds of question which appear in different versions in Figure 5.2 and feature in much more detail in 'Questions to Ask about Experiments' in Part 4 of this book:

- Were the subjects really similar in the ways they should be similar and/or really different in the ways they should be different?
- Were the treatments really different in the ways they should be different and/or similar in the ways they should be similar?
- Were any other influences at play which should have been excluded, actually excluded from having an effect on the outcomes?

Only if all these questions can be answered in the affirmative can the results of an experiment be accepted with confidence. These same questions, or something like them, arise wherever someone makes a claim that doing such and such has such and such an outcome. In the absence of experimental control they are very difficult questions to answer convincingly.

12   The external validity of experiments

A research study may be valid in its own terms – internally valid – but none the less what happened in the experiment might not happen anywhere or anytime else; its results may not be generalisable; they may lack external validity.

   The way in which experiments control variables is what makes them good designs for studying causality. Unfortunately in the real world variables may not be controlled, or controllable. Thus the artificiality of the experiment can become a problem when attempts are made to generalise from the experiment to situations beyond it. The success of physics and chemistry in producing knowledge with everyday applications does not come entirely from using the experimental method, but also from transforming the world so that what happens in the laboratory can be made to happen outside it. High tech machine medicine works because it makes hospitals more like experimental laboratories where variables can indeed be brought under greater control. Thus when it comes to making a judgement about the generalisability of research findings the question is whether enough of the circumstances under which the experiment was performed could be reproduced in practice to ensure that similar results are obtained. Some kinds of interventions, drug treatments for example, do often seem to travel quite well, whereas the outcomes of others seem to depend very much on who does them, where, to whom and under what circumstances. Table 5.1 suggests the characteristics of topics with regard to which research might produce more or less generalisable knowledge about effectiveness.

   Another issue about the generalisability of experimental research concerns the representativeness of the people involved as subjects. In

Table 5.1   **Topics for which research is more or less likely to produce sound generalisations**

The characteristics of topics about which research is more likely to produce generalisable knowledge about effectiveness	The characteristics of topics about which research is less likely to produce generalisable knowledge about effectiveness
Where the entities being studied have robust, reliable and predictable properties: for example, materials, forces, muscles, bones, cells, genes	Where the entities being studied do not have robust, reliable and predictable properties; for example, emotions, interpretations, meanings, relationships, group dynamics
Where interventions are simple and standardised and can be much the same irrespective of which practitioner carries them out; for example, administering a drug	Where interventions are complex and differ from client to client and/or where the same named intervention differs according to which practitioner carries it out; for example, counselling
Where there is a strong consensus (or an enforcement) of some criteria of effectiveness	Where there are multiple and contradictory criteria of effectiveness
Where there is little ambiguity as to what evidence counts as meeting the criteria of effectiveness	Where there is considerable ambiguity as to what evidence counts as meeting criteria of effectiveness

fact, it is relatively rare for RCTs in health and social care to start with representative samples. They usually use 'grab' or 'convenience' samples: just the people who happen to be around when subjects are needed. Or they may be samples selected so that any effect of different treatments will show clearly in the results. For example, Tudor Hart (1993) notes that most trials for hypertension management involve people who are suffering from nothing other than hypertension. But 90 per cent of people suffering from hypertension are suffering from something else as well. Selecting those with hypertension alone gives the best chance of achieving clear unambiguous results not muddled by other conditions from which subjects might be suffering. But since such people are unlike most of those with hypertension who crop up in routine practice, it will be difficult for practitioners to know how far what worked for people suffering only from hypertension will work for people suffering from a diversity of other conditions as well – people like their own patients.

Practitioners do not recruit their own clients by representative sampling either, so for most practical purposes it is not too important that an experiment has subjects who are unrepresentative of some wider population. What is important is that researchers publish enough details about the subjects so that practitioners can extrapolate the results to their own distinctive client mix. Statements about indications and contraindications are particularly useful in this regard.

Differences of client mix and of practice circumstances together may mean that what 'worked' in the research will not work in practice.

Research in the cost-effectiveness field is particularly sensitive to context, because doing something in one place very rarely costs the same as doing it in another, to say nothing of the problem that the cost-base of practice is likely to change quite quickly through time (see also Chapter 7, section 12). Thus economic analyses have a two-way problem of generalisability. The relative effectiveness of two treatments shown under research conditions may not be the same as can be achieved in some practice setting, *and* the relative costs of two interventions demonstrated in the research may not be the same as happens in practice, even in the same practice after a period of time.

A further problem with regard to generalisation comes from the interpretations made by subjects and practitioners. Blinding can prevent such interpretations affecting outcomes for one arm of the trial more than another. But it cannot prevent such interpretations influencing the outcomes for (at least some) subjects in *all* arms of the trial. In routine practice clients are not blinded to the treatment they receive, and this makes it possible that some effects that occur because people are blinded, or some that occur because people know they are part of an experiment, will not be reproduced in practice. Or again, under experimental conditions it may be possible for practitioners to ensure a high degree of compliance with a treatment – much higher than would be possible in routine practice. Similarly, staff may be particularly punctilious, or enthusiastic or otherwise different in an experiment compared with their counterparts in routine practice. The term *Hawthorne effect* is often used to refer to the tendency for people to behave differently because they know they are being researched or involved in research (Sapsford and Abbott, 1992: 105), while the term *experiment effect* may be used to include this, and any other things that are more likely to happen in an experiment than under naturally occurring circumstances. This is one reason for the sensitivity analysis carried out by Shepperd et al., in the exemplar study in Chapter 3 (see also Chapter 7, section 12).

13 Single subject experiments

The fact that experiments typically produce results for groups of people often makes it difficult for practitioners to apply the results to individual clients, because what is 'effective' for a group may be beneficial to some of them, have no effects on others, and adverse effects on yet others. The techniques of n-of-1 experiments in medicine and single case evaluations in social work and clinical psychology take the experimental approach down to the individual level.

The 'n' in the n-of-1 refers to the number of subjects in the experiment, which is one person. But sometimes several are conducted in parallel with different patients, making the term n-of-1 slightly misleading.

The more usual kinds of randomised controlled trial provide predictions about what is likely to happen among a group of people subject to a treatment, but do not provide enough information to predict what will happen to any patient in particular. In this sense n-of-1s bridge the gap between knowledge about groups and knowledge about individuals. One way of looking at n-of-1 trials is as their being a more systematic version of the kinds trial and error procedures used by clinicians when, for instance, they attempt to stabilise a drug dose for a patient, or to establish the cause of a food allergy by systematically excluding items of diet. N-of-1 trials are usually based on what has been found effective *on average* for groups, where what is unknown is the effectiveness of the treatment for the individual patient.

Box 5.2 provides an example of a typical n-of-1 trial, or rather of a set of n-of-1s being conducted alongside each other.

These are double-blind randomised controlled experiments with cross-over (see Box 5.1). However, it is not patients who are randomly allocated to different treatments but different treatments which are allocated to the *same* patient in a random sequence (two different treatments, or a treatment and a placebo). Where there is indeed only one trial going on, the only purpose of randomisation is the double-blinding (see section 5 above). With a series of n-of-1 experiments, randomisation will also control for the effects of the order in which treatments are given. Such control of order-effects will apply only to the results of all the trials, and not to the result of any one of them.

This is a 'same-subject(s) cross-over' design where the individual patient constitutes his or her own 'control' in the sense that what happens to the patient when receiving one treatment, is compared with what happens to the same patient when receiving the alternative treatment (the cross-over) (see Figure 5.5 in Box 5.2). This limits the use of n-of-1 experiments to the kinds of interventions which have only transitory effects. Pain control is a particularly common area. As always, the purpose of an experimental approach is to control variables that might influence outcomes, other than the intervention which is given an opportunity to effect outcomes. In any RCT there is always a possibility that other things happening in a patient's life will affect their response to treatment. Where there are many patients in the trial, as in the usual RCT, then there is a good chance that these extraneous variables will balance out between the arms of the trial. But in an n-of-1 trial there is only one patient who has, in random sequence, to be in both arms of the trial. Since the primary purpose of the trial is to establish what works for this particular patient the clinician will want to discover the treatment which works best, extraneous factors and all. Extraneous factors that are persistent in the patient's life, or show a consistent time trend do not constitute a research problem, but extraneous factors that come and go may well do so. Thus if the administration of the active drug coincided with a particularly stressful period at work, and the placebo with the patient's holidays, this may well give misleading results. Hence a run of several alternations (or cycles) of treatments is important, despite the strong temptation to discontinue the trial when the patient feels better, or feels particularly ill. Drop out is particularly common in n-of-1s. Group RCTs can survive drop outs, but drop out from an n-of-1 experiment is the end of the affair.

Series of n-of-1 trials demonstrate the diversity of responses to treatments. They may provide useful data about indications and contraindications which can be used by practitioners in their own decision-making. With the pressure towards 'evidence based practice'

Box 5.2   N-of-1 trials comparing a non-steroidal anti-inflammatory drug (NSAID) with paracetamol for osteoarthritis (based on March et al., 1994)

Paracetamol has a risk of accidental or intended overdose. NSAID drugs carry a risk of gastrointestinal complications, occasionally fatal. Thus it is important to choose the drug which, for the particular patient, gives the lowest risk for the optimum pain control. Where equally effective, paracetamol is usually to be preferred as the drug which carries the lower risk for most patients.

Main objective: to evaluate individual patient responses to paracetamol and a non-steroidal anti-inflammatory drug (NSAID) in terms of pain relief, immediate side effects and general well-being.

Subjects: 25 patients from general practice experiencing painful osteoarthritis with no contraindications for non-steroidal anti-inflammatories and no corticosteroid injection in the previous four weeks. Five patients dropped out very early, five dropped out before the end, but after a clinical decision had been made as to the best treatment for them.

Procedure: each patient was treated in three cycles of four weeks. Each cycle consisted of two weeks taking a non-steroidal anti-inflammatory drug and two weeks taking paracetamol. The order of this was determined for each patient at random. Both drugs appeared visually identical to the patient and researcher/practitioner and both were blind to which drug was in use. Patients were allowed to use paracetamol as 'escape' analgesic, whichever other treatment they were experiencing.

Measures: Patients completed a daily diary for pain and stiffness using visual analogue scales (see Figure 5.5) and a weekly checklist of 11 symptoms known to be associated with NSAID drugs. There was weekly monitoring of ability to perform activities selected according to which joints were inflamed. The use of escape analgesia was recorded. The most important outcome was the evidence necessary to make an informed clinical decision of the drug of choice acceptable to the patient.

Figure 5.5 Daily visual analogue scores for pain and stiffness for a patient who benefited most from the **NSAID** drug (March et al., 1994: Fig. 3: 1043)

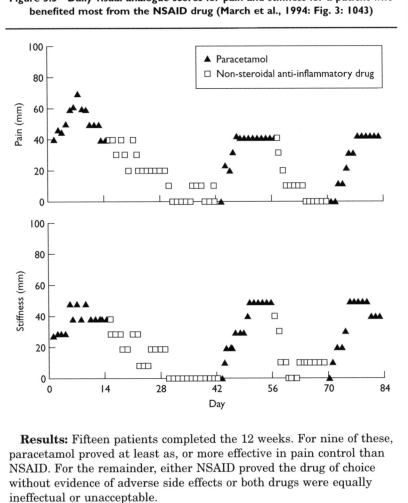

Results: Fifteen patients completed the 12 weeks. For nine of these, paracetamol proved at least as, or more effective in pain control than NSAID. For the remainder, either NSAID proved the drug of choice without evidence of adverse side effects or both drugs were equally ineffectual or unacceptable.

some clinicians have seen the n-of-1 experiment as something which should be adopted in routine practice where possible, as a way of customising to the individual the knowledge derived from effectiveness research on groups (Campbell, 1994).

The human genome project has, on the one hand, thrown some doubt on the standard RCT in medical research, and on the other has directed interest towards n-of-1 experiments as an alternative. The source of the doubt is the way that the human genome project draws attention to the genetic diversity which must exist among any group of subjects for an RCT and hence to the possibility of a large field of uncontrolled variables. The larger the diversity, the larger a sample needs to be to allow randomisation to produce two groups of subjects similar to each other in ways relevant to the experiment. Insofar as genetic differences do make a difference to the results of medical interventions, it is likely that the results of RCTs will reflect pre-existing genetic differences between subjects which have been inadequately randomised between the arms of an experiment if the sample has been too small. As the mapping of the human genome proceeds, it will become more and more possible to see what genetic differences do exist between people and to attempt to relate these differences to different responses to treatments. Knowing an individual's genome will also make it possible to control for genetic differences by starting with a pool of subjects selected for their genetic similarity in ways relevant to the experiment, and then randomising these between the arms of the experiment. This is a long established procedure in RCTs in agriculture and in medical research using animal subjects. In both fields experimenters usually start with a pool of subjects bred to be genetically very similar to each other. N-of-1 experiments offer a different way of controlling for genetic diversity since the same person is alternately 'experimental subject' and 'control'.

As with an n-of-1 trial in medicine, a single case evaluation is a same-subject(s) cross-over design and a way of discovering whether an intervention is effective for a particular client. Randomisation in the n-of-1 design is largely for the purpose of blinding. Thus it is not useful where it is neither feasible nor desirable to prevent clients and practitioners knowing which treatments are being administered. What is left of an n-of-1 structure when randomisation is removed is the alternation of interventions, or the alternation of a period of intervention with a period of non-intervention. That essentially is what a single case evaluation is. The technique has mainly been used in conjunction with cognitive behavioural interventions in social work and clinical psychology (Bloom and Fischer, 1982; Sheldon, 1983; Barlow and Hersen, 1984; Johannessen, 1991; Thyer, 1993; Kazi and Wilson, 1996). Box 5.3 gives an example.

Figure 5.6 in Box 5.3 shows that AR's attendance improves at the beginning of an intervention period, and then drops off, and that it deteriorates markedly when the intervention is withdrawn. During each intervention phase his attendance is on average higher than in the preceding phase of non-intervention. Overall there is a ratchet effect such that as time goes on his attendance during the period of non-intervention improves.

It does seem as if progress has been made with AR's attendance. That, of course, might have been due to factors other than the intervention made. However, alternating intervention and non-intervention and carefully recording the results provides evidence which suggests

Box 5.3 An example of single case evaluation in social work: an ABABA design

Figure 5.6 AR's school attendance (percentage of possible attendance per week) (based on Kazi and Wilson, 1996: Fig. 7: 707)

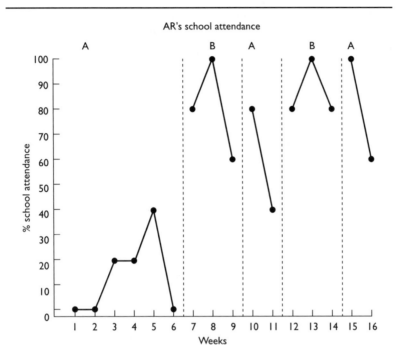

Figure 5.6 above records alternate phases of non-intervention (conventionally called 'A') and intervention (conventionally called 'B') with regard to AR, a 14-year-old referred to educational social work for persistent absenteeism by a Scottish High school. The interventions (Bs) consisted of counselling for both AR and his family, building better home–school links, and providing encouragement for AR in school. The measure used was the school register which was completed twice a day.

that the improvement is attributable to the intervention. Unless there were evidence that something other than the intervention caused the improvement in attendance, common-sense suggests that the evidence in Figure 5.6 should be accepted as evidence of effectiveness. This is particularly so if similar patterns of response are shown for the same procedures applied to other truants.

The intervention in the example was a complex one, and it is difficult to know which aspect of it was the effective ingredient; family

or individual counselling, better home–school links, more encouragement for AR in school, or indeed AR's perceptions that his absence
might be more easily spotted. And each of these is again made up of
many components. To investigate this further it is imaginable that
a whole series of single case evaluations featuring AR might be
mounted, each featuring only one aspect of the intervention. However,
this does not seem desirable or feasible. First, the main purpose of
single case evaluation is to solve the problem. Explaining how the
trick was done is only a secondary objective. Second, while the outcome measure chosen here was school attendance, absenteeism was
not the only problem being addressed. No doubt counselling, better
home–school liaison and so on, are also addressing other issues, and in
ways that would not be closely reflected in the school attendance
record. Third, it is to be hoped that the problem would have been
resolved in a period much shorter than would be required to test the
intervention bit by bit.

Single case evaluation not only lends itself well to incorporation into
routine practice but is likely to improve practice by requiring practitioners to specify targets carefully and to look for ways of measuring
their attainment. Measures need to be valid and reliable (see Chapter
6), but since this is as much practice as research, measurement data
also need to be of the kind which can be acquired with minimum effort
by practitioners. It is usually beneficial if they are meaningful to the
subject of the evaluation. In this example AR had the goals and the
measurements foisted on him. But there is no reason why this
approach should not be directed towards achieving goals chosen by the
client and measured by indicators meaningful to him or her. This
makes the approach particularly applicable to various kinds of 'brief
intervention' counselling, or methods using contracts in social work or
probation work.

There is a potential problem of 'false measurement'. In the example
in Box 5.3, for instance, an improvement in school attendance might
be accompanied by an increase in AR's misery. But given the nature of
the intervention, this seems unlikely to go unnoticed.

14 Questions to ask about controlled experiments

In Part 4 of this book there is a checklist of questions to use in
critically appraising pieces of experimental research. The questions
step through the issues raised in this chapter, and some which are
raised in Chapters 6 and 7. There are two kinds of questions: one kind
is concerned with internal validity – does the research seem true in its
own terms? The other kind relates to external validity or generalisability: is it likely that what happened in the experiment could be
made to happen elsewhere, if so where, and would this be desirable?

You might like to use the checklist as a way of appraising the research reported in Chapters 1 or 2, or for appraising other published experimental research more closely related to your own interests.

15 Further reading on controlled experiments in health and social care research and cost-effectiveness studies

A good place to start is with Ann Bowling's *Research Methods in Health* (1997), or the chapter on RCTs by Shepperd et al. (1997), both of which also provide access to a wide range of more technical literature. Pocock's *Clinical Trials* (1983) is a standard reference for medical research. Campbell and Stanley (1996) provide a more than usually adequate account of quasi-experimental designs. Since the 1950s social work has been rather hostile to experimental research, though pre-war experimentalism was more common in social work than in medicine. Something of the contemporary debate is captured in Oakley and Fullerton (1996) and in the papers in Williams et al. (1999).

For single subject experiments, the original sources from which the examples in the chapter were drawn are themselves worth reading in their entirety (March et al., 1994; Kazi and Wilson, 1996). In addition, Johannessen (1991) is a useful source on n-of-1 trials; and see Sheldon (1983) and Thyer (1993) on single case evaluations.

Cost-effectiveness studies

Experimental designs are often used as a basis for judging the cost-effectiveness of interventions. Watson (1997) provides an introduction to this kind of analysis. Jefferson et al. (1996) is a more comprehensive guide. There are references on costing services at the end of Chapter 7.

References and further reading

Barlow, D. and Hersen, M. (1984) *Single Case Experimental Designs: Strategies for Studying Behaviour Change*, 2nd edition. London: Pergamon Press.

Bloom, M. and Fischer. J. (1982) *Evaluating Practice: Guidelines for the Accountable Professional*. Englewood Cliffs, NJ: Prentice Hall.

Boseley, S. (1999) 'Trial and error puts patients at risk', *Guardian*, Tuesday 27th July, p. 8.

Bowling, A. (1997) *Research Methods in Health: Investigating Health and Health Services*. Buckingham: Open University Press.

British Medical Journal (1998) 'Dealing with Research Misconduct in the United Kingdom', *British Medical Journal*, 316: 1726–33.

Brugha, T. and Glover, G. (1998) 'Process and health outcomes: need for clarity in systematic reviews of case management for severe mental disorders', *Health Trends*, 30 (3), 76–9.

Campbell, M. (1994) 'Commentary: n-of-1 trials may be useful for informed decision making', *British Medical Journal*, 309: 1044–5.

Campbell, T. and Stanley, J. (1996) *Experimental and Quasi-Experimental Designs for Research*. Chicago: Rand McNally.

Dennett, D. (1995) *Darwin's Dangerous Idea: Evolution and the Meanings of Life*. London: Allen Lane.

Jefferson, T., Demicheli, V. and Mugford, M. (1996) *Elementary Economic Evaluation in Health Care*. London: BMJ Publications.

Johannessen, T. (1991) 'Controlled trials in single subjects', *British Medical Journal*, 303: 173–4.

Kazi, M. and Wilson, J. (1996) 'Applying single-case evaluation in social work', *British Journal of Social Work*, 26: 699–717.

March, L., Irwig, L., Schwartz, J., Simpson, J., Chock, C. and Brooks, P. (1994) 'n of 1 trials comparing a non-steroidal anti-inflammatory drug with paracetamol in osteoarthritis', *British Medical Journal*, 309: 1041–6.

Newman, F. (1994) 'Disabuse of the drug metaphor: introduction', *Journal of Consulting and Clinical Psychology*, 62 (5): 941.

Oakley, A. and Fullerton, D. (1996) 'The lamp-post of research: support or illumination?', in A. Oakley and H. Roberts (eds), *Evaluating Social Interventions*. Essex: Barnados, pp. 4–38.

Pocock, S. (1983) *Clinical Trials: a Practical Approach*. New York: John Wiley.

Roberts, C. and Sibbald, B. (1998) 'Randomising groups of patients', *British Medical Journal*, 316: 1898.

Rosenthal, R. and Rubin, D. (1978) 'Interpersonal expectancy effects: the first 345 studies', *The Behavioural and Brain Sciences*, 3: 377–415.

Sapsford, R. and Abbott, P. (1992) *Research Methods for Nurses and the Caring Professions*. Buckingham: Open University Press.

Schultz, K., Charmers, I., Hayes, R. and Altman, D. (1995) 'Empirical evidence of bias: dimensions of methodological quality associated with estimates of treatment effects in controlled trials', *Journal of American Medical Association*, 273: 408–12.

Schwartz, S., Flamant, R. and Lellouch, J. (1988) *Clinical Trials* (trans. M. Healy). London: Academic Press.

Senn, S. (1997) 'Regression to the mean', *Statistical Methods in Medical Research*, 6: 99–102.

Sheldon, B. (1983) 'The use of single case experimental designs in the evaluation of social work', *British Journal of Social Work*, 13: 477–500.

Shepperd, S., Doll, H. and Jenkinson, C. (1997) 'Randomized controlled trials', in C. Jenkinson. (ed.), *Assessment and Evaluation of Health and Medical Care: a Methods Text*. Buckingham: Open University Press. pp. 6–30.

Shepperd, S., Harwood, D., Jenkinson, C., Gray, A., Vessey, M. and Morgan, P. (1998) 'Randomised controlled trial comparing hospital at home care with inpatient hospital care. I: three month follow up of health outcomes', *British Medical Journal*, 316: 1786–91.

Thyer, B. (1993) 'Single-system research designs', in R. Grinnerll (ed.), *Social Work Research and Evaluation*, 4th edition. Itasca, Ill., F.E. Peacock, pp. 94–117.

Tudor Hart, J. (1993) 'Hypertension guidelines: other diseases complicate management', *British Medical Journal*, 306: 1337.

Watson, K. (1997) 'Economic evaluation of health care', in C. Jenkinson (ed.), *Assessment and Evaluation of Health and Medical Care: a Methods Text*. Buckingham: Open University Press. pp. 129–50.

Williams, F., Popay, J. and Oakley, A. (1999) *Welfare Research: a Critical Review*. London: UCL Press.

CHAPTER 6

RESEARCH INSTRUMENTS IN EXPERIMENTAL RESEARCH

Introduction — 1 The use of standard instruments — 2 Cultural specificity and instruments — 3 Data levels and qualities — 4 Instruments and data distributions, data transformations, floor and ceiling effects — 5 Validating instruments for their reliability — 6 Reliability tests — 7 Validating the validity of instruments — 8 Questions to ask about research instruments — 9 Further reading on research instruments — References and further reading

Introduction

Experiments usually entail the use of some kind of data collection instrument to produce quantitative data which are then analysed statistically. The instrument used, the measurements made and the way the data are analysed shape the results. In appraising research it is important to know how the instruments and statistical tests shaped the results.

Any device that is used to aid data collection can be called an 'instrument' in research, ranging from thermometers and their associated temperature charts to questionnaires used in surveys. For research purposes, 'having a fever' may be scoring above a certain level on a thermometer, and 'being satisfied with the NHS' may be ticking a particular box on a questionnaire (see Chapter 8). Any instrument structures the data it collects. Thus looking at the design and use of such instruments is an extremely important aspect of appraising research.

Figure 6.1 gives an example of a research instrument: it shows one of the panels of the Dartmouth COOP charts used in the research by Shepperd and colleagues which is presented as the exemplar study in Chapter 3 of this volume. Table 3.1 in Chapter 3 gives data resulting from the use of the whole set of COOP charts.

Figure 6.1 gives a simple illustration of what a measurement instrument of this kind does, which is to turn ideas into numbers which can then be mathematically manipulated. It also hints at the kinds of queries this manoeuvre gives rise to. For example, what, exactly, is being measured? Nominally this is 'feelings over the past

FEELINGS

During the past 4 weeks...
  How much have you been bothered by
  emotional problems such as feeling anxious,
  depressed, irritable or downhearted and blue?

Not at all		1
Slightly		2
Moderately		3
Quite a bit		4
Extremely		5

4 weeks'. But does the instrument capture these adequately? Will
respondents understand 'feelings' as the kinds of feelings which practitioners and researchers believe are relevant to health? Questions of
this sort are questions of *validity*. These also include questions about
whether people respond to such instruments as intended, or perhaps
as a way of making complaints, or issuing compliments to their carers.

This particular chart also presents a problem of *retrospective (or recall) bias* which arises because people reconstruct their memories according to later events, or to fit the circumstances in which they are asked about them.

There are also questions of *reliability*. Does everyone mean the same thing by 'slightly'? Would the same person confronted with the same instrument on another occasion, feeling just as good, or bad, give the same answer? Would it make a difference if the questions were asked by a key-worker, or a trained interviewer, or if the answers were given anonymously?

Questions like these arise however information is collected. The problems are just more noticeable when research instruments are used. And where instruments are used the problems are more investigable. In interview research where data are collected without the use of a research instrument (save perhaps for a checklist and a tape recorder) it is extremely difficult to know how the research process shaped the data produced, unless full transcripts of the interviews are made available (see Chapter 16). Where research instruments are used, it is possible to investigate this shaping process by testing the instruments under different circumstances. This testing is referred to as *validation*.

1 The use of standard instruments

Validation is very time-consuming. This encourages researchers to use instruments that have already been validated. For example, much research in health care in the UK uses instruments where people report on their own health and well-being irrespective of any particular diagnosis: *generic health measures*. Rather than inventing new instruments here most researchers choose one of the four widely used and well-validated instruments (Essink-Bot et al., 1997):

- the Nottingham Health profile – NHP (Jenkinson, 1994b; Bowling, 1995: 281–5);
- the Medical Outcomes Study 36 item Short-form Health Survey – the SF-36 (Brazier et al., 1992; Wright, 1994) (see Figure 6.2);
- the Dartmouth COOP/WONCA charts (see Figure 6.1) (Nelson et al., 1990);
- the EuroQol questionnaire (EuroQol Group, 1990; Kind et al., 1998).

In this volume, the research by Sasha Shepperd and colleagues presented in Chapter 3 uses both the COOP charts and the SF-36. There are also many instruments for recording baselines and outcomes in experiments which are specific to particular medical conditions: see, for example, the deviant behaviour rating scale used in

Chapter 2, and the World Health Organisation Angina Questionnaire used in Chapter 9.

The use of the same instruments in different pieces of research also produces results that can be compared directly with each other. Where two pieces of research on the same topic use different instruments there is always a puzzle as to whether any differences in results are real, or just the result of using different data collection instruments and measurement procedures. Chapter 4 features a systematic review of a number of different experiments on home visiting schemes and their impact on child injury rates. One of the problems encountered by the reviewers was that the different studies used different ways of measuring child injury.

Some instruments originally designed for research purposes are used to provide measures in routine health and care practice, and vice versa. For example, the *Barthel Index* used to measure the degree of assistance someone needs in order to carry out basic tasks of daily living (Bowling, 1995: 182–5) is used in both research and in routine practice. The Barthel was used by Sasha Shepperd and colleagues (Chapter 3). While two practitioners saying that their clients improved in their daily living abilities does not mean much, one practitioner saying that on average their clients improved by 10 Barthel index points, and another that theirs improved by 15 has a precise and common meaning. Thus the use of a common set of measuring instruments provides something of a common language enabling research to be applied to practice, and practice to be interpreted in the light of research findings.

2   Cultural specificity and instruments

Changes in linguistic habits may render any instrument out of date. There are obvious problems also of translating instruments from one language to another (including from American to British English), and of using instruments with sub-cultural groups. Instrument designers hit a particular problem here. In attempts to make instruments 'user-friendly' designers often use colloquial language (as in the COOP chart in Figure 6.1). But colloquial language is much more exclusionary than formal language for people of different generations, ethnic or dialect groups and it dates much more quickly. Consider, for example, the use of 'quite a bit', or 'blue' in Figure 6.1.

3   Data levels and qualities

Different instruments produce data of different kinds, or 'levels'. Box 6.1 explains what this means.

Box 6.1   Levels of data

Different kinds of data are classified into different levels, the higher levels containing more information than the lower levels. It is possible to treat higher level data as if they were lower level data, by ignoring some of the information they contain. But it is not permissible to treat lower level data as if they were data of a higher level. Different statistical tests are appropriate for different levels of data (see Chapter 7, section 6).

- **Nominal or categorical data** – entities are classified into types and counted; for example, males and females, Yeses and Nos. No mean (average) nor median (mid-score) can be calculated: you can't have an 'average' gender. The mode or most common category is the only measure of central tendency possible.*
- **Ordinal level data** – scores can be rank ordered, but without the distances between the ranks being measureable: for example, NHS Trust positions in a league table, clients' ranked preferences for particular kinds of services. No mean (average) can be calculated, but a median (mid-score) can be.*
- **Interval level data and ratio level data** – scores can be placed on a scale where the difference between them can be measured precisely: for example, areas of ulcerated tissue, ages of clients, numbers of delinquent episodes. Ratio level data differ from interval level data in deriving from scales with a true zero. Both allow for the calculation of a mean (average), median (mid-point) and standard deviation.*

Nominal and ordinal level data are often called 'qualitative data' by statisticians and medical researchers, and interval and ratio data 'quantitative data'. This is not the same quantitative/qualitative distinction which is made more generally in the methodology of the social sciences (see Chapter 16).

* For modes, means and medians and standard deviations, see Chapter 7, section 9.

Measures of time, temperature, pressure, length, area, weight and orientation allow for the use of instruments that produce the higher level interval or ratio data. But many instruments used in health and care research do not produce higher level data, or do not do so without controversy. This is almost always so when the data concern the opinions of clients, and often when they concern the judgements of practitioners.

The COOP chart in Figure 6.1 produces data which reach the *ordinal* level. That means that scores can be put in (rank) order on a five-point scale from 'not at all' to 'extremely.' Strictly speaking, the instrument will not produce *interval* level data, since there is no way of knowing whether the gap between 'moderately' and 'slightly' is the same size as the gap between 'moderately' and 'quite a bit' – for everyone, or for anyone in particular. Taking a purist line, the appropriate measure of central tendency for ordinal level data is not the mean (average) but the median (Chapter 7, section 9). The median expresses the point below which 50 per cent of all scores and above which 50 per cent of all scores fall – the middle score. On the same principle, distributions can be described in terms of *percentiles*, where the median is the 50th percentile, where 20 per cent of scores fall below the 20th percentile and so on. Non-parametric statistics (Chapter 7, section 6) are the appropriate tests to use since these get by on comparing either the rank order of two samples, or the profiles of two samples according to the percentages of each score. Parametric tests by contrast always entail calculating a mean (average) and usually a standard deviation (see Chapter 7, section 9).

The COOP instrument (Figure 6.1), and other generic health status measures listed earlier (section 1), actually produce data no higher than ordinal. But the data are very often analysed as if they were at an interval level. Thus it will be said, perhaps, that the mean (average) score from this COOP chart for a particular population is 1.88. But that is derived from adding together '1s' which are not necessarily equal to each other nor necessarily half the value of '2s', and '4s' which are not necessarily twice the value of '2s' and so on, and dividing the total by the number of respondents. Treating data as if they were of an interval level allows for the use of the more powerful parametric statistical tests (see Chapter 7, section 6). There is controversy in general as to whether this is a sensible practice. The consensus is that sometimes it will lead to misleading results, and sometimes not, according to the instrument, the test, the sample size and whatever it is that is being measured (Pett, 1997: 32–4).

4   Instruments and data distributions

Instruments also produce data that have particular shaped distributions. The ideal data distribution for statistical analysis is a *normal distribution*, meaning that when the instrument is used with a large sample, a graph of the results will take the shape of a 'bell-curve' with most results in the middle clustered around the mean/average. But many instruments used in measuring health and welfare give *skewed* distributions. This may arise when they are designed to distinguish only between degrees of unwellness, and hence tend to clump all the people who regard themselves as well together at one end of the graph. Figure 6.2 shows the distribution of scores derived from the use of the SF-36 health questionnaire with a random sample from general

Figure 6.2   A skewed distribution: distribution derived from using questions on physical functioning from the SF-36 with a random sample of general practice patients (Brazier et al., 1992: 163)

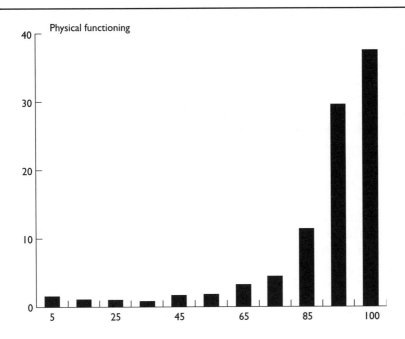

practice. The SF-36 was one of the instruments used by Shepperd and colleagues in the RCT which is the preliminary to the economic analysis in Chapter 3. From Figure 6.2 it seems that nearly 40 per cent of respondents have no problems of physical function. This kind of *skew* is common in generic health measures (section 1). There are two issues here.

Data transformations

One has to do with the possibilities for subjecting skewed distributions to statistical analysis, since the more powerful (parametric) statistical procedures depend on the properties of a normal (unskewed) distribution (Chapter 7, section 6). This can sometimes be solved by *transforming* the scores so that they do take something much more like a normal distribution. Thus, for example, the distribution in Figure 6.2 might take on a bell-shaped curve if instead of the raw scores, their square roots, their logarithms, or their inverses were substituted (Pett, 1997: 37, 52–4). Several of the exemplar studies use transformations for this purpose (Marshall et al., in Chapter 2; Shepperd et al., in Chapter 3; Roberts et al. in Chapter 4). (For further notes on data transformations, see Chapter 7, section 6).

The second issue has to do with the purpose of the research. Someone who was interested in mapping feelings of anxiety, depression and irritability in the general population by doing a survey would be missing the more subtle differences among 40 per cent of the population if they used the COOP chart (Figure 6.1). However, someone doing an experiment who was particularly interested in measuring changes just among people who were ill might regard the difference between a score of 2 and a score of 3 as a threshold between 'health' and 'dis-ease'. On one side of the threshold differences would be clinically interesting and important (differences among the 'suitable cases for treatment'). On the other side of the threshold any such differences might be regarded as unimportant and uninteresting.

Floor and ceiling effects

This matter is sometimes discussed in terms of *floor* and *ceiling* effects. The COOP chart produces data with a strong ceiling effect but only a small floor effect: meaning that the data *discriminate* poorly between people without serious problems, but fairly well between people with serious problems. Which is termed the 'floor' and which the 'ceiling' is an arbitrary matter.

Whether floor and ceiling effects matter depends on the uses to which an instrument is put. For example, using nominal level data to compare the effectiveness of bandaging systems for leg ulcers reduces measurement to the two categories 'healed' and 'not healed'. This produces acute floor and ceiling effects. In the study in Chapter 1, two bandaging systems were judged as equivalent, since they both produced similar rates of 'healing'. But some differences in effectiveness might be hidden below the floor, or above the ceiling of measurement if the data were nominal. In fact the authors of this study did also use additional more discriminating means of measuring and this was not the case.

5 Validating instruments for their reliability

A weighing machine which kept giving different weights for the same package would be regarded as *unreliable*. It is easy enough to imagine one way of checking its reliability: keep on weighing the same package. *Test–retest* reliability means that using the instrument a second time with the same subjects will produce the same results (so long as nothing has changed between occasions of use).

In experimental work it is common for assessments by practitioners to provide baseline and/or outcome measures. There is a huge amount of research on the judgements of practitioners in most fields of health and social care. Most of it shows that in normal practice practitioners are very *unreliable* judges in the sense that different practitioners faced with the same case make diverse judgements about the nature of the case, the diagnosis, the severity and so on. This is so even with apparently simple procedures such as taking temperatures or blood pressures (Bloor, 1978; Bloor et al., 1987; Gau and Diehl, 1982; Jenkins et al., 1985; Sackett et al., 1991). The same seems to be as true for social work as for medicine (Packman et al., 1986; Campbell, 1991). Thus, experiments that rely on practitioners making judgements 'as usual' have to be regarded with suspicion. Most experimental research using practitioner judgements attempts to enforce reliability on practitioners by providing them with a protocol or guidelines for making judgements. The protocol is, of course, the 'instrument'. It is often in a questionnaire format. An example is the MRC Needs for Care Schedule used in the study reported in Chapter 2, guiding, in this case, a psychiatrist and a psychiatric nurse in rating the care needs of subjects on entry to the experiment and after 7 and 14 months. Such instruments are validated for their reliability by testing them to see whether different practitioners using the same instrument come to the same conclusions with regard to the same cases: an *inter-rater reliability test*. Occasionally an *intra-rater reliability test* is used to see whether the same practitioner using the same instrument comes to the same conclusions when presented with the same case on two, or more, different occasions.

A different kind of reliability is *internal consistency reliability*. If an instrument has internal consistency reliability there will be a statistical correlation between those parts of the instrument allegedly measuring the same thing. In an examination that also awarded marks for grammar and spelling, for example, we would expect the same student to score much the same for this on each question answered. Many research instruments include several different ways of measuring what is allegedly the same thing, precisely for judging internal consistency.

6 Reliability tests

Test–retest, inter- and intra-rater tests are usually analysed for *correlation* – sometimes called 'agreement', using a correlation co-efficient called *Kappa* (Pett, 1997: 237–48), though other statistics might be used instead. Most correlation co-efficients express perfect agreement as +1 and no agreement at all as 0 and completely contrary judgements about the same matter as -1. Perfect positive or negative correlations are rare and 0.8 is regarded as a high degree of agreement, and -0.8 as a high degree of disagreement.

Correlation co-effecients are usually tested for statistical significance. This is dealt with in more detail in the next chapter (sections 1
and 2), but the issue is whether or how far an agreement might have
occurred by chance. Thus for inter-rater reliability, between two
judges who can only opt for 'yes' or 'no', there is already a 50 per cent
chance of agreement if they merely answered at random. For three
judges there is only a 25 per cent chance of agreement by chance (**YYY,**
YYN, YNY, YNN, NYY, NYN, NNY, **NNN**). An 80 per cent agreement
between three judges would be much more impressive than an 80 per
cent agreement between two.

A Kappa, or κ test is often used in this context:

> The weighted κ for the agreement between the two assessors was 0.94 for
> adequacy of allocation concealment, 0.51 for the extent to which the
> analyses were based on all randomised participants, and 0.78 for blinding.
> (Chapter 4, p. 40)

Here we are being told that two assessors independently assessed the
quality of a set of research studies on three criteria. The extent to
which they agreed is expressed by values of κ (Kappa). Conventionally,
a κ of between 0.4 and 0.6 is a 'fair' level of agreement (possibly due to
chance but unlikely to be so), 0.6 to 0.75 are 'good' and values greater
than 0.75 are 'excellent' (Fleiss, 1971).

Internal consistency is usually measured using a co-efficient called
Cronbach's alpha – the higher the alpha, the greater the consistency
(Cronbach, 1951).

7 Validating the validity of instruments

Broadly speaking, the validity of an instrument refers to whether it
measures what it is supposed to measure. There is little difficulty in
agreeing that measuring changes in the area of ulcerated tissue is
validly measuring whether leg ulcers are healing or not (Chapter 1).
Often matters are not as simple as this. For example, the experiment
featured in Chapter 2 examines which of two different ways of
providing a service to people with severe mental health problems is
more effective in promoting mental health. In order to measure this it
is necessary for the researchers to take a position on the meaning of
'mental health', since 'mental health' and 'mental illness' are highly
contested ideas. The position they adopt is a psychiatric one, and
the scales they use measure matters which psychiatrists and most
community mental health team members consider to be important
aspects of mental health – severity of psychiatric symptoms, episodes
of deviant behaviour and so on. Two of the instruments captured the

subjects' own opinions, but according to an agenda set by psychiatric ideas.

The important point here is that if the researchers had adopted a different view as to the nature of 'mental health' they would have chosen different things to measure and different instruments to measure them with, and perhaps would have produced research with different results. For example, viewed from the perspective of some self-styled 'survivors' of the mental health system, what psychiatrists would term 'deviant behaviour' could be viewed as acts of political resistance to psychiatric control. Subjects losing touch with mental health services might be viewed in terms of liberation rather than in terms of a failure of mental health care (Romme and Escher, 1993).

There are two different issues here. One is a fundamental one as to what meaning should be given to ideas such as 'health', 'illness', 'intelligence', 'social adjustment', 'equity', 'empowerment', or 'satisfaction' (as in 'consumer satisfaction'). These are all highly contested ideas, and there is no way in which research can determine their 'true' meaning. Rather researchers have to start off with some idea as to what they mean. At this fundamental level what might be a valid way of measuring mental health from a psychiatric viewpoint, would be invalid from an anti-psychiatry viewpoint, and *vice versa*

The second issue then, is whether, once having decided what such fundamentals mean, researchers adopt a suitable way of studying them. At this level, someone antipathetic to psychiatric ideas might grudgingly concede that 'if you think that psychiatric ideas about mental health are right, then the way you are measuring it is appropriate'.

All this impacts particularly on research designed to measure 'effectiveness'. Rightly or wrongly, that term implies more than investigating the effects of doing something, and has the implication that what is 'effective' is what is also desirable. Since there may be dispute about what are more or less desirable outcomes in health and care practice, there may be disputes about what kinds of outcome measures to feature in research. One axis of the debate here is about *who* should define desirable outcomes: practitioners or service users? Much experimental research includes instruments that elicit the opinions of research subjects – as with the COOP/WONCA charts (Figure 6.1). But such information may not necessarily reflect what is of particular importance to the person from whom it is elicited. During the 1990s considerable progress was made in tempering professional judgements about desirable outcomes with the opinions of service users (see, for example, Greenhalgh et al., 1995). However, whether instruments are derived from the ideas of practitioners or from the ideas of service users, to be useful in experimental research they always have to meet standards of reliability and validity.

There are at least four different notions of validity used in the validation of research instruments. People often find it easier to understand these through the example of scholastic examinations:

- **Face validity** – the questions on the examination paper seem to be relevant to the course studied by the students and to the aims of the course they followed. The questions on the COOP chart (Figure 6.1) seem to be about the kinds of feelings which are of interest in judging morale. This is a very weak criterion for validity.
- **Content validity** – together all the questions on the examination paper cover most of the content and most of the aims of the course. Together the nine COOP charts seem to cover most dimensions of health-related quality of life, which is what they are supposed to measure.
- **Criterion validity** entails comparing results on one instrument with results on another allegedly measuring the same thing. For criterion validity there should be a correlation between what students achieved in the examination and what they achieved on continuously assessed work. The group who score most healthy on the COOP charts will also be the group who are judged as most healthy by practitioners. Criterion validity is particularly important where a cheap and easy to use instrument is used instead of an expensive or intrusive investigation, as in many screening procedures.
- **Construct validity** – the results achieved from using the instrument predict those matters which the theory underlying the instrument's design says they should predict. For example, if the purpose of an examination is to differentiate students according to their ability in general terms, then those who score most highly should, as a group, be the more successful in later life. There is a self-fulfilling prophecy problem in this example, however. If the theory underlying the use of the COOP charts is that ill people with higher morale will get better quicker, then better scores on the 'feelings' chart now (Figure 6.1) should predict better scores on all the charts later. Chapters 9 and 11 deal with deprivation indices, which are validated in terms of how well they predict all the things which are associated with deprivation: death rates, morbidity rates, accident rates, low birth weights, crime rates and so on.

Judgements with regard to the last three of these criteria are usually made in terms of the strength of statistical correlations, which are explained in more detail in Chapter 10, section 10. The stronger the correlation, the better the instrument. However, it is worth noting that it is very difficult to design an instrument which is excellent in terms of all criteria of reliability and validity; a good showing on one criterion is often achieved by a poorer showing on another. It is not enough for researchers to write that an instrument has been validated. They should say in what ways it has been validated and in terms of which criteria.

8 Questions to ask about research instruments

In textbook explanations the different criteria for validity above are commonly differentiated. But in real research contexts they are often difficult to distinguish from each other, and indeed, often difficult to distinguish from issues of reliability. It may be better to think of the issues here in terms of two generic questions to ask about the validity and reliability of instruments:

- What is the instrument supposed to measure?
- What evidence is there that it measures this, rather than something else?

Part 4 of this book includes a checklist of 'Questions to Ask about Data Collection Instruments'. This refers to some matters not dealt with above. For example, there are questions about whether the instrument is acceptable to the people it is used with, and whether it is appropriate for use in the context in which it is used. At first sight these may seem to be issues different from those of validity and reliability. Actually they are not, since an unacceptable instrument or one inappropriate for the context is most unlikely to produce valid results.

9 Further reading on research instruments

Ann Bowling's two books, *Measuring Disease* (1995) and *Measuring Health* (1991), both explain the theory of measurement and instrumentation and both provide comprehensive catalogues of a large range of research instruments used in health research, reviewing their validation history to date of publication. Crispin Jenkinson's compilation *Measuring Health and Medical Outcomes* (Jenkinson, 1994a) is particularly useful with regard to generic health status measures. His article with Hannah McGee (1997) is a lucid, though shorter, treatment of the same field. Any research paper using a validated instrument should give references to its validation pedigree, and those that do not should be regarded with some suspicion, though not with as much suspicion as those that use novel and unvalidated instruments.

References and further reading

Bloor, M. (1978) 'On the routinised nature of work in people-processing agencies: the case of adeno-tonsillectomy assessments in ENT outpatient clinics', in A. Davis (ed.), *Relationships between Doctors and Patients*. Farnborough: Saxon House.

Bloor, M. (1991) 'A minor office: the variable and socially constructed character of death certification in a Scottish city', *Journal of Health and Social Behaviour*, 32: 273–87.

Bloor, M., Samphier, M. and Prior, L. (1987) 'Artefact explanations of inequalities in health: an assessment of the evidence', *Sociology of Health and Illness*, 9(3): 231–64.

Bowling, A. (1991) *Measuring Health: a Review of Quality of Life Measuring Scales*. Buckingham: Open University Press.

Bowling, A. (1995) *Measuring Disease*. Buckingham: Open University Press.

Brazier, J., Harper, R., Jones, N., O'Cathain, A., Thomas, K., Usherwood, T. and Westlake, L. (1992) 'Validating the SF-36 health survey questionnaire: a new outcome measure for primary care', *British Medical Journal*, 305: 160–4.

Campbell, M. (1991) 'Children at risk: how different are children on child abuse registers?', *British Journal of Social Work*, 21: 259–75.

Cronbach, I. (1951) 'Coefficient alpha and the internal consistency of tests', *Psychometrika*, 16: 297–334.

Essink-Bot, M.-L., Krabbe, P., Bonsel, G. and Aaronson, N. (1997) 'An empirical comparison of four generic health status measures', *Medical Care*, 35 (5): 522–37.

EuroQol Group (1990) 'EuroQol – a new facility for the measurement of health-related quality of life', *Health Policy*, 16: 199–208.

Fleiss, J. (1971) 'Measuring nominal scale agreements among many raters', *Psychological Bulletin*, 76: 378–82.

Gau, D. and Diehl, A. (1982) 'Disagreement among medical practitioners regarding cause of Death', *British Medical Journal*, 284: 239–40.

Greenhalgh, J., Georgiou, A., Williams, D., Dyas, J. and Long, A. (1995) *Measuring the Outcomes of Diabetes Care*. Outcome Measurement Reviews No.4. Leeds: University of Leeds, Nuffield Institute for Health, UK Clearing House on Health Outcomes.

Jenkins, R., Smeeton, N., Markinder, M. and Shepperd, S. (1985) 'A study of the classification of mental ill-health in general practice', *Psychological Medicine*, 15: 403–9.

Jenkinson, C. (ed.) (1994a) *Measuring Health and Medical Outcomes*. London: UCL Press.

Jenkinson, C., (1994b) 'Weighting for ill-health: the Nottingham Health Profile', in C. Jenkinson, (ed.), *Measuring Health and Medical Outcomes*. London: UCL Press. pp. 77–88.

Jenkinson, C. and McGee, H. (1997) 'Patient assessed outcomes: measuring health status and quality of life', in C. Jenkinson (ed.) *Assessment and Evaluation of Health and Medical Care: a Methods Text*. Buckingham: Open University Press. pp. 64–84.

Kind, P., Dolan, P., Gudex, C. and Williams, A. (1998) 'Variations in population health status: results from a United Kingdom national questionnaire survey', *British Medical Journal*, 316: 736–40.

Nelson, E., Langraf, J. and Hayes, R. (1990) 'The COOP Function Charts: a system to measure patient function in physicians' offices', in M. Lipkin (ed.), *Functional Status Measurement in Primary Care: Wonca Classification Committee*. New York: Springer-Verlag.

Packman, J., Randall, J. and Jacques, N. (1986) *Who Needs Care? Social Work Decisions about Children*. Oxford: Blackwell.

Pett, M. (1997) *Non-Parametric Statistics for Health Care Research: Statistics for Small Samples and Unusual Distributions*. London: Sage.

Romme, M. and Escher, S. (1993) *Accepting Voices*. London: Mind.

Sackett, D., Haynes, R., Guyatt, G. and Tugwell, P. (1991) *Clinical Epidemiology – a Basic Science for Clinical Medicine*. London: Little, Brown and Co.

Shepperd, S., Harwood, D., Jenkinson, C., Gray, A., Vessey, M. and Morgan, P. (1998) 'Randomised controlled trial comparing hospital at home care with inpatient hospital care: I: three month follow up of health outcomes', *British Medical Journal*, 316: 1786–91.

Wright, L. (1994) 'The long and the short of it: the development of the SF-36 General Health Survey', in C. Jenkinson (ed.), *Measuring Health and Medical Outcomes*. London: UCL Press. pp. 89–109.

CHAPTER 7

READING THE RESULTS OF EXPERIMENTAL RESEARCH

Introduction

This chapter provides information to help in deciphering the numerical presentation of research results, which people often find daunting.

1 Statistical significance

The results of experiments are usually tested for statistical significance. Results that are statistically significant are results that are most unlikely to have arisen by chance. Your friend deals you ten red playing cards from what she says is a standard shuffled pack. You know that this is very unlikely but not impossible. Having shuffled the pack again she deals you four reds. How suspicious would you be now? In fact, of all four-card deals 5.5 per cent of them will be all reds. One such deal should come up roughly every 18 deals. Ten reds running will only occur once in 3,333 deals. Knowing these odds, you know that ten reds is much more unlikely to be a chance deal than four reds is likely to be.

Testing for statistical significance is a matter of checking what actually happened against an estimate of how often it might have happened by chance. The principle is easy to understand, but lots of people get bogged down in the mechanics.

2 χ^2 as an example of a statistical significance test

The most transparent of all tests is one used in the research featured in the exemplar study for Chapter 1. It is called χ^2 and pronounced 'Ki-square'. How it is calculated is demonstrated below.

The Observed (or 'O') figures are what actually happened. The O figures in Table 7.1 show that of 35 ulcers 16 healed. Eight of these were treated with one kind of bandage and eight with another. It should be fairly obvious from 'eye-balling' the data that the differences in healing rates (8/17 and 8/18) are just the kind which might have occurred by chance with two treatments of equal effectiveness. Though this is obvious, the text below will show how the same conclusion can be reached statistically.

The Expected (or 'E') figures are what would be most expected to happen by chance. In this case they are calculated simply on a fair-shares basis, sharing out the healings, non-healings and withdrawals proportionately between the two bandaging systems. Thus 7.77 = seventeen thirty-fifths of 16, which is the Charing Cross 'fair-share' of all healings. Fair-shares is what would be most expected if the results were due to chance. The further calculation is simple:

For each pair of cells calculate $\dfrac{(O - E)^2}{E}$

Then add up all the results:

$$\frac{(8 - 7.77)^2}{7.77} + \frac{(8 - 8.23)^2}{8.23} + \frac{(5 - 6.32)^2}{6.32} + \frac{(8 - 6.69)^2}{6.69} + \frac{(4 - 2.91)^2}{2.91} +$$

$$\frac{(2 - 3.08)^2}{3.08} = 1.3 = \chi^2$$

In this calculation the subtractions are the comparisons between the actual figure (O) and what is most to be expected to happen by chance (E). Logically then, the bigger the resulting figure the more

Table 7.1 A χ^2 calculation with the data from the leg ulcer bandaging trial
(Chapter 1)

	Charing Cross Bandaging System		Trial Bandaging System		
	Observed	Expected	Observed	Expected	Total
Healed	8	7.77	8	8.23	16
Not healed	5	6.32	8	6.69	13
Withdrawn	4	2.91	2	3.08	6
Totals	17	17.00	18	18.00	35

$\chi^2 = 1.3$; df = 2; $p = 0.51$.

different the observed figures will be from the expected figures and the less likely the results were due to chance.

The figure for χ^2 is then looked up in a ready-reckoner table, two rows of which are given below as Table 7.2

In Table 7.2 df stands for 'degrees of freedom'. There are two degrees of freedom in Table 7.1, since once the row totals and the column totals are filled in, filling in *two* of the remaining O cells determines all the content of all the others: think of crossword puzzles. The content of two cells are free to vary; hence two degrees of freedom. Usually the formula for calculating degrees of freedom is (columns − 1) × (rows − 1) = df: in this case (2 − 1)(3 − 1) = 2.

The *p* stands for probability and the *p* values provide an estimate of the likelihood of a particular value of χ^2 occurring by chance. In terms of the card deals referred to in section 1, four reds running would have a probability of just a bit more than 20 per cent ($p = 0.20$) and 10 reds running have a probability of just over 1/3000. Usually this latter would be expressed as $p < 0.001$ (less than one in one thousand). Probability values are ubiquitous in tables of experimental results and the top line of Table 7.2 will serve as a useful resource for you if you find it difficult to remember what *p* values mean.

Table 7.2 shows that, at two degrees of freedom, a value for χ^2 of 13.82 or more will occur by chance less than once per 1000, i.e. $p = 0.001$. If we had a result like that we could be very confident that it was not due to chance. It would be a highly statistically significant result.

A value of 5.99 or more will occur less than 5 times in 100, i.e. $p = 0.05$. By convention statisticians will not accept as significant any value of *p* greater than 0.05 (or 'the 5% level'). The question to be asked about the value of χ^2 obtained in the calculation above is 'is it equal to or bigger than the 0.05 value?'

The 0.05 (5%) value is 5.99. The value given by the calculation was 1.3. This is much, much smaller. This tells us what we already knew, that the result is not statistically significant. It also tells us how

Table 7.2   Critical values of χ^2 level of significance for a two-tailed test*

p =	0.90	0.70	0.50	0.20	0.10	0.05	0.02	0.01	0.001
	90%	70%	50%	20%	10%	5%	2%	1%	1/1000
	likely by chance	likely by chance	likely by chance	likely by chance	likely by chance	likely by chance	likely by chance	likely by chance	likely by chance
df = 1	0.02	0.15	0.45	1.64	2.71	3.84	5.41	0.64	10.83
df = 2	0.20	0.71	1.39	3.22	4.61	5.99	7.38	9.21	13.82

* 'Two-tailed' means that we are interested in a difference in any direction. In terms of Table 7.1 that means any difference whether this is in favour of the Charing Cross bandages or in favour of the trial bandages. Most significance testing is two-tailed (Wright, 1997: 39)

statistically *in*significant it is. It lies between the value where $p =$ 0.70 and where it equals 0.50. So if χ^2 equals 1.3 then differences of this size would crop up as chance variations somewhere between 50 and 70 per cent of times if the experiment were repeated again and again.

3 Tests, questions and hypotheses

Researchers often frame their questions in terms of hypotheses. In the leg ulcer bandaging trial (Chapter 1) the so-called *null hypothesis* (or H_0) would have been that: 'there is no difference in effectiveness between the two bandaging systems greater than might have been expected by chance'. The so-called *experimental hypothesis* (H_E) would be that there is a statistically significant difference in effectiveness between the two bandaging systems. Saying that results show no statistical significance is the same as saying that the null hypothesis should not be rejected, and that the experimental hypothesis falls.

There is actually an opportunity for two null hypotheses here:

H_{0i} – there is no difference in drop-out rates as between the two bandaging systems greater than might be expected by chance.

H_{0ii} – there is no difference in healing rates as between the two bandaging systems, greater than might be expected by chance, when the effect of drop-out has been accounted for.

The way the calculation above (Table 7.1) was done tested both null hypotheses in a single test. But there might have been a statistically significant difference in drop out rates between the two bandaging systems, but no significant difference in healing rates for those ulcers remaining in the trial, *or* no significant difference in drop out rates, but a significant difference in healing rates for those ulcers remaining in the trial. In fact this is not so, but it is important to note that a single statistic, χ^2 in this case, may be measuring several differences at once. To compare the two bandaging systems for drop out rates only it would be necessary to use a two row table amalgamating the healed and the not-healed ulcers. Then the only difference visible to the statistical test would have been that between withdrawals and non-withdrawals. The lesson here is that the way the data should be set up for testing will depend on the hypothesis being tested.

4 Confidence intervals

The TV pathologist says 'Time of death twelve midnight, give or take two hours either side'. The 'give or take two hours' defines a confidence interval. Similarly, experimental results are always regarded as estimates of the true state of affairs and are usually cited with confidence limits. The 95% confidence intervals are those most usually used, but the 99% intervals are not uncommon. The assumption being made is that if the experiment were repeated again and again and again it would produce a series of different results, but 95% of these would fall within the 95% confidence limits. For example, for the leg ulcer bandaging trial it can be calculated that 95 per cent of such results would fall between 5 healings for the Charing Cross Bandages and 11 for the Trial Bandages at one extreme, and 11 healings for the Charing Cross Bandages and 5 for the Trial Bandages at the other extreme. This is another way of saying that in this trial one bandaging system would have to show at least 7 more healings than the other to be regarded as superior, which is much the same as saying that anything less than a difference of 7 out of 16 here would not be statistically significant at the 0.05 (5%) level.

5   Confidence intervals and meta-analyses

Confidence intervals are particularly useful for making 'at a glance' judgements about the meaning of experimental results. This is shown particularly when they are used in meta-analyses, but you can regard this section as an illustration of how to interpret confidence intervals however they are used.

Meta-analyses involve bringing together the findings of a number of experiments or trials and comparing the results. They are dealt with in further detail in Chapter 4. Very often they include a diagrammatic synopsis of results, like Figure 7.1, which puts confidence intervals to good use.

Figure 7.1   The effect of home visiting in preventing childhood injury: eight randomised controlled trials reviewed by Roberts et al., 1996: odds ratios and 95% confidence intervals (see Chapter 4)

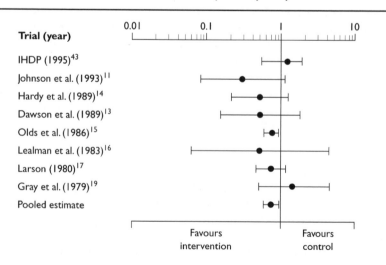

Figure 7.2   First two lines from Figure 7.1 annotated

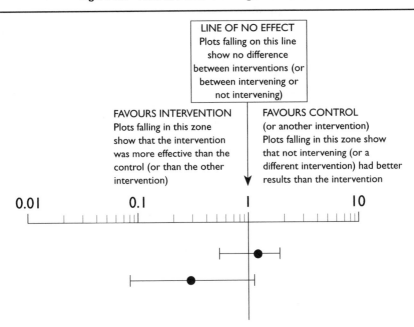

Each of the trials involved comparing rates of injury for children who were and children who were not visited as part of a visiting scheme. The diagram shows the differences between the children visited and the controls as odds ratios for each of the trials reviewed. Odds ratios are explained in section 10.4, but understanding odds ratios is not necessary for understanding diagrams like this.

The first line on Figures 7.1 and 7.2 is for a trial conducted as part of the USA Infant Health and Development Program (IHDP) in 1995. The dot, or 'plot' on the line gives the actual result. It falls to the right of the vertical line on the side marked 'Favours Control'. In this trial there was less childhood injury among those who were not visited, than among those who were. The vertical line is called 'the line of no effect'. If the actual results of a trial fell on this line this would indicate that there was roughly the same amount of childhood injury among those who were visited as among those who were not: no greater difference than might have been expected to occur by chance. The next trial on the diagram has its results well to the left of the line of no effect, on the side which 'Favours Intervention'.

The plots show the actual results of the trials. But the results of a trial are always regarded as estimates, on the assumption that had the trial been conducted over and over again in the same way its results would tend to cluster round a mid-point, but would not be identical. The horizontal lines (or whiskers) show how wide the estimates are. In this case the estimates are the 95% confidence limits (see section 4). What the limits suggest is that we can be 95% certain that the true result lies somewhere on the horizontal line. Sometimes 99% confidence intervals are used instead.

The plot for the IHDP study was to the right of the midline, favouring not visiting (Figure 7.2). But one of the whiskers strays over the line into the area favouring intervention. Maybe if the IHDP study had been done again in exactly the same way except that the intervention and the control groups were made up of different families, its results would be to the left of the line rather than to the right, favouring intervention. Confidence limits that stray across the midline indicate that no confident judgement can be made as to whether two interventions are different in their effects.

For relatively rare events such as childhood injury the sample sizes for each trial here are rather small. The IHDP is the largest, with 345 visited and 551 controls, and the smallest is Gray et al., with 26 visited and 25 controls. Small samples tend to give wide confidence intervals – long whiskers, and hence imprecise estimates. Figure 7.1 shows seven of the eight trials with confidence intervals crossing the line of no effect. The last entry on Figure 7.1 pools the results of all trials. It treats all the trials together as if they were just one randomised controlled trial involving several thousand subjects. The plot for the pooled results falls to the left, favouring intervention. But, more importantly, its confidence intervals fall entirely to the left, so that there is a 95 per cent chance that the results of all the trials together indicate in favour of visiting rather than not visiting, though the benefits of visiting schemes still seem to be rather small.

The same logic can be used in interpreting confidence intervals where effects are shown in different ways. But it is important to be clear as to how the different ways of reporting results differ in expressing equivalence. With odds ratios and risk ratios (section 10.4) equal effectiveness is expressed as 1, and the line of no effect (Figure 7.2) runs through the 1s. But where effects are shown by subtracting averages (section 10.1), or subtracting proportions (section 10.2), or using a standard deviation (section 10.3), equivalent effectiveness is shown as zero. Hence with these other ways of interpreting effects it is 0 (as it were) which marks the 'line of no effect', and confidence intervals which stray over that line are likely to indicate non-significant results.

6   Non-parametric and parametric statistics

Statistical tests are divided into two kinds:

- Non-parametric tests, which are the only kinds which should be used with nominal data (see Box 6.1 in Chapter 6). Using non-parametric tests with higher level data is possible, but non-

parametric tests cannot 'see' all the information included in inter-val or ratio level data.
- Parametric tests, which should not be used with nominal level data, which are, but perhaps should not be, used with ordinal level data, and which make the best use of all the information contained in interval and ratio level data.

Parametric tests should only be used when a number of conditions are satisfied. These include that:

- A sample is drawn from a population in which the characteristic of interest is *normally distributed*. If it were graphed it would show a bell-shaped curve, with the mean or average somewhere very close to the middle of the range. Some of the complicated statistical manoeuvres to be found in the literature derive from converting non-normally distributed data into normally distributed data: for example, by using the logarithms or square roots of scores rather than the scores themselves. In Chapter 4, for example, Roberts et al. quote their results in terms of 'an inverse variance weighted average of the study specific odds ratios'. The 'inverse variance weighted average' is a way of converting scores that are not norm-ally distributed into scores that are, so that they are amenable to processing using parametric statistics.
- When comparing two samples of dissimilar size, the variance of the two samples should be similar. Roughly speaking, the statistical concept of variance refers to the degree of variability *within* samples (see section 9).

In Chapter 2 Marshall, Lockwood and Gath write: 'The data were first evaluated to ensure normality of sampling distributions, linearity and homogeneity of variance.' This means that they checked to see whether it was permissible to use the parametric statistics they proposed to use.

7 Sample size

The extent to which confident conclusions can be drawn from experi-ments depends on sample size. Unfortunately, it is very difficult to lay down general rules as to what is an adequate sample size, but Table 7.3 gives some rules of thumb for judging whether a sample size was adequate.

Most of the discussion of sample size revolves around the second item in Table 7.3: the size of the difference which can be detected in

Table 7.3   Some considerations in judging adequate sample size

A sample size of 40 would be adequate if:	A larger, sometimes much larger, sample would be needed if:
The experiment only has two arms and there are no less than 20 in each arm	The experiment has more than two arms (20 for each arm would be a usual minimum)
There is no interest in differences smaller than 10 per cent	There is an interest in differences smaller than 10 per cent
And/or the events of interest are common	And/or the events of interest are rare (an experimental evaluation of a suicide prevention scheme would require a very large sample, since suicide is rare even among those of highest risk)
The subjects very similar to each other in the ways relevant to the experiment	The subjects are very diverse in ways relevant to the experiment – then a large sample is needed to ensure the same range of characteristics in each arm of the experiment (see Chapter 5, section 3 on forming comparison groups)
The interventions are highly standardised within each arm	The interventions within each arm are diverse. A 'two arm' trial with diverse interventions within each arm is not really a 'two arm trial' but a many armed trial and there should be at least 20 subjects for each of the diverse interventions *within* an arm
There is no interest in what happens to sub-groups within the different arms of the trial	There is an interest in what happens to sub-groups. The logic here is to think of the trial as having as many arms as there are sub-groups, e.g. male controls, female controls, males treated, females treated. In that case there should be at least 20 in each group, disregarding other considerations in this table
The range of possible outcomes is limited and/or the measuring scale to be used has a limited number of measurement categories	There is a large array of possible outcomes/the measuring scale has a large number of categories. Obviously if 100 grades of outcome are possible a sample of 40 is too small

an experiment with a sample of a given size, which is the idea of 'statistical power'.

8   Statistical power

Table 7.4 shows that two different kinds of errors can occur in interpreting the results of statistical tests. For example, there may really be no significant difference in the healing power of two bandaging systems, but it is assumed erroneously that there is – a type I error. Or there may really be a difference and it is assumed erroneously that there is not: a type II error. In the leg ulcer bandaging trial (Chapter 1) this is the more likely error because of the small sample size.

The more one kind of error is avoided, the more likely the other is to be committed. However, researchers would prefer not to make any

Table 7.4   Type I (alpha or α) and type II (beta or β) errors

	We assume that:	
	There is no difference (we do not reject the null hypothesis)	There is a difference (we reject the null hypothesis)
In reality there is no difference	Our judgement is correct	We make a type I error (an alpha error): we reject the null hypothesis when we should uphold it
In reality there is a difference	We make a type II error (a beta error): we do not reject the null hypothesis when we should reject it	Our judgement is correct

errors at all. There is something of an art about choosing both a sample size and a statistical test which will produce the optimum balance in avoiding both kinds of error, while at the same time not requiring a sample size which is prohibitively expensive.

Improving the power of a test means lowering the risk of failing to detect real differences – that is lowering the risks of making type II errors. This might be done in various ways:

- Increasing the sample size.
- Using a higher level of data (see Box 6.1 in Chapter 6).
- Using a more powerful statistical test.
- Improving the design of the experiment.

But usually the power is set by choosing an appropriate sample size. The calculation of an appropriate sample size involves the researcher:

- Declaring the size of the risk he or she is willing to take of making a type I error: the error of assuming a difference when really there isn't one. The choice is often 5 per cent (the 95 per cent limits again). In this context this is often called the alpha level.
- Declaring the size of the difference of interest. In health and social care often only largish differences will be of practical significance. No one is going to invest large sums of money, or undertake large scale service reorganisations, to boost their success rate by 1 per cent for non-life-threatening matters.
- Declaring the size of the risk he or she is willing to take of committing a type II error: the error of mistaking a real difference for a non-significant one – setting the beta level.

Sometimes you will read something like this:

Sample size for patients having a hysterectomy had a power of 80% with an α of 0.05, to detect a change of 10 points on a physical functioning domain of the SF-36, based on a standard deviation of 18.7. (Shepperd et al., 1998: 1787; see also Chapter 3 in this volume)

This means that the researchers have decided that they are not interested in differences of less than 10 points on part of a standard instrument called SF-36 which measures health and well-being (Chapter 6, section 1). Ten points was chosen as being a *clinically* important difference: the kind of outcome difference which, if it were shown between two different treatments, would be a persuasive case for choosing the better one. The SF-36 is a very widely used instrument and usually produces results with a standard deviation of around 18.7 (see section 9). The authors are willing to take a 5 per cent risk of mistaking a chance difference for a real one: α is 0.05 But they want to be 80 per cent certain that they will not mistake a real difference of 10 points for a chance difference. The minimum sample size is set by entering all this information into a calculation (Cohen, 1988; Altman, 1991). For readers this information is useful insofar as it warns them not to take too much notice of any comments by the researchers about differences smaller than those nominated – here smaller than 10 points on this scale, because their research design makes it unlikely that they can say anything sensible about differences smaller than this. It also tells readers that if there are real differences of 10 points or more then the researcher has an appropriate sample size for detecting them.

Decisions about power are not just about statistical significance. They are also about *substantive*, or 'clinical' significance. The appropriate power depends on the practical implications of making a decision on the basis of results that turn out to be wrong. For example, making the assumption that there is no difference in survival rates between two clinical operations, when there really is a difference – a type II error – may have very serious consequences if a clinician then chooses to use the technique with the higher death rate. In an experiment providing data for making a decision like this it would be wise to set a high beta level to give the best chance of detecting any difference between the treatments. By contrast, in situations where the consequences of making the wrong decision are not particularly serious, or where it would take a big difference to persuade someone to change their practice, experiments with relatively little power may be quite adequate.

9   Measures of central tendency, dispersion and diversity: modes, medians, means, variance and standard deviation

Measures of central tendency express the extent to which results cluster, or the extent to which they are spread out. The arithmetical average or 'mean' is the most familiar of these – add up all the scores and divide by the number of scores. However, quoting the average/ mean can sometimes be misleading, for the following reasons.

- A handful of very small or very large scores can skew the mean so that most results fall above or below it. With a skewed distribution it is often better to cite the *median* – which is the score below which 50 per cent of scores fall, and above which 50 per cent of scores fall. Sometimes when the median is used, statistical calculations are done only with the *inter-quartile* range, that is with the middle 50 per cent of scores: the 25 per cent of all scores which fall immediately above and the 25 per cent of all scores which fall immediately below the middle score: 25 per cents are 'quartiles'. The reason for doing calculations with the score in the inter-quartile range is that the further scores are from the median the more erratic they are likely to be. For an example see the paper by Shepperd et al. in Chapter 3 of this volume (Table 3 on p. 30).
- A measure of central tendency has little meaning without reference to the *range*, which is the distance between the highest and lowest scores.

The other main measure of central tendency is the *mode*, which is the most commonly occurring datum. This is the only measure of central tendency possible with nominal level data (see Box 6.1, Chapter 6). In Table 1 in Chapter 1, for example, the mode for all ulcers is 'healed', as it is for the Charing Cross bandages alone. The outcome for the Trial bandages is bimodal, with 8 healed and 8 not healed. The mode is rarely a very useful statistic.

The *variance* is a measure of how variable the data are in terms of whatever is being measured. The *standard deviation* combines in one statistic both a measure of how much scores are clustered around the mean, and how much they are dispersed: the smaller the standard deviation, the more clustered the scores are around the mean. The calculation of the standard deviation is embedded in most statistical tests and cited in many tables of results (SD, sd, s, S or δ) and is involved in calculations of statistical power. Any standard statistics textbook will explain how these are calculated. You don't have to know how to calculate the variance or standard deviation in order to read research as a practitioner. However, the two statistics do give some 'at a glance' information which is useful. For example:

- If all the subjects had the same score then the variance and the standard deviation would be zero. In comparing two groups of subjects, the one with highest variance or standard deviation is the one showing most diversity in scores. Thus, if two groups of subjects in an experiment show much the same mean, but very different standard deviations or variances, then they differ from each other in that one group is more homogeneous than the other. Knowing this can be important in judging the possibility of regression to the mean effects (see Chapter 5, section 6) and judging whether it is permissible to use parametric statistics (section 6 above).

● With variables that show a normal distribution the figure for the standard deviation can be used to calculate the confidence intervals. The 95% confidence limits will lie at the mean plus two standard deviations and at the mean minus two standard deviations. Thus if the mean were 62 and the standard deviation were 22, the 95% confidence limits would be 18 and 106 respectively, and it would be a reasonable expectation that 95 per cent of all scores would fall in that range. The 99% confidence limits are the mean plus and minus three standard deviations. Though they are rarely used, the 68% confidence limits are the mean plus and minus one standard deviation.

10   Expressions of effect size

Experiments are usually designed to demonstrate the size of the effect of doing one thing rather than another. For example, it might be the difference between treating and not treating, or the difference in outcomes between two treatments. Some of the more usual ways of expressing effect size are given below (sections 10.1–10.5). Note, however, that a large effect size is not necessarily a significant effect size. A small effect shown by comparing two large groups will be more significant (and probably more real) than a large effect shown by comparing two small groups. To be important effect size needs to be both statistically significant and to be important in a practice-relevant way.

10.1   *Showing effect size by subtracting averages*

The simplest way of expressing an effect is to subtract the average results of a group who have been treated in one way from the average results of a group who have been treated in another. This is the approach adopted by Marshall et al. in the exemplar study in Chapter 2. Two lines of their table of results are reproduced below as Table 7.5. Column 6 is the result of subtracting group averages.

In Table 7.5 REHAB GB (column 1) is a rating scale for observations of social competence, the observations being conducted by observers trained to do so. Several observers were involved so this raises issues about inter-rater reliability (see Chapter 6, sections 5 and 6). There are two arms to the experiment, hence two groups: a control group receiving ordinary mental health care and a group experiencing case management (column 2). Baseline scores (column 3) refer to the

Table 7.5   Outcomes of a trial comparing case management and normal practice in mental health care (see Chapter 2)

1	2	3	4	5	6	7	8
Measure	Group	Baseline score (n)	Change at 7 mth (n)	Change at 14 mth (n)	Mean difference at 14 mth (95% CI)	F	Clinically relevant difference
REHAB GB	Control	44.7 (40)	4.3 (35)	4.9 (30)	4.3 (−4.9 to +13.4)	0.87	15
	'Case-man.'	42.2 (40)	5.3 (34)	7.5 (31)			

average score on REHAB GB for each group, with the number of subjects in each group in brackets – 40 each at this stage. Columns 4 and 5 show changes to these average scores, which are improvements for both groups, though greater for the case managed group. But these columns also show drop out, so that by 14 months there were only 30 controls and 31 case managed clients left in the experiment. Improvements might be due to those least likely to recover disappearing (see Chapter 5, section 8). The improvements quoted here will not be improvements for all 40 in each group, but improvements on the average baseline scores of just those left in the trial in each group. Column 6 subtracts the mean scores of the two groups at 14 months. Those left in the case managed group showed a greater improvement than those left in the control group to the extent of 4.3 REHAB GB points. As always, the results are regarded as an estimate. The 95% confidence limits quoted suggest that there is only a 5 per cent chance that the true figure lies beyond 13.4 points greater improvement for the case managed group on the one hand, or beyond 4.9 points greater improvement for the controls on the other. Since the confidence interval spans scores which would show more improvement for the controls, and scores which would show more improvement for the case managed group, the conclusion to draw is that there is no significant difference in improvement between the two groups. The statistic for F (column 7) is akin to χ^2: the result of a test for statistical significance, which can be looked up in a ready-reckoner of critical values for F (similar to Table 7.2). At 0.87, F is not statistically significant, this being shown (as is often done) by the absence of any note to say it is, although sometimes researchers will give p values for non-significant results (for p values see section 2). Hence the difference between the two groups on this line of the table is within the range that might be expected to have occurred by chance. Column 8 gives a figure for the size of the difference between groups which practitioners would regard as clinically important – a statement of substantive, rather than statistical significance. Roughly speaking, this means that practitioners would think something important had happened if someone improved their REHAB score by 15 points. The measured difference between the two groups was only 4.3 points, and 15 is not even within the confidence limits range. From a practitioner's point of view the two groups were just as much like each other at the end as they were at the beginning in terms of social competencies.

10.2   Showing effect size by subtracting proportions and rates

Another way of expressing effects is to convert results to proportions, such as percentages or rates out of 1000, and subtract. Thus one of the trials contained in the meta-analysis diagram (Figure 7.1 section 5) showed that there were eight head injuries among the 131 visited, and 15 among the 132 controls. This converts to injury rates of 6.1 and 11.36 per 100 children respectively. Subtracting yields 2.7. This might be interpreted by saying that home visiting may have reduced the injury rate by 5.26 per 100 children; or by 5.26 per cent.

10.3   Showing effect size using standard deviation

This is sometimes simply called 'effect size'. It is calculated with the formula

$$\frac{\text{(Mean of change shown by treatment group)} - \text{(Mean of change shown by alternative treatment/control group)}}{\text{Standard deviation of mean change shown by alternative treatment/control group}}$$

There is no example of this calculation in the studies in this volume, but if you do encounter it, a result of zero means no difference. Assuming that improvement is shown in terms of higher scores, a result of 0.2 would be a small difference in favour of the treatment group, a result of 0.5 a medium sized difference, and one of 0.8 or more, a large difference. Minus figures indicate that the control or alternative treatment group has fared better than the treatment group. The smaller scores might or might not be statistically significant depending on the result of a test of statistical significance.

10.4   Showing effect sizes using risk ratio and odds ratio

Using the figures for home visiting trials again, as above (section 10.2):

Risk ratio
(number to whom event happened in one group divided by total in group) divided by (number to whom event happened in the other group divided by total in group)

$(8/131) / (15/132) = 0.061/0.1136 = 0.537 = 0.54 = \text{Risk ratio}$

Odds ratio

(number to whom event happened in one group divided by number to whom event did not happen in that group) divided by (number to whom event happened in the other group divided by number to whom event did not happen in that group)

(8/123) / (15/117) = 0.065/0.128 = 0.508 = 0.51 = Odds ratio

Neither of these statistics is particularly easy to describe in non-numerical terms, but odds ratios are a particularly common statistic for expressing the results of experimental work. In either case a ratio of 1 would mean that there was no difference between the two groups. A ratio of 1 would put the results on the line of no effect in a diagram summarising a meta-analysis (see Figures 7.1 and 7.2). Where an intervention group is being compared with a control group it is usual, though not universal, to divide the results for the intervention group by the results for the control (as above). Then ratios of less than 1 suggest that something was less likely to happen to the intervention group, and ratios above 1 mean that something was more likely to happen to the intervention group. In the example above there were fewer injuries in the group visited, hence the ratio was less than 1, and this was evidence in favour of home visiting. However, this trial was about preventing something happening. Thus if these figures had come from a trial to see whether a drug cured an illness, a ratio of less than 1 would be evidence against the drug's effectiveness. Where two treatments are being compared with each other, it is important look carefully to see what has been divided into what.

In the leg ulcer bandaging trial (Chapter 1) the authors cite an odds ratio of 1.11, which is short for 1.11 healings for the Charing Cross bandages for every 1 of the trial bandages, or '1 to 1.11'. If you look at Table 7.1 you will not be surprised to see that this is the result of comparing 8 out of 17 with 8 out of 18. The authors also cite confidence intervals of 0.24 to 5.19. Since the limits fall on either side of 1, the 'true' result might be in favour of either bandaging system (see Section 5 for the way this interpretation is made).

10.5 Numbers needed to treat (NNT)

For practitioners, one of the most useful expressions of effect size is the calculation of the numbers needed to treat (NNT) (Chattelier et al., 1996). This is a measure of how many people would, on average need to be treated to produce *one additional* successful outcome by comparison with the alternative treatment. In the trials on home visiting and childhood injury (Chapter 4) this is the question of how many families would need to be visited in order to prevent one injury, since the alternative is simply not visiting at all. One of the trials showed that there were 8 head injuries among the 131 visited, and 15 among the 132 controls. This converts to injury rates of 6.1 and 11.36 per 100 children respectively. But in this case the interest is in *non-injury* rates, which are 93.9 and 88.64 respectively.

The calculation for NNT is:

100 divided by (percentage or rate of desired outcome in intervention group) minus (percentage or rate of desired outcome in non-intervention group)

$100/ (93.9 - 88.64) = 19$

Thus this particular trial suggests that 19 families (of the kinds featured in the trial) need to be put on the visiting list to prevent one head injury; that visiting 100 families might prevent between 5 and 6 injuries. Or, put another way, visiting one of these families would reduce the chances of a child there experiencing a head injury by 1 in 19, or by 5.26 per cent.

NNT figures should be interpreted with care. If a practitioner had a case mix identical to that featured in the research and was able to do precisely what was done in the research then the NNT figure would provide a close estimate of the number of these clients who would have to be treated in this way to produce an additional benign outcome. However, it is highly likely that any particular practitioner will have a case mix that is different from that which featured in the research, and may not be able to do exactly what was done in the research.

11   Counting costs

NNT calculations convert the results of an experiment into a form where the cost per desirable outcome can be calculated. If the NNT is 95 then the additional cost of getting one additional benign outcome by adopting this intervention will be the cost of intervening 95 times. The exemplar study in Chapter 3 illustrates the way in which the costs of services are calculated, and the further reading for this chapter gives a list of useful sources.

12   Sensitivity analysis

Experiments are always to be regarded as producing estimates as to the true state of affairs. Confidence intervals (sections 4 and 5) provide some purchase on the extent to which experimental results are likely to be misleading because of the play of chance factors. However, experimental research may also provide a misleading basis for practice decision-making because the circumstances under which the research was conducted are unlike those in some practice setting

(Chapter 5, section 12). A *sensitivity analysis* is a 'what if' analysis. The researcher says, 'things were thus and thus in the research, what if they had been different?' Sometimes sensitivity analyses are conducted as a way of managing the problem of subjects lost to an experiment. The researcher will say, 'if there were data for these lost subjects it might be like this, and then the results would be thus, or alternatively it might be like that, and then the results might be like this.' However, sensitivity analyses are most common as accompaniments of economic analyses. Chapter 3 in this volume is an economic analysis, which compares the cost-effectiveness of a hospital at home scheme with inpatient care. The first phase of the study, which is not reprinted in this volume, was a randomised controlled trial showing that both modes of postoperative care were equally effective, leaving the way clear to choose the one with the lowest cost. In fact, the study found that inpatient care was cheaper than hospital at home care. However, costs depend on a great many factors, such that costs in one place may be different from costs in another and change quickly over a period of time (Briggs and Gray, 1999). In their study, Shepperd et al. (1998) carry out a number of sensitivity analyses to investigate this. Table 7.6 gives part of one of these by way of illustration.

The research found that care was delivered for a much longer period to hospital at home patients than to inpatients. This made it more expensive. The researchers were suspicious that this was an 'experiment effect' (see Chapter 5, sections 5 and 12) arising from the staff delivering care at home behaving differently because they were involved in an experiment. If this were so, then the results of the research might be misleading insofar as staff delivering hospital at home care routinely, and not as an experiment, might discharge patients quicker and provide a cheaper service. Table 7.6 gives a number of estimates for the relative costs of hospital at home and inpatient care according to different lengths of time spent in hospital at home care.

Table 7.6 Sensitivity analysis of relative costs of inpatient care and hospital at home (HaH) care varying average length of hospital at home treatment: hysterectomy patients only (see Chapter 3)

Cost per case of hospital at home care, above or below cost of inpatient care	
+£92.40 (HaH is more expensive than inpatient care)	Average time as actually recorded
−£21.75 (HaH would be cheaper than inpatient care)	Estimate if HaH was on average one day shorter
−£80.84 (HaH would be much cheaper than inpatient care)	Estimate if HaH was on average two days shorter

13　Further reading on understanding the results of research

On the way experimental data are analysed and presented

There are many excellent textbooks on the statistics relevant to research in health and social care. Coolican (1994) is recommended for its user-friendliness and as a good primer on research methods as well, and Wright (1997) provides some accessible commentary on the theory and philosophy of statistics in addition to basic information. Most recent textbooks assume readers have access to computer software for doing statistical calculations. The *Statistical Package for the Social Sciences* (SPSS) is most widely used by sociologists and psychologists and very widely used in medical and nursing research as well (Norusis, 1993). Computer packages often turn out to be an easy way of producing results which are incomprehensible to the user. Wright (1994) and Pett (1997) (and many other writers) explain how to interpret the computer print-outs. For a book that is specifically a tutor on how to use SPSS, readers might try the book and disk kit by Babbie and Halley (1994). Pett (1997) is a particularly useful text for dealing with the problems of small samples and unusual distributions and takes its examples from health care.

Two widely used texts for the statistics of medical research are Altman (1991) and Bland (1995).

On costings

Netton and Beecham (1993), Clark and Lapsley (1996) and Yates (1996) all provide details about costing methodologies. Jefferson et al. (1996) is a good primer on economic analysis in health and social care generally.

The Further Reading in Chapter 5 includes references to conducting cost-effectiveness research.

References and further reading

Altman, D. (1991) *Practical Statistics for Medical Research*. London: Chapman & Hall.

Babbie, E. and Halley, H. (1994) *Adventures in Social Research: Data Analysis using SPSS®*. London: Pine Forge Press.

Bland, M. (1995) *An Introduction to Medical Statistics*. Oxford: Oxford University Press.

Briggs, A. and Gray, A. (1999) 'Handling uncertainty in economic evaluations of healthcare interventions', *British Medical Journal*, 319: 635–8.

Chattelier, G., Zapletal, E. and Lemaitre, D. (1996) 'The number needed to treat: a clinically useful nonogram in its proper context', *British Medical Journal*, 312: 426–9.

Clark, C. and Lapsley, I. (eds) (1996) *Planning and Costing Community Care*. London: Jessica Kingsley Publishers.

Cohen, J. (1988) *Statistical Power Analysis for the Behavioral Sciences*, 2nd edn. Hillsdale, NJ: Lawrence Erlbaum.

Coolican, H. (1994) *Research Methods and Statistics in Psychology*, 2nd edn. London: Hodder and Stoughton.

Jefferson, T., Demichelli, V. and Mugford, M. (1996) *Elementary Economic Evaluation in Health Care*. London: BMJ Publishing Group.

Netton, A. and Beecham, J. (1993) *Costing Community Care*. Canterbury: PSSRU University of Kent.

Norusis, M. (1993) *SPSS for Windows Base Systems: Users' Guide*. Chicago: SPSS Inc.

Pett, M. (1997) *Non-Parametric Statistics for Health Care Research: Statistics for Small Samples and Unusual Distributions*. London: Sage.

Shepperd, S., Harwood, D., Jenkinson, C., Gray, A., Vessey, M., and Morgan, P. (1998) 'Randomised controlled trial comparing hospital at home care with inpatient hospital care: I. three month follow up of health outcomes', *British Medical Journal*, 316: 1786–91.

Wright, D. (1997) *Understanding Statistics: an Introduction for the Social Sciences*. London: Sage.

Wright, L. (1994) 'The long and the short of it: the development of the SF-36 General Health Survey', in C. Jenkinson, (ed.), *Measuring Health and Medical Outcomes*. London: UCL Press. pp. 89–109.

Yates, B. (1996) *Analyzing Costs, Procedures, Processes, and Outcomes in Human Services*. Thousand Oaks, CA: Sage.

SURVEY RESEARCH

CHAPTER 8

SURVEYS, SAMPLES AND QUESTIONS: CONSUMER SATISFACTION WITH THE NHS

Cohen, Geoff, Forbes, John and Garraway, Michael (1996) 'Can different patient satisfaction survey methods yield consistent results? Comparison of three surveys', *British Medical Journal*, 313: 841–4

What you need to understand in order to understand the exemplar
The idea of representative sampling and ways of selecting representative samples. *See Chapter 10, section 1*
Age-weighting and re-weighting. *See Chapter 11, sections 1 and 2*
The importance of an adequate sample size for a survey. *See Chapter 10, sections 6 and 7*
Survey non-response and ways of managing it. *See Chapter 10, section 8*
Testing the results of surveys for statistical significance. *See Chapter 7, sections 1 and 2*
The importance of reliability in survey research. *See Chapter 10, section 14*
For any terms which are unfamiliar, try the index.

Introduction

Three surveys produce different results for similar populations for much the same topics. Is this because the populations questioned were really more different than they seemed, due to the surveys drawing samples differently, or due to the surveys using different questions administered in different ways? These are the possibilities investigated by Geoff Cohen, John Forbes and Michael Garraway in the exemplar reading for this chapter, which concerns two runs of the all-Scotland *NHS Users' Survey* and another NHS consumer survey in Lothian.

The exemplar illustrates some of the manoeuvres involved in validating research instruments: here questionnaires. The results of using one questionnaire are compared with the results of using another. Although they use the term 'reliability', what the authors do is akin to the idea of testing for criterion validity as explained in Chapter 6, section 7. As noted there, it is often very difficult to distinguish between the idea of reliability and the idea of validity.

The study also illustrates how survey researchers investigate the structure of non-response, and hence estimate the extent to which a sample deviates from representativeness, and it shows the way in which what look like minor differences in question wording and ways of administering questionnaires can make large differences to the results.

The reading is particularly pertinent at a time when central government has initiated annual consumer satisfaction questionnaires to monitor the performance of NHS agencies. Readers might like to consider to what extent the choice of wording in a questionnaire might determine an NHS Trust's position in a performance league table, independently of how well it catered for its patients.

CAN DIFFERENT PATIENT SATISFACTION SURVEY METHODS YIELD CONSISTENT RESULTS? COMPARISON OF THREE SURVEYS

Geoff Cohen, John Forbes and Michael Garraway

Abstract

Objective: To examine the consistency of survey estimates of patient satisfaction with inter-personal aspects of hospital experience.

Design: Interview and postal surveys, evidence from three independent population surveys being compared.

Setting: Scotland and Lothian.

Subjects: Randomly selected members of the general adult population who had received hospital care in the past 12 months.

Main outcome measures: Percentages of respondents dissatisfied with aspects of patient care.

Results: For items covering respect for privacy, treatment with dignity, sensitivity to feelings, treatment as an individual, and clear explanation of care there was good agreement among the surveys despite differences in wording. But for items to do with being encouraged and given time to ask questions and being listened to by doctors there was substantial disagreement.

Conclusions: Evidence regarding levels of patient dissatisfaction from national or local surveys should be calibrated against evidence from other surveys to improve reliability. Some important aspects of patient satisfaction seem to have been reliably estimated by surveys of all Scottish NHS users commissioned by the management executive, but certain questions may have underestimated the extent of dissatisfaction, possibly as a result of choice of wording.

Introduction

NHS reforms have increased pressure on health care providers and purchasers to monitor patient satisfaction. Though there are many processes by which patients' views can be explored and brought to bear on improving health care,[1,2] there has been disenchantment with structured questionnaire surveys as appropriate instruments. Not only are the problems of ensuring adequate coverage, a high response, and reliable questions often addressed inadequately[3] but the patient populations surveyed may be far too heterogeneous to generate information relevant to the needs of specific client groups.[4] Despite these reservations it seems likely that structured questionnaires will continue to be used in the health sector as a fairly inexpensive way of eliciting opinions, views, and preferences of patients and the general public.

Patient satisfaction surveys often report remarkably high levels of contentment or satisfaction with health services. For some components of care this may indeed be a valid reflection of patient views and not simply an artefact of survey design and conduct. However, it has long been acknowledged that the wording and presentation of questions may influence responses.[5] We examined consistency among three patient satisfaction surveys. We considered a repeated interview survey of the population of all users of the NHS in Scotland and a postal survey of the general adult population of one Scottish region. Both surveys were wide ranging but we chose to deal only with questions on the experience of hospital patients in relation to communication of information, personal treatment by staff, and the degree to which they felt involved in their care. These components of care have repeatedly been evaluated as extremely important by patients.[6-8]

Populations and methods

Survey design

In 1992 the management executive of the NHS in Scotland commissioned a population survey of NHS users' experiences.[9,10] Topics included waiting times, information given to patients, involvement of patients in decisions about their care, and treatment of patients as individuals. Though maternity, community and general practitioner services were covered, this paper is concerned only with respondents' experiences as inpatients or day cases, outpatients, or accident and emergency cases. A random sample of 2539 adults was selected from the postcode address file in a three stage design with stratification of primary sampling units (enumeration districts) by health board, population density, and social class profile. Respondents were interviewed for about 30 minutes on average.

The survey was repeated in 1994 using the same design and questionnaire.[11] A random sample of 2643 adults was selected with booster samples of users of accident and emergency and maternity services selected by quota sampling.

In 1993 Lothian Health, the health purchasing authority for Lothian region in south-east Scotland, commissioned a general population health survey.[12] One objective was to examine selected aspects of patient satisfaction with hospital experience. The sampling frame was the community health index, a centrally held file on all Lothian residents registered with a general practitioner. A non-proportional sampling design was used, with equal sized random samples taken from the age groups 16–44, 45–64, 65–74 and 75 years and over. Just under 10,000 postal questionnaires were despatched in May 1993.

Here we consider only respondents who said they had been in hospital in the past year as an inpatient, day case, outpatient, or emergency case. There were 2569 such respondents in the Lothian survey, 1187 in the 1992 users' survey, and 1498 in the 1994 survey.

Choice and style of questions

NHS users' survey included a series of similar modules on 'information', 'involvement', and 'treatment as an individual' referring to respondents' most recent experience of each category of service. The information module contained a card with a set of negative statements, such as 'I was not given enough information' and 'I was not encouraged to ask questions', and the interviewer asked: 'Thinking about the information you were given at the hospital, did any of these things happen at your visit?' Respondents were then asked to indicate the seriousness of any problem identified (on a five point scale) and, finally, asked how satisfied or dissatisfied they were overall with the amount of information they had been given. The involvement module included such negative statements as 'I was not encouraged to get involved in the decisions about my treatment,' 'Nobody listened to what I had to say,' and 'There was not enough time for me to be involved.' The module on treatment as an individual had statements such as 'My privacy was not respected' and 'The staff were insensitive to my feelings' and also included the neutral question, 'Did you feel you were treated as an individual or just another case?'

Of the 17 negative statements in the three modules, 13 were of similar if not identical content with questions in the Lothian survey. However, the Lothian questions consisted of two distinct sets of positive and negative statements. Positive statements were preceded by 'Thinking generally about your experience in hospital in the last year, please tell us if you agree or disagree with the statements below' and included statements like 'Your privacy was respected,' 'Staff were sensitive to your feelings,' and 'You were encouraged to ask questions about your treatment.' Negative statements were preceded by 'The National Health Service in Scotland published a booklet called *Framework for Action*. They listed some of the things that upset patients. In your experience of hospitals in Lothian are any of these things a cause of concern?' Among the negative items were 'Doctors who have no time to listen', 'Doctors who ignore what you say', and 'Feeling you are seen as a medical condition, not as a whole person.' All the Lothian questions allowed a 'don't know or not applicable' response, and these are included in the denominators of the dissatisfaction rates.

Analysis

The Lothian sample was deliberately designed to represent older age groups disproportionately; hence for estimating overall population percentages it was necessary to reweight the age specific sample estimates. Three age weightings were compared: the 1992 age distribution of non-psychiatric, non-obstetric hospital discharges in Lothian and the 1992 age distributions of people who had been hospital inpatients the previous year or had visited outpatient or casualty departments in the previous three months as reported by the British general household survey.[13] There was very little difference between the overall estimates produced by these weightings, so the average of the two general household survey weightings was used. This weighting mitigates to some extent the effects of non-response bias by age and social class. The results of the NHS users' surveys were reweighted by sex, age, region, urban or rural composition, and household size.

Results

Response rates were 76% in the 1992 users' survey, 80% in the 1994 users' survey and 78% (6212/7976) in the Lothian survey. Response was lower in the younger age groups, and in the 1994 survey men were underrepresented; the Lothian survey obtained lower response rates in the poorer wards of the region. However, after weighting by age, all three surveys gave estimated population rates of inpatient and outpatient attendance that agreed well with the findings of the general household survey and with statistics compiled by the Scottish morbidity record schemes.[14] Thus there was no evidence of differential response according to hospitalisation experience.

For the questions considered here there were no significant differences in dissatisfaction rates between the inpatient or day case, outpatient, and accident and emergency users in the Scottish surveys, and the changes between 1992 and 1994 were also small and non-significant. Table 1 therefore presents pooled results for the two Scottish surveys compared with the Lothian survey. Results are also pooled for some questions within each survey with similar content and closely similar dissatisfaction rates. For example, the Lothian items 'You were given enough time to ask questions about your treatment' and 'Doctors who have no time to listen' had dissatisfaction rates of 12.8% and 12.2%; the average of these was compared with the average of the two Scottish users' survey items 'Not enough time was made available' (in the information module) and 'There was not enough time for me to be involved' (in the involvement module), which had dissatisfaction rates of 3.7% and 4.1%.

No regional breakdown of the results of the NHS users' survey has been published, probably because the sizes of the regional subsamples with hospital experience was rather small. However, we obtained the raw data for the Lothian subsamples of the NHS users' surveys. Results were generally similar to those of the whole Scottish sample (Table 1).

Where comparisons were possible across the three surveys the Lothian health survey consistently recorded more patient dissatisfaction compared with the NHS

Table 1   Patient dissatisfaction rates in three population surveys. Values are age
weighted percentages of respondents[†]

Statement no.	Aspect of patient care	Lothian health survey (1993)	NHS users' surveys (1992–4)	Lothian subsample of NHS users' surveys[‡]
1	Respect for patients' privacy	3.4	2.7	1.6
2	Respect for patients' dignity	3.2	3.0	4.8
3	Sensitivity to patients' feelings	6.3	5.2	7.2
4	Treated as a individual or whole person	9.0	5.7	8.8
5	Treated like a child and patronised	10.6	§	§
6	Clear explanation of care or enough information	8.7	7.1	6.4
7	Understanding of what doctor is saying	6.4	2.4	2.6
8	Encouraged to ask questions*	23.9	5.6	4.2
9	Given time to ask questions or be involved*	12.5	3.9	3.1
10	Listened to by doctors or staff*	12.5	3.2	2.3
11	Explanation of right to second opinion	22.1	§	§
12	Not knowing whom to ask about options	7.5	§	§
13	Not given any choices about treatment	§	6.4	5.8
	Sample size[¶]	2058	2685	310

* Differences between Lothian health survey and NHS users' surveys significant at $P < 0.01$.
† See text.
‡ Figures relate to 1992 for first four rows and 1992 and 1994 combined for remaining rows.
§ No exactly corresponding question in survey.
¶ Sample size for Lothian survey was average number of subjects who answered these questions (including 'don't know or not applicable' responses). Sample size for NHS users' surveys was sum of inpatient, day case, outpatient, and accident and emergency samples from 1992 and 1994.

users' surveys. For survey items concerned with respect for patients' privacy and dignity levels of patient dissatisfaction were both low (<5%) and in close agreement. Slightly more dissatisfaction was expressed about sensitivity to patients' feelings and whether a clear explanation of care was offered, but again there was very close agreement across the surveys.

The greatest differences between the surveys emerged in relation to communication between patient and doctor. There was large (threefold to fourfold) and statistically significant disagreement on levels of dissatisfaction with being encouraged and given time to ask questions, being listened to by doctors, and understanding what the doctor was saying. Nearly one-quarter of respondents in the Lothian health survey expressed dissatisfaction with being encouraged to ask questions compared with only 6% in the NHS users' surveys.

Discussion

The Scottish surveys of all NHS users were explicitly designed to give quality assurance with regard to the undertakings in the patient's charter.[10,11] Among the promises relevant to this paper were (a) that patients would be given accurate, relevant and understandable explanations and (b) that patients would be involved as far as practicable in making decisions about their own care and whenever possible given choices. On the whole, the conclusions drawn from these surveys by the management executive of the NHS in Scotland were favourable. After both surveys it was reported that 'nearly 9 out of 10 people were satisfied with the amount of information they were given', though users of accident and emergency services were rather less satisfied than users of other services.[10,11] A similar picture was painted of users' views on involvement and choice and treatment as an individual.

After the 1994 survey the management executive asked health boards to develop plans for improving those aspects of health services in which a need had been identified and suggested that boards and trusts might wish to carry out local surveys using the same questionnaire.[11] However, our comparisons with the Lothian survey show that some elements of this questionnaire lead to notably lower estimates of dissatisfaction than alternative question wordings. Though the use of a consistent tool is necessary to investigate change in quality of service over time or variation across different geographical areas, the instrument chosen could by virtue of its wording tend to highlight some areas of need at the expense of others.

It seems implausible that differential non-response bias could account for the larger differences in satisfaction between the surveys. Age was the demographic factor most highly associated with non-response in both surveys. If a greater degree of dissatisfaction is necessary in order to persuade a younger person to respond than an older person, then this could partially account for the similar association between age and satisfaction observed in both surveys. On this hypothesis non-respondents in each survey would, on average, be both younger and more dissatisfied than respondents, but there seems little reason to suppose that the degree of bias differed substantially between the surveys. Given the reasonably high response rates such differential bias would have to be extremely large to account for the larger differences in Table 1. More important, the use of weighting by age and sex is likely to remove a good part of the bias due to demographic factors, as is indicated by the good agreement with external measures of hospital utilisation.

Responses may vary with approach

The most striking area of disagreement was in response to the items about being encouraged to ask questions. Whereas only 5.6% of respondents in the Scottish users' surveys agreed with the statement 'I was not encouraged to ask questions', 23.9% of the Lothian respondents disagreed with the statement 'You were encouraged to ask questions about your treatment.' Thus substantially different conclusions can be obtained if patients are presented with a negative statement about care and asked to agree that something 'bad' happened, as opposed to presenting them with a positive statement and asking them to disagree that something 'good' happened.

It seems unlikely that the other wording differences in the above questions accounted for these contrasting results. For example, in response to the statement 'I was not encouraged to get involved in decisions about my treatment' 6.4% of the Scottish users' surveys respondents agreed, a very similar proportion to the other item discussed above. In the Lothian survey when presented with the negative item 'Not knowing whom to ask about the options for your treatment' only 7.5% of patients gave this as a major concern.

Another reason for the apparently lower levels of dissatisfaction detected in the Scottish users' surveys could be a greater reluctance on the part of patients to express negative attitudes openly in a face to face interview. The users' survey interview entailed showing a card with a series of negative statements and asking the interviewee if any of these things happened during his or her last hospital visit. It would be quick, easy and non-confrontational for the respondent in such a situation just to say 'no' to the whole card and get on with the next question. That the interviewer's schedule had the instruction 'Multicode OK' might also tend to encourage the interviewer to pass on quite quickly unless the respondent had definite feelings about a negative item.

Several items in both surveys asked if patients thought they had been given enough time to ask questions or be involved in their treatment. Again the levels of agreement with the negative items in the Scottish survey were notably lower than the levels of disagreement with the positive items in the Lothian survey.

However, in the case of items concerning respect for privacy, treatment with dignity, and sensitivity to feelings levels of dissatisfaction were very similar in the two surveys despite the contrasting use of positive and negative statements. Though this makes less persuasive the arguments advanced above, there is no reason why agreement with negative statements and disagreement with positive statements should always produce different results irrespective of the content. The sensitivity of dissatisfaction rates to question wording may quite plausibly vary according to the content of the question. Arguably the good agreement on these particular questions supports the conclusion that the estimated levels of satisfaction with these aspects of patient experience are reliable. But it is clear that taken together our results are open to different interpretation and further research would be required to settle the matter.

In conclusion, it is worth emphasising that there is no 'gold standard' measure of patient satisfaction.[15] But this study suggests that it is possibly easier to frame reliable questions on respect for patients' privacy, dignity, and feelings than questions concerning communication of information or involvement in care. Over-reliance on negative statements to elicit information about users' perceptions and views may provide a misleading picture and poor foundation for informing policy directed at improving the quality of care.

References

1 Hopkins A, Gabbay J, Neuberger J. Role of users of health care in achieving a quality service. *Qual Health Care* 1994; 3: 203–9.

2 Audit Commission. *What Seems to be the Matter? Communication between Hospitals and Patients.* London: HMSO, 1993.

3 Carr-Hill RA. The measurement of patient satisfaction. *J Public Health Med* 1992; 14: 236–49.

4 Hopkins A. *Measuring the Quality of Medical Care.* London: Royal College of Physicians, 1990.

5 Belson WA. *The Design and Understanding of Survey Questions.* Aldershot: Gower, 1981.

6 Simpson M, Buckman R, Stewart M, Maguire P, Lipkin M, Novack D, *et al.* Doctor-patient communication: the Toronto consensus statement. *BMJ* 1991; 303: 1385–7.

7 Hall JA, Dornan MC. What patients like about their medical care and how often they are asked: a meta-analysis of the satisfaction literature. *Soc Sci Med* 1988; 27: 935–9.

8 Williams SJ, Calnan M. Convergence and divergence: assessing criteria of consumer satisfaction across general practice, dental and hospital care settings. *Soc Sci Med* 1991; 33: 707–16.

9 Capewell S. What users think: a survey of NHS users in Scotland in 1992. *Health Bull* 1994; 52: 26–34.

10 National Health Service in Scotland. *The Patient's Charter: What Users Think, 1992.* Edinburgh: Scottish Office, 1993.

11 National Health Service in Scotland. *The Patient's Charter: What Users Think, 1994.* Edinburgh: Scottish Office, 1994.

12 Cohen G, Forbes JF, Garraway M. *Lothian Health Survey – Summary of Initial Findings.* Edinburgh: University Department of Public Health Sciences, 1994.

13 Office of Population Censuses and Surveys. *General Household Survey, 1992.* London: HMSO, 1994.

14 National Health Service in Scotland. *Scottish Health Statistics, 1994.* Edinburgh: Information and Statistics Division of Common Services Agency for NHS in Scotland, 1994.

15 Fitzpatrick R. Surveys of patient satisfaction: 1–important general considerations. *BMJ* 1991; 302: 887.

What you might do now

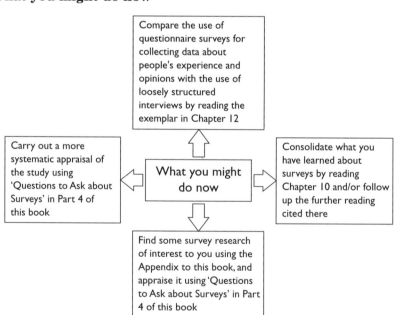

Compare the use of questionnaire surveys for collecting data about people's experience and opinions with the use of loosely structured interviews by reading the exemplar in Chapter 12

Carry out a more systematic appraisal of the study using 'Questions to Ask about Surveys' in Part 4 of this book

What you might do now

Consolidate what you have learned about surveys by reading Chapter 10 and/or follow up the further reading cited there

Find some survey research of interest to you using the Appendix to this book, and appraise it using 'Questions to Ask about Surveys' in Part 4 of this book

CHAPTER 9

AN EQUITY AUDIT IN CORONARY CARE

EXEMPLAR Payne, Nick and Saul, Carol (1997) 'Variations in use of cardiology services in a health authority: comparison of coronary artery revascularisation rates with prevalence of angina and coronary mortality', *British Medical Journal*, 314: 257–61

What you need to understand in order to understand the exemplar
The term 'prevalence'. Here this means the number/proportion of people in an area suffering from a condition (angina) at a point in time or over a given time period.
The idea of representativeness and ways of selecting representative samples. *See Chapter 10, section 1*
The importance of an adequate sample size for a survey and how to read the confidence intervals given. *See Chapter 10, sections 6 and 7*
Age standardisation. *See Chapter 11, sections 1 and 2*
Standardised Mortality Ratios. *See Chapter 11, section 3*
Deprivation Indices. *See Chapter 11, section 4*
Correlation, correlation co-efficients, regression and scatterplots. *See Chapter 10, section 10*
For any terms which are unfamiliar, try the index.

Introduction

The inverse care law was formulated by Tudor Hart in 1971, stating that there is an inverse relationship between the need for care and the availability of care: the people who need care most are those least likely to get it. In the exemplar reading for this chapter, Nick Payne and Carol Saul demonstrate this for cardiology services in Sheffield in the late 1990s. Their research involved:

- A community sample survey using a postal questionnaire charting the prevalence and social distribution of symptoms of heart disease.
- The use of a deprivation index to rank electoral wards in Sheffield on a scale of deprivation and affluence.
- The use of a standardised mortality ratio for deaths from coronary heart disease to show the relationship between death from this cause and area deprivation, after discounting for the effects of different wards having different age profiles.
- The correlation of deprivation, severally with early death, coronary symptoms and treatments provided, analysed by regression analysis expressed in terms of a correlation co-efficient (Pearson's Product Moment) and scatterplots.
- The validation of data collected by service agencies against data collected by a survey.
- The comparison of the pattern of 'need' as established by the research, as against the pattern of services actually delivered, which showed that poorer areas had more people in need of cardiology services, but fewer people in these areas received them.

Payne and Saul describe their study as an 'equity audit', as indeed it is, since the research evaluates whether services are being delivered on an equitable basis. However, much of what they did could equally well be used in an exercise of epidemiologically based needs assessment designed to prioritise different areas of an authority for additional resourcing or for special exercises to improve access to services.

VARIATIONS IN USE OF CARDIOLOGY SERVICES IN A HEALTH AUTHORITY: COMPARISON OF CORONARY ARTERY REVASCULARISATION RATES WITH PREVALENCE OF ANGINA AND CORONARY MORTALITY

Nick Payne and Carol Saul

Abstract

Objective: To explore the relation between rates of coronary artery revascularisation and prevalence of angina to assess whether use of health services reflects need.

Design: Prevalence of angina symptoms determined by postal questionnaire on 16,750 subjects (18 to 94 years). Comparison of data on use of coronary artery revascularisation with prevalence of symptoms and mortality from coronary heart disease.

Setting: Health authority with population of 530,000.

Subjects: Patients admitted to hospital for coronary heart disease; patients who died; and patients undergoing angiography, angioplasty, or coronary artery bypass graft. Cohort of 491 people with symptoms from survey.

Main outcome measures: Pearson's product moment correlation coefficients for relation between variables.

Results: Overall, 4.0% (95% confidence interval 3.7% to 4.4%) of subjects had symptoms. Prevalences varied widely between electoral wards and were positively associated with Townsend score ($r = 0.79$; $P < 0.001$), as was mortality, but the correlation between admission rates and Townsend score was less clear ($r = 0.47$; $P < 0.01$). Revascularisation rate and Townsend score were not associated. The ratio of revascularisation to number experiencing symptoms was inversely related to Townsend score ($r = -0.67$; $P < 0.001$). The most deprived wards had only about half the number of revascularisations per head of population with angina than did the more affluent wards. In affluent wards 11% (13/116) of those with symptoms had coronary angiograms compared with only 4% (9/216) in poorer wards ($\chi^2 = 4.96$; $P = 0.026$). Townsend score also inversely correlated with revascularisations per premature death from coronary heart disease ($r = -0.55$; $P < 0.01$) and revascularisations per admission for myocardial infarction ($r = -0.47$; $P < 0.01$).

Conclusion: The use of interventional cardiology services is not commensurate with need, thus exhibiting the inverse care law.

Introduction

Tudor Hart enunciated the sad fact that 'the availability of good medical care tends to vary inversely with the need for it in the population served'; often summarised as the inverse care law.[1] More recent work has suggested health authorities should carry out 'equity audits' to determine whether health care resources are being utilised in accordance with need.[2]

In the treatment of angina, increased availability of coronary artery revascularisation, such as coronary artery bypass graft and angioplasty, has been recommended.[3] There is, however, distinct national and local variation in rates of treatment.[4,5] While some have shown poor access to services among residents of deprived areas[6] others have found no such relation.[7]

In general, utilisation of revascularisation treatment for angina will be influenced by the following: firstly, need – epidemiology of disease that, even after differences in age and structure are considered, varies substantially from place to place, at both national and local levels;[8] secondly, supply – the availability of cardiologists and centres carrying out revascularisation procedures has been shown to be a substantially important predictor of utilisation;[4,9] thirdly, demand – in turn affected by patients' consultation thresholds, general practitioners' referral thresholds, and cardiologists' referral and intervention thresholds.

We examined the prevalence of symptoms of angina at small area level within a city, Sheffield, no part of which is more than 20 km from a major cardiological centre.

Methods

Sheffield has a population of 530,000, living in both rural and urban areas. It has 29 electoral wards ranging in size from 12,400 to 31,800 residents. Specialist cardiological investigation and treatment is carried out at the Northern General Hospital, which is located closest to some of the wards with the highest standardised mortality ratios for coronary heart disease. This hospital also provides specialist cardiological services to the surrounding districts in South Yorkshire and North Derbyshire, thus serving a population of around 1.5 million.

Determining prevalence of angina

After we obtained ethical approval we used the health authority's population register to generate a random sample, stratified for age and sex, of residents registered with general practitioners. The stratification was by six age and sex bands: men or women and ages 18–34, 35–54 and 55–94 years. A postal questionnaire to determine the prevalence of a range of common symptoms was sent to this sample of 16,750 residents in March 1994.

The sample was also stratified at the electoral ward level, such that the prevalence of the various conditions studied could be estimated with reasonable confidence limits for each of the 29 electoral wards.

We used a slightly simplified form of the World Health Organisation (Rose) angina questionnaire[10] to assess the prevalence of angina symptoms (D. Cook, personal communication). To improve the specificity only those with more severe symptoms were included. Up to two reminders (one full questionnaire and one postcard) were sent to those who failed to respond. By preserving a unique patient number we directly linked questionnaire data from individual respondents with health event data such as hospital admissions and procedures.

Health event and census data

The health authority's database was used to examine hospital admission activity at electoral ward level – all these data were based on hospital admissions not consultant episodes, which can be multiple within a single admission. We calculated overall admission rates (emergency and elective) for coronary heart disease (ICD-9 (International Classification of Diseases, ninth revision) codes 410–414), myocardial infarction (code 410), coronary artery bypass graft (codes K40–K47 in the fourth revision of Office of Population Censuses and Surveys classification of operations[11]), and angioplasty (codes K49–K50.1). At individual level, particular attention was paid to admissions for angiography (codes K63–K65), coronary artery bypass graft, and angioplasty from 1 April 1991 to 31 December 1995, the time period just before and after the survey. For survey respondents, linked activity data were examined at the individual patient level, thus multiple admissions of the same patient were counted only once.

We used the 1991 census to calculate the Townsend score[12] for each electoral ward. This score is designed to be high in areas of increased deprivation.

Data handling and analysis

Survey data were analysed with EpiInfo.[13] When appropriate we standardised individual ward data directly by using the England and Wales population as the reference. Data were plotted as scatter plots, and Pearson's product moment correlation coefficients were calculated.

Results

Of the 16,750 questionnaires sent out, 12,240 (73%) were completed and returned. After we excluded a further 1160 that were returned without reaching the person for whom they were intended, the response rate was 79%. Table 1 shows the prevalence of symptoms of angina by age and sex for Sheffield as a whole.

Overall, 4.0% (95% confidence interval, 3.7% to 4.4%) experienced symptoms of pain or discomfort in the chest when walking at an ordinary pace on the level. The proportion was 4.6% (4.0% to 5.2%) in men compared with 3.6% (3.2% to 4.0%) in women and was substantially higher in older age groups.

Table 1   Prevalence of symptoms of angina[10] by sex and age band

Sex and age (yr)	No. (%) of patients
Men:	
18–34	32/1711 (1.9)
35–54	45/1758 (2.6)
55–94	172/1975 (8.7)
18–94	249/5444 (4.6)
Women:	
18–34	22/2027 (1.1)
35–54	48/2079 (2.3)
55–94	172/2689 (6.4)
18–94	242/6795 (3.6)

Prevalence of symptoms and mortality from coronary heart disease compared with deprivation

There was wide variation in the age standardised prevalence of symptoms of angina between electoral wards; it ranged from under 2% in some to over 6% in others. Figure I shows that there was a strong positive relation ($r = 0.79$; $P < 0.001$) between the Townsend score of the electoral ward and the prevalence of symptoms.

Figure 2 shows a similar relation when we plotted premature mortality (<65 years) from coronary heart disease against Townsend score. Again, there was wide variation in the mortality between electoral wards, and mortality was strongly and significantly correlated with Townsend score ($r = 0.78$; $P < 0.001$).

Unlike symptoms of angina or mortality from coronary heart disease, admission rates for coronary heart disease varied only twofold between the highest and lowest electoral wards. There was still a significant correlation between admission rates and Townsend score ($r = 0.47$; $P < 0.01$), but it was now smaller than for prevalence of angina symptoms or mortality from coronary heart disease. There was, however, no relation at all between the rates of coronary artery revascularisation (angioplasty and coronary artery bypass graft) and Townsend score.

To determine whether utilisation of coronary artery revascularisation was uniformly related to need we calculated the ratio of revascularisations to the number in the electoral ward estimated to have symptoms of angina. Figure 3 shows

Figure I   Prevalence of angina symptoms compared with Townsend deprivation score

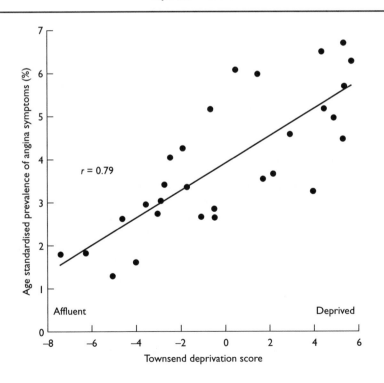

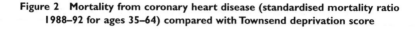

Figure 2   Mortality from coronary heart disease (standardised mortality ratio 1988–92 for ages 35–64) compared with Townsend deprivation score

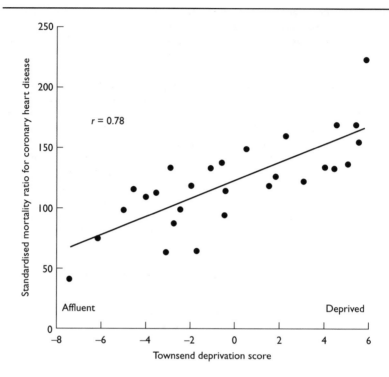

this index plotted against Townsend score. There was a clear variation between electoral wards in these ratios: deprived wards had only about half the numbers of revascularisations per head of population estimated to have angina symptoms than did affluent wards ($r = -0.67$; $P < 0.001$).

Proxy measures of prevalence of angina

As health symptom surveys may overestimate the true prevalence of angina, two proxy measures were compared with the coronary artery revascularisation rate. Figure 4 shows a similar inverse relation between revascularisations per premature death (<65 years) from coronary heart disease and Townsend score ($r = -0.55$; $P < 0.01$). Figure 5 shows that the same was true when revascularisations per myocardial infarction were compared with Townsend score ($r = -0.47$; $P < 0.01$).

Linkage data for survey and service utilisation

It may not be valid to assume that relations found at small area level exist at the level of the individuals who make up those areas (the 'ecological fallacy'). We also considered, therefore, data at both small area and individual level.

Figure 3   Coronary artery revascularisations per number with symptoms of angina compared with Townsend deprivation score

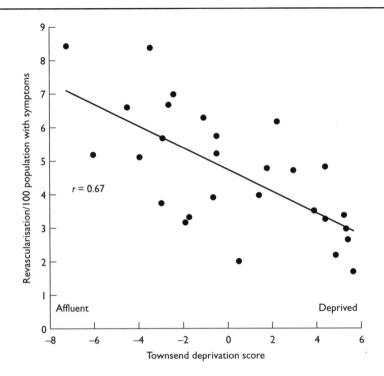

Individual survey results from respondents who had angina symptoms were linked to health event data to determine whether they had been admitted to hospital for angiography in the three years before and 21 months after the survey. Validation showed 100% linkage accuracy – that is, no relevant records were lost in this process. The angiography rate was found to be 20 times higher in those with angina identified through the survey (19.7/1000 population) compared with the rate in the general population (1.0/1000 population). Table 2, however, shows that there was substantial difference between more affluent and less affluent electoral wards: in the 10 most affluent wards 11.2% (13/116; 95% confidence interval 5.5% to 16.9%) had had angiography compared with 4.2% (9/216; 1.5% to 6.9%) in the 10 most deprived electoral wards ($\chi^2 = 4.96$; $P = 0.026$). Finally, 6.9% (22/321) of those aged under 70 years with angina symptoms had had an angiogram compared with only 1.2% (2/170) of those aged 70 and over ($\chi^2 = 6.53$; $P = 0.01$).

Discussion

Our results show a large local variation in both mortality from coronary heart disease and prevalence of angina as determined by a population survey. Both mortality and prevalence of symptoms were strongly correlated with material deprivation, as estimated by the Townsend score, at electoral ward level. We found that the ratio of rates of coronary artery revascularisation to the prevalence of

Evaluating Research in Health and Social Care

Figure 4   Coronary artery revascularisations per death from coronary artery disease compared with Townsend deprivation score

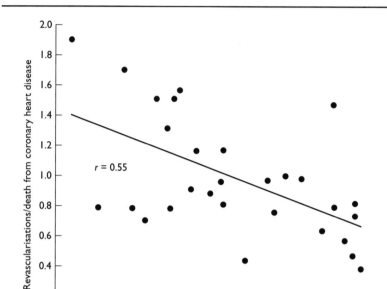

angina symptom varied substantially across the city and was inversely proportional to deprivation. Thus, use of services was not commensurate with need and seemed to exhibit the inverse care law,[1] even though the availability of care is the same.

The data on rates of coronary artery revascularisation refer only to procedures undertaken within the NHS, and private sector activity may add another 10–20% to this.[14] Given that private sector activity is likely to be higher for more affluent wards, however, and indeed that private insurance coverage in professional groups is much higher than in unskilled manual groups (23% compared with 2%[15]), the differences in use in relation to need for these services between the affluent and deprived populations may be even greater than described.

Response rates to the electoral ward survey varied between 63% and 88%, with affluent wards tending to have highest response, and this might have influenced the results. All but five of the 29 wards, however, had a response rate of over 70%. Moreover, the lower response rates in deprived electoral wards are only of concern if they result in deprived respondents being less representative of the deprived population than affluent respondents are of the affluent population; there is no evidence that such response bias exists.

Problems have been identified regarding the utility of the angina questionnaire,[10] particularly regarding its specificity in women.[16,17] The health survey for England,[18] which used similar questionnaire and survey methodology, gave an overall prevalence of 3.1% (95% confidence interval 2.7% to 3.6%) in an equivalent age group.

Figure 5 **Coronary artery revascularisations per admission for myocardial infarction compared with Townsend deprivation score**

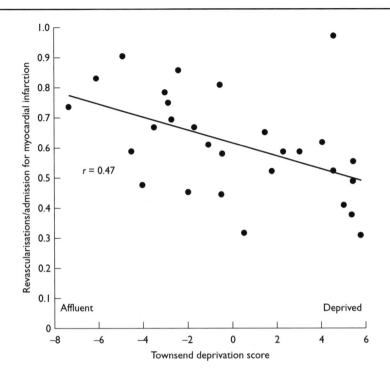

Table 2 **Proportions of subjects who reported symptoms of angina and had undergone angiography**

Wards	No. of subjects	Proportion (%) (95% CI)
Ten most affluent	13/116	11.2 (5.5 to 16.9)
Ten most deprived	9/216	4.2 (1.5 to 6.9)

Even in their 18–34 year group the estimated prevalence was about 1%. The same survey, by using diagnosis as reported by patients, produced estimates of 4.3% in men and 3.4% in women; broadly similar to our results. Other estimates are lower, at 1.6% in men and 1.2% in women, but these are derived only from numbers of patients consulting general practitioners in a single year.[19] Although these methodological problems may have implications for the absolute values of symptoms of angina, however, there is no evidence that specificity and sensitivity rates are likely to vary according to level of deprivation, so any impact on the comparison between affluent and deprived populations is probably insignificant. Prevalence of other symptoms (for example, hip pain) examined in our survey and elsewhere[20] showed little or no relation to deprivation, thus failing to support the notion that people in lower socioeconomic groups complain more about symptoms. Moreover, the relation shown between mortality from coronary heart disease and deprivation strongly reinforces our finding with respect to the distribution of angina symptoms.

The hospital data on admissions, like other routine data, have limitations,[21] but the data used for this study have been subject to local validation between provider and purchaser and suffer from these problems much less than most hospital episode statistics datasets.

Patients who smoke are known to have poorer results after revascularisation procedures,[22–24] and though this has led to considerable debate, many clinicians are reluctant to perform these procedures unless patients have stopped smoking.[25] One possible explanation for the findings reported here is that they are related to the prevalence of smoking, which is higher among less affluent groups. If we assumed that prevalence of smoking among angina sufferers is twice as high in the more deprived parts of Sheffield, however, this would explain only half of the observed difference in the difference of the revascularisation to prevalence ratio between electoral wards. To illustrate, the angiography rate in those with angina identified through the survey was found to be 11% (13/116) in the 10 most affluent wards and 4% (9/216) in the 10 most deprived wards. National and local data suggest that about 83% of affluent populations are likely to be non-smokers but only 65% of deprived populations.[26 27] Even if the smokers had been excluded from treatment (that is, from the numerator) and if the denominator was adjusted to reflect the likely number of non-smokers, the angiography rate in affluent wards would still be twice that in deprived wards – that is, 13% (13/(116 × 0.83)) v 6% (9/(216 × 0.65)), respectively. In future studies, however, smoking prevalence and measures of comorbidity from hospital activity datasets could be controlled for directly. This would also be important in the investigation of our finding of differential revascularisation rates between older and younger patients as age alone should not be a determining factor in selection of patients for this treatment. Selection of elderly patients for angiography is more complex than for younger patients, but it has been argued that symptomatic benefit is similar for younger and older patients and that earlier referral and investigation might yield a population with lower operative risk.[28]

Recommendations for action

We recommend an audit of referral of angina patients, particularly seeking to redress this apparent inequity. If consultation thresholds are higher in the less affluent areas it should be determined whether education of patients is required to encourage consultation by those with symptoms suggestive of angina. General practitioners should be aware of referral recommendations and potential benefits of treatment for those with angina. Detailed discussion of these results with cardiologists suggests that once patients have been referred for angiography those needing revascularisation are prioritised only on the basis of the severity of their disease. Finally, if cardiology services are expanded, steps should be taken to ensure that those in less affluent parts of the city receive a fairer share of these health services.

References

1 Tudor Hart J. The inverse care law. *Lancet* 1971; i: 405–12.
2 Variations Subgroup of the Chief Medical Officer's Health of the Nation Working Group.

Variations in Health. What can the Department of Health and the NHS do? London: Department of Health, 1995.

3 Working group of the British Cardiac Society. A report of the working group of the BCS: cardiology in the district hospital. *Br Heart J* 1994; 72: 303–8.

4 Clinical Standards Advisory Group. *Coronary Artery Bypass Grafting and Coronary Angiography: Access to and Availability of Specialist Services.* London: HMSO, 1993.

5 Ben-Shlomo Y., Chaturvedi N. Assessing equity in access to health care provision in the UK: does where you live affect your chances of getting a coronary artery bypass graft? *J Epidemiol Community Health* 1995; 49: 200–4.

6 Azeem Majeed F., Chaturvedi N., Reading R., Ben-Shlomo Y. Monitoring and promoting equity in primary and secondary care. *BMJ* 1994; 308: 1426–9.

7 Kee F., Gaffney B., Currie S., O'Reilly D. Access to coronary catheterisation: fair shares for all? *BMJ* 1993; 307: 1305–7.

8 Central Health Monitoring Unit. *Coronary Heart Disease; an Epidemiological Overview.* London: HMSO, 1994.

9 Wennberg D., Dickens J., Soule D., Kellett M., Malenka D., Robb J., et al. Invasive cardiac procedures: the relationship between resource supply and utilisation. In: *Conference Abstracts of Scientific Basis of Health Services.* London: Department of Health, 1995.

10 Rose G.A., McCartney P., Reid D.D. Self administration of a questionnaire on chest pain and intermittent claudication. *Br J Prev Soc Med* 1977; 31: 42–8.

11 Office of Population Censuses and Surveys. *Tabular List of the Classification of Surgical Operations and Procedures.* 4th rev. London: HMSO, 1990.

12 Townsend P. Deprivation. *J Soc Policy* 1987; 16: 125–46.

13 Dean A.G., Dean J.A., Burton A.H., Dicker R.C. *EpiInfo Version 5: a Word Processing, Database and Statistics Programme for Epidemiology on Microcomputers.* Stone Mountain, Georgia: USD, 1990.

14 Audit Commission. *Dear to Our Hearts? Commissioning Services for the Treatment and Prevention of Coronary Heart Disease.* London: HMSO, 1995.

15 Office of Population Censuses and Surveys. *General Household Survey 1982.* London: HMSO, 1984.

16 Garber C.E., Carleton R.A., Heller G.V. Comparison of Rose questionnaire on angina to exercise thallium scintigraphy: different findings in males and females. *J Clin Epidemiol* 1992; 45: 715–20.

17 Harris R.B., Weissfeld L.A. Gender differences in the reliability of reporting differences in symptoms of angina pectoris. *J Clin Epidemiol* 1991; 44: 1071–8.

18 Colhoun H., Prescott-Clarke P. *Health Survey for England 1994.* London: HMSO, 1996.

19 McCormick A., Fleming D., Charlton J. *Morbidity Statistics from General Practice: Fourth National Study 1991–1992.* London: HMSO, 1995.

20 Payne J.N., Coy J., Milner P.C., Patterson S. Are deprivation indicators a proxy for morbidity? A comparison of the prevalence of arthritis, depression, dyspepsia, obesity and respiratory symptoms with unemployment rates and Jarman scores. *J Public Health Med* 1993; 15: 161–70.

21 McKee M. Routine data: a resource for clinical audit? *Quality in Health Care* 1993; 2: 104–11.

22 Cavendar J.B., Rogers W.J., Fisher L.D., Gersh B.J., Coggins C.J., Myers W.O. Effects of smoking on survival and morbidity in patients randomised to medical or surgical therapy in the coronary artery surgery study (CASS): 10 year follow up. *J Am Coll Cardiol* 1992; 20: 287–94.

23 Cameron A.A., Davis K.B., Rogers W.J. Recurrence of angina after coronary artery bypass surgery: predictors and prognosis (CASS registry). *J Am Coll Cardiol* 1995; 26: 895–9.

24 Voors A.A., van Brussel B.L., Plokker T., Ernst S.M., Ernst N.M., Koomen E.M., et al. Smoking and cardiac events after venous coronary bypass surgery: a 15 year follow-up study. *Circulation* 1996; 93: 42–7.

25 Underwood M.J., Bailey J.S., Shiu M., Higgs R., Garfield J. Should smokers be offered coronary artery bypass surgery? *BMJ* 1993; 306: 1047–50.

26 Thomas M., Goddard E., Hickman M., Hunter P. *General Household Survey 1992.* London: HMSO, 1994. (OPCS Series GHS No 23.)

27 Roberts H., Dengler R., Zamorski A. *Trent Health Lifestyle Survey Report to Sheffield Health Authority 1993/94.* Nottingham: Department of Public Health Medicine and Epidemiology, 1994.

28 Elder A.T., Shaw T.R.D., Turnbull C.M., Starkey I.R. Elderly and younger patients selected to undergo coronary angiography. *BMJ* 1991; 303: 950–3.

What you might do now

Read Chapter 10, section 9 on case control studies. Compare this approach with that adopted by Payne and Saul in investigating the relationship between deprivation and coronary heart disease. What are the relative advantages and disadvantages of the two methods?

Carry out a more systematic appraisal of the study using 'Questions to Ask about Surveys' in Part 4 of this book

What you might do now

Consolidate what you have learned about the use of deprivation indices by reading Chapter 11 or follow up the further reading cited there

Find some epidemiological survey research of interest to you using the Appendix to this book, and appraise it using 'Questions to Ask about Surveys' in Part 4 of this book

CHAPTER 10

SURVEYS AND CASE CONTROL STUDIES

Introduction — 1 Sampling and representativeness — 2 Sampling frames — 3 Stratified (or non-proportional) samples — 4 Cluster sampling — 5 Staged sampling and phased sampling — 6 Confidence intervals and surveys — 7 Selecting a stratified sample of adequate size: an example — 8 Under- and over-representation and their management — 9 Case control (or case comparison) studies — 10 Correlation, co-efficients, regression and scatterplots — 11 Correlation, causes and statistical control — 12 Contemporaneous and longitudinal surveys — 13 The ecological fallacy in interpreting survey results — 14 Questionnaires, reliability and meaningfulness — 15 Questions to ask about surveys — 16 Further reading on surveys and case control studies — References and further reading

Introduction

This volume contains two exemplar studies with surveys as important components. Chapter 8 offers an exercise by Geoff Cohen and his colleagues in validating the sampling procedures and the instruments (questionnaires) used in Scottish surveys of consumer satisfaction with the NHS. General remarks about the validation of instruments are made in Chapter 6. Chapter 9 presents an exemplar of service evaluation by Nick Payne and Carol Saul using, among other research techniques, a survey to chart the social distribution of angina symptoms. This chapter now provides some general comments about survey technique and how to read the results of surveys.

The purpose of a survey is to chart frequency distributions in a population. These might be the percentages of people in the population of the UK of different ages with limiting and long-standing disabilities or perhaps the numbers of people of different types who are satisfied with the primary care they receive (Chapter 8). Such data may be put to use in:

- Planning services, for example, how many people of what different types would benefit from and appreciate this kind of care?
- Evaluating policies and interventions, for example, how many people of what types engaged in health-damaging behaviours before the health promotion campaign and how many afterwards

(Tudor Smith et al., 1998)? Are the people receiving a service also those with the greatest need for the service (see Chapter 9)?

- Measuring time trends, for example repeating the same survey after a period of time to see whether people are more or less satisfied with the NHS (see Chapter 8). A *repeated survey*, such as the NHS Users' survey, usually repeats the same survey with different people at different time periods.

- Investigating causality, for example, is there something about being black in Britain which undermines mental health (Nazroo, 1997)?

It is perhaps worth noting that in medical and nursing research surveys are sometimes described as *observational studies*. This is part of a classification of research methods which distinguishes experimental research on the one hand from survey and qualitative research on the other, both of the latter being called 'observational'.

1 Sampling and representativeness

Most surveys are *sample surveys*. The major exceptions are the national ten-year censuses which attempt to collect data about everyone, and in-house evaluation exercises where an agency will attempt to poll all its clients. For a sample survey, the sample needs to be selected so that it represents some wider population. If this is accomplished successfully the survey researcher can claim that what was found in the sample will be true also of the population from which the sample was drawn; that is, the results will be *generalisable* to that population, at least at some point in time close to when the survey was carried out. Box 10.1 gives a synopsis of various techniques used to select representative samples. The same techniques might be used to select samples for experiments, although experiments often use convenience samples (see Chapter 5, section 12).

Representativeness is not an all or nothing matter. A relatively small sample can be representative of, for example, the sex ratio in a wider population. Here a random sample of 384 would be sufficient to find the sex ratio of a population of one million, to an accuracy of plus or minus 5 per cent with a 95 percent chance of being right (see Table 10.4 below).

The size a sample needs to be in order to achieve representativeness depends on the level of diversity which is of interest to the researcher. The minimum sample size is thus given by the number of possible unique combinations of responses which the survey will generate and in which the researcher is interested. Thus, for instance, in a three-question questionnaire, each with two possible responses (say, Yes and No), there are eight possible permutations of answers: YYY, YYN, YNY, YNN, NYY, NYN, NNY, NNN. But if the researcher is interested

Box 10.1   Representative samples for surveys

There are two basic ways in which representative samples for surveys are collected and variations on these.

1. Probability samples (random and systematic sampling) (Bowling, 1997: 163–6; Alston and Bowles, 1998: 83–9). Each person in the population of interest has an equal chance of being chosen – or as near equal as possible. This presupposes some listing (or *sampling frame*) from which people can be chosen which lists everyone in the population. Since complete sampling frames are rare, some kinds of people get excluded at the outset, reducing the representativeness of the sample. **Random selection** is usually done with a table of random numbers or a computer program that generates random numbers. Sometimes **systematic sampling** is used: for example, every seventeenth name on a list (Layte and Jenkinson, 1997: 48–51). In this example, 17 would be the **sampling interval**. So long as there is no feature of the list which makes, say, every seventeenth name more or less likely to be a particular kind of person, systematic samples are as good as random samples, and they have an added advantage of spreading the sampling evenly within the population (Arber, 1993: 79–80).

Since not all people chosen will be contactable and not all will cooperate, a sample which starts out as representative may become unrepresentative through **non-response**. Deviation from representativeness is often checkable by comparing the sample of respondents with the population from which it was drawn in terms of the known demographic characteristics of the population, such as its age profile or gender ratio.

Very large **unmodified** (or **simple**) **probability samples** are needed to represent diversity within subgroups or to recruit adequate numbers of people to represent groups which are in the minority in the population. To ensure adequate representation of minority groups **random stratified sampling** (or **non-proportional random sampling**) is sometimes used: for example, collecting samples of the same size from each ethnic group in the area, even though some ethnic groups only make up a small percentage of the population (Layte and Jenkinson, 1997: 48–51). The same principle may be used to ensure that the sample adequately represents people across a geographical area, or represents people from a wide range of agencies.

Two advantages of probability sampling over quota sampling (below) are that the probability sample is more likely to be representative with regard to previously unknown characteristics and that results can be subjected to statistical analysis in ways that those from quota samples cannot.

2 Quota Sampling (Bowling, 1997: 166–7; Alston and Bowles, 1998: 91–2). Researchers need to have a good knowledge of the structure of the population in advance of doing the research. Quotas are lists specifying the respondents who need to be recruited in order to build a sample that is a small-scale model of the population. Thus, if the population has 5 per cent black males between the ages of 15 and 25 then the instruction will be to find the number of such people needed to make up 5 per cent of the sample. Filling the quotas is on a first-found, first-in basis, so there is no non-response. Despite this, however, there are problems of deciding how far those who fit the criteria for a quota and are included are representative of all those who would fit the criteria of a quota. For example, those who become respondents may be unrepresentative in being more accessible or more cooperative than others, and in other ways associated with their accessibility or cooperativeness. The problem of representing minorities adequately in a quota sample can be solved by setting quota percentages disproportionate to percentages in the population, creating the same effect as random stratified sampling (see above).

See also **cluster sampling** (section 4), **staged sampling** and **phased sampling** (section 5).

---

in the distribution of these permutations between people of different genders, there are 8×2 possible unique permutations, and if interested in the pattern of answers by gender, age (five age groups), social class (three classes) and by ethnicity (five ethnic groups), that is $8 \times 2 \times 5 \times 3 \times 5 = 1,200$. If each of these permutations cropped up with equal frequency in the population, then a sample size of around 60,000 would be needed to represent the frequencies with which these patterns were to be found in the wider population. But if some permutations were rare, and they were none the less of interest to the researcher, then an even larger sample would be needed to give rare permutations a chance of being captured by simple random sampling. But a sample of 60,000 is already much larger than most survey researchers can afford, and few restrict themselves to asking just three questions, or allowing only two answers each. There are two main approaches to this problem.

1   A survey may be analysed as if it were a series of surveys all conducted at the same time with the same sample: one survey studying the relationship between responses and gender, one between responses and age, one between responses and ethnicity: or one survey looking at age, gender and ethnic differences in responses to question 1, one looking at these factors in relation to question 2, and so on; the analysis being unable to say what relationships exist between giving a particular combination of answers on questions 1, 2 and 3, and being, say, male, African Caribbean and between 25 and 45 years old.

2   Survey researchers may (and may have to) concentrate on broad patterns and ignore fine detail; for example, by looking only at common answers and consigning the remainder to the category 'other answers', and/or looking only at larger groups and consigning the remainder to the category 'other groups', as in White/African-Caribbean/South Asian/Other.

Table 10.1 gives a synopsis of the more common kinds of problems which may arise from the unrepresentativeness of samples. In each

Table 10.1   Problems of representativeness in surveys

Shortcomings in design	Problems in interpreting the results
Poor selection of clusters in cluster sampling – often adopted as a way of avoiding the expense of interviewing large numbers of people scattered widely across the country (see section 4)	There is usually a problem in deciding how far the clusters are representative of the wider population of areas, agencies, institutions etc., which they are supposed to represent, and hence a problem of deciding how far individuals selected from within clusters make up a representative sample of the wider populations of individuals
An incomplete sampling frame. Those omitted might be different in significant and relevant aspects from those included (see section 2) A sample drawn in a way other than those which ensure representativeness (see Box 10.1): for example, a convenience sample of clients known to services presented as standing for all people with a particular problem, or a poll of members of a service user pressure group presented as standing for all service users. Case control studies show these problems too (see section 9) A high non-response rate. The non-responders may be different in significant and relevant respects from the responders (see section 8) Non-reponse to some questions Attempts to generalise from the sample to a population that is not the population from which the sample was drawn (see also **cluster sampling** above)	There will be problems about generalising the results of the survey to the population from which it was drawn. That is, what was true for the sample *will not be true* for the population at which the generalisation is directed. The extent of the problem will depend on the size and composition of the group who should have been included, but were excluded, and/or the extent of the difference between the population and the sample. Problems arising from non-response to some questions apply to those questions only
A sample too small adequately to represent the population with regard to relevant characteristics (see sections 6 and 7) Asking questions allowing for more responses than sample size will cater for	The necessary size of a sample depends on the degree of diversity made relevant by the analysis attempted (see this section and section 7). The more sub-categories the sample is to be divided into, and/or the more options are available for answers, and/or the smaller the differences of interest between categories, the bigger the sample needs to be

case the problem is one of generalisability because only insofar as a sample is representative of the population from which it is drawn can the results for the sample be regarded as true for the population (within the confidence limits cited). On a smaller scale only if a sample is representative for its sub-groups will what is true for the sub-groups in the sample be true for the same sub-groups in the population.

2   Sampling frames

A *sampling frame* is a listing from which a sample can be chosen. The comprehensiveness and accuracy of the list influences who might be included in the sample. For example, in the Lothian survey reviewed in Chapter 8, the sampling frame was a listing of all adults registered with GPs. That would exclude the 4 or 5 per cent of people not registered, as well as include some people who were dead or had moved away where this had not been corrected on the register. Since these would be uncontactable, they would become part of the non-response of the survey (see section 8).

Two of the most common kinds of sampling frame used in health and social care research are various service registers (including GP practice lists and medical registers) and the Post Code Address File (PAF) maintained by the post office (Wilson and Elliot, 1987). Researchers tend to use the sub-set of the PAF called the 'Small User File', which identifies addresses receiving mail, but receiving less than 25 items per day, thus excluding most business addresses. This was used as the sampling frame for the NHS Users' Survey reviewed in Chapter 8. The sampling unit for the PAF is an address, hence a further sampling decision has to be made as to which person living at the address becomes the respondent. A 'Kish grid' is the tool usually used to make a random selection of household members (Kish, 1965). Post code addresses can be identified with the territorial units from which census (and other) data are collected. It is census data from which deprivation indices are constructed (see Chapter 11, section 4). Thus, using the PAF as a sampling frame makes it convenient to stratify a sample in order to include a range of addresses representing the spectrum from very affluent to very poor areas (section 4). This was the way in which the NHS Users' survey (Chapter 8) stratified respondents by social class.

3   Stratified (or non-proportional) samples

Probability sampling (Box 10.1) is more widely used in health and social care research than quota sampling, because of the amenability of the results to statistical analysis. The principle of probability sampling is that each member of the relevant population has an equal chance of being chosen. However, this means that minorities in a population have a lesser chance of being included in the sample. In a population of 50,000 where there are only 500 Chinese people, a sample of 1,000 only gives 10 chances for a Chinese person to be included in the sample. It is impossible for ten Chinese people to be representative of all Chinese people in the population in terms of age, gender, opinions and so on. This problem is often handled by *stratifying* the sample, that is by taking non-proportional random samples. Thus the problem of getting an adequately sized sub-sample of Chinese people could be solved by stratifying by ethnicity.

The large scale Office of Population, Censuses and Surveys (OPCS) survey of psychiatric morbidity (Meltzer et al., 1995) did not stratify by ethnicity. The overall sample size was over 10,000, but this still only included about 460 from all ethnic minorities of colour. This accurately represents the number of such adults in the population of Great Britain (about 4.6 per cent), but it is much too small a sample to give meaningful results when this category is subdivided by ethnic group, gender and mental health status. By contrast, Nazroo's survey (1997), which was designed to emulate features of the OPCS survey, did stratify by ethnicity, selecting a random sample of 5,106 members of ethnic minorities of colour, and another of 2,867 white people. Even so, the sample was too small to provide an adequate representation of people of Chinese origin, or of white people with family origins outside Britain. The NHS consumer surveys reviewed by Cohen and his colleagues (Chapter 8) also used stratified approaches to recruiting samples. For example, the sample for the Scottish Users' survey was stratified by health board areas. This was to ensure a sample giving adequate coverage to all the health boards equally in the face of the fact that some have bigger populations than others. It was also stratified by social class, to ensure an equal representation of people from different social classes when different social classes make up different percentages of the population.

When sampling involves stratification, it is important to check whether the results are quoted for the sample as recruited or after re-weighting them back to proportionality. For example, the Lothian health survey reviewed in Chapter 8 recruited equal-sized samples from a range of age groups, despite the fact that these age groups made up different percentages of the Lothian population. In order to compare the results of this survey with that of the all-Scotland NHS Users' survey, Cohen and his colleagues had to *(re-)weight* the results of the Lothian survey so that each age group only contributed to the overall results in proportion to the percentage of the population each constituted.

Stratification in sampling is sometimes referred to as 'weighting'. However, as Box 10.2 shows, this term is used in a variety of ways in survey research.

Box 10.2   'Weighting' in survey research

The term 'weighting, as in 'age-weighting', is used in at least four different ways in survey research:

- Weighting a sample to ensure that important categories of respondent get included in sufficient numbers – this is better termed *stratification* or *disproportionate sampling* (see above).
- (Re-)weighting the results of a survey to compensate for higher levels of non-response by some categories of respondents (see section 8).
- Weighting the results of a survey in order to apply the results to another area with different demographic characteristics. Where this involves a reference population this is better referred to as *standardisation* (see Chapter 11).
- Weighting the results of a survey in order to control for the effects of some variable; better referred to as *statistical control* (see section 11 of this chapter and Chapter 11).

A case study of stratified sampling is given in Section 7.

4   Cluster sampling

Imagine a researcher wanting to select a national sample of 2,000 people living in nursing homes. Using an unmodified probability sample (Box 10.1) would produce a list of people to be interviewed scattered across the UK. The scatter might be no problem if postal questionnaires, or telephone interviewing were to be used, but if the research required face-to-face interviewing the scatter of respondents would make the research very costly. Similarly, the time and effort required to get research approved by research ethics committees is a considerable cost against research budgets. A simple probability sample of 2,000 might require gaining permissions from several hundred ethics committees. Even without ethics committees there may be a need to negotiate access to respondents via service managers and/or clinicians. To reduce such problems *cluster samples* are some-times used. For the nursing home example, perhaps, a selection would be made first of nursing homes and then a selection would be made of residents only within those nursing homes selected. All individuals for interview would then be in one of a few clusters selected. The selection of nursing homes might be made on a quota basis (see Box 10.1), with quotas defined by criteria such as size, statutory, voluntary or private

---

Box 10.3   The trade-off between cost and precision with cluster sampling

Aim: To select a nationally representative sample of 2,000 hospital
   nurses
First stage: Select hospitals
Second stage: Select nurses within sample hospitals
Options available:

Number of hospitals selected	Number of nurses selected within each	
5	400	lower cost, lower precision
10	200	
20	100	
40	50	
50	40	
80	25	
100	20	
200	10	
400	5	higer cost, higher precision

Source: After Arber, 1993: 89

---

status, speciality or generality, urban or rural catchment areas, or on
a random basis – simple or stratified. However, with cluster sampling
it is very difficult to ensure a sample of respondents who are representative of all such people in the population, when the opportunities
for selecting individuals have already been severely limited by the
selection of clusters. Box 10.3 shows the trade-off between the convenience of clustering on the one hand and the loss of 'precision' on
the other. Here precision means the extent to which results from the
survey can be taken as accurate for the population as a whole.

While stratification (section 3) improves the extent to which a
sample can be representative of a population, clustering makes this
less likely to be achieved. In terms of the table in Box 10.3, a sample of
2,000 nurses drawn from five hospitals is only doubtfully representative of all hospital nurses because five hospitals are unlikely to be
representative of all hospitals, in terms of their recruitment patterns,
the experiences they provide for nurses, and so on. The table in Box
10.3 might be extended upwards to suggest a sample of 2,000 nurses
from one hospital. Putting aside the fact that this would have to be a
very large hospital, and unrepresentative in this regard, this illustrates a different kind of trade-off. Such a study would be a *case study*.
Because of the clustering of nurses in one hospital, it would be
possible to use their responses to build up a detailed picture of the
experience of nursing in that hospital. But it would remain a puzzle as

to how far the nursing experience in that hospital was representative of other hospitals elsewhere. Alternatively, a sample of 2,000 nurses drawn from 400 hospitals would have a better claim to represent the nursing experience nation-wide, but since the hospitals selected would be very diverse, it would be difficult to read the results as representative of the nursing experience in any one of them in particular.

In some texts a study involving interviews done in, say, five agencies might be described as a 'multi-site case study' (Yin, 1994), and in others the same design might be described as a 'survey with a two stage sampling design' – the first stage establishing clusters in the shape of five agencies, and the second consisting of interviews with people selected from within each agency.

5 Staged sampling and phased sampling

Sampling is sometimes said to be *staged*, as in 'two-stage', 'three-stage' or 'multi-stage' sampling. Box 10.3 gives an example of two-stage sampling, where the first stage is the selection of a cluster sample and the second, perhaps, a simple random sample of nurses within each hospital. Or, with a small number of hospitals, the second stage might be a random stratified sample of nurses designed to represent both genders and all grades. A staged sampling design might involve any combination of cluster sampling, stratified sampling, simple probability sampling and/or quota sampling (see Box 10.1).

Sometimes the term 'stage' is used as a synonym for 'phase'. More narrowly defined, however, a *phased* sampling design is one in which the first phase includes a search for respondents of particular kinds, and the second phase is the collection of data about them, rather than about other kinds of respondents. This strategy is often used where the respondents of interest are rare and there is no convenient way of identifying them apart from using survey technique. For example, the OPCS national survey of psychiatric morbidity (Meltzer et al., 1995) was designed to estimate the prevalence of mental illness irrespective of whether the cases were known to services or not. That objective in itself made it important to use a sample drawn from the general population, rather than to rely on health service case records. However, the survey was also interested in details about people who had symptoms of severe mental illness. Thus the first phase of the survey identified people as having mental health problems or not, and the associations between this and age, gender, socio-economic status and so on. The first phase also served to *screen* respondents in terms of their mental health and hence allowed for the selection of a sub-sample of people with more severe problems for more detailed investigation. In this survey the sub-sample were invited for a second interview, which included a clinical assessment.

Although the term 'phase' may not be used, phased designs of this kind are very common in survey work, with a little information being collected from a large number of people at one phase, and, at another phase, more information being collected from a sub-sample selected on the basis of information collected in the earlier phase. Sometimes the effect of phasing is accomplished within a single interview or questionnaire by using screening or routing questions which select some respondents to answer more or different questions from others.

6 Confidence intervals and surveys

Most of what appears in Chapter 7 (sections 1 to 9) on testing experimental results for their statistical significance applies equally to surveys and will not be repeated here. If you have not read sections 4 and 5 of Chapter 7 it would be a good idea to read them before you proceed further.

As with the results of experiments, so the results of surveys should always be regarded as estimates as to the true state of affairs, estimates that are likely to be influenced by chance factors associated with sampling – *sampling bias*. The results are often cited with confidence intervals. These indicate the frequency with which various results might have been expected had the survey been repeated again and again with different probability samples of the same size. The confidence intervals provide a quick check as to whether the sample size was adequate. However, it seems to be fairly common that where sample sizes are large and more than adequate, survey researchers do not bother to provide confidence limits; they rely on their readers knowing enough about sampling to see at a glance that a sample size is big enough to produce very narrow confidence limits; that is, very precise estimates of the frequency of some phenomenon in the population. Thus, in Chapter 8 Cohen and his colleagues are working with sample sizes that are much larger than the minimum necessary and they present their results without confidence intervals. However, they do present enough data for anyone interested to calculate them for themselves (Box 10.4).

As with experiments (Chapter 7, section 8), so with surveys, sample size will determine the *statistical power* of a piece of research. With surveys, statistical power refers to the capacity of a research design to distinguish between those differences between sub-groups shown for a sample which reflect real differences for the same sub-groups in the population, and those differences between sub-groups in the sample which simply result from the chanciness of sampling. All other things being equal, a bigger sample allows for the more confident detection of smaller differences. Wide confidence intervals indicate too small a sample. Accuracy, however, comes expensive. A sample size of 384

Box 10.4   How to calculate and interpret confidence intervals in surveys

Table 10.2 below repeats part of Table 1 in the exemplar presented in Chapter 8, which is a study of NHS consumer satisfaction surveys by Cohen and colleagues.

Table 10.2   Patient dissatisfaction rates in three population surveys[a]

Statement no.	Aspect of patient care	Lothian Health Survey (1993)	NHS Users' survey (1992 and 1994 combined)
3	Sensitivity to patients' feelings[b]	6.3%	5.2%
8	Encouraged to ask questions*	23.9%	5.6%
Sample size		2,058	2,685

[a] For example, 6.3% means that 6.3% of the Lothian sample were dissatisfied about the sensitivity with which patients' feelings were treated.
[b] No statistically significant difference between the Lothian Health survey and the NHS Users' survey.
* Statistically significant difference between the Lothian Health survey and the NHS Users' survey at $p < 0.01$.

The actual result obtained is treated as an estimate. A confidence interval expresses the likely extent to which the estimate is wrong.

The formula for calculating the 95% confidence interval for percentages is:

$$1.96 \times \sqrt{\frac{(P \times Q)}{N}}$$

Where 1.96 is the 'magic number' for the 95% confidence intervals. P is the percentage you are interested in. (Don't confuse this with p meaning probability (see Chapter 7, section 2).) Q is $100 - P$ (all the percentages in which you are not interested), and N is the size of the sample. Thus for item 3 (for Lothian: $P = 6.3$, $Q = 100 - 6.3 = 93.7$ and $N = 2058$. The calculation goes as follows:

$P \times Q = 6.3 \times 93.7 = 590.31$	(1)
$(P \times Q)/N = 590.31/2058 = 0.28684$	(2)
Square root of $(P \times Q)/N = 0.53557$	(3)
$1.96 \times$ square root of $(P \times Q)/N = 1.96 \times 0.53557$	
$\qquad\qquad\qquad\qquad\qquad = 1.0497258$ rounded to 1.05	(4)

The confidence interval is 1.05

Now for the confidence limits. The actual result was 6.3% The estimate is thus 6.3% plus or minus 1.05%:

$6.3 + 1.05 = 7.35$ and
$6.3 - 1.05 = 5.25$

The confidence limits are from 5.25 to 7.35, meaning that we can be 95 per cent sure that the true percentage for the population lies somewhere between these two points.

The corresponding confidence limits for the NHS Users' survey were 5.2 plus or minus 0.84 = 4.36 to 6.04. The confidence limits for the two figures overlap (Figure 10.1).

Figure 10.1 Confidence limits for the Lothian Health survey and the NHS Users' survey separately and for combined results for Statement No. 3, illustrating a difference that is not statistically significant

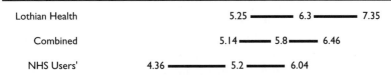

Lothian Health		5.25 ——— 6.3 ——— 7.35
Combined		5.14 ——— 5.8 ——— 6.46
NHS Users'	4.36 ——— 5.2 ——— 6.04	

The middle line on Figure 10.1 shows what happens when the results for Lothian and the NHS Users' surveys are combined with a sample of 4,743 and a dissatisfaction rate of 5.8 per cent.

Note (b) to Table 10.2 says that there is no statistically significant difference in dissatisfaction rates for this issue between the Lothian Health and the NHS Users' survey. That conclusion came from doing a statistical test (see Chapter 7, sections 1 and 2), but the same conclusion might be drawn from looking at the way the confidence intervals overlap. The logic goes as follows. If the difference between the Lothian Health survey and the NHS Users' survey is just due to chance (not statistically significant), then the confidence intervals for both should overlap with the confidence intervals for the combined results of both surveys. In statistical texts this is often expressed in terms of the differences between the two being no greater than might be expected to occur in 95 per cent of probability samples drawn from the same population. Thus, here there might be a single population with a dissatisfaction rate of 5.8 per cent from which two probability samples were drawn, one giving a dissatisfaction rate of 5.2 per cent and one of 6.3 per cent, both of which scores are within the 95% confidence intervals for the whole population.

By contrast, the other line on Table 10.2 shows results that are highly statistically significant. Plotting the confidence limits, as in Figure 10.2, shows no overlap.

Figure 10.2 Confidence limits for the Lothian Health survey and the NHS Users' survey separately and for combined results for Statement No. 8, illustrating a statistically significant difference

NHS Users'	4.7·5.6·6.5	
Combined	12.5 — 14 — 15.5	
Lothian Health		22.0·23.9 = 26

In Figure 10.2 there is no overlap of the confidence limits at all. We can be 95 per cent sure that neither the NHS Users' survey result of 5.6 per cent dissatisfaction, nor the Lothian Health survey result with 23.9 per cent dissatisfaction, were random samples drawn from a population with a 14 per cent dissatisfaction rate.

would produce an estimate of the sex ratio (or any other two-value variable) in a population plus or minus 5 per cent, but it would need a sample of 1,536 to be 95 per cent sure of getting it right plus or minus 2.5 per cent (Bernard, 1994: 75–80).

Care must be taken in interpreting confidence limits when quoted for the results of a staged sampling design (section 5) using clustering (section 4). For a survey along the lines of that suggested in Box 10.3, with random samples of nurses within hospitals as a second stage, the confidence intervals would only give an estimate of how accurate the results would be *for nurses in the hospitals chosen*, and not for nurses in all hospitals. Introducing clustering divides a sample into as many samples as there are clusters and confidence interval calculations should really be done for each cluster, rather than for the grand sample. Since each cluster will be a smaller sample, the confidence intervals for each cluster will be wider, and the estimates shown will be less precise than would be the case for confidence interval calculations done at the level of the sample as a whole. This reflects the reality of the situation, but it is not uncommon to find researchers using clustering and misleadingly citing confidence intervals for the grand sample.

7   Selecting a stratified sample of adequate size: an example

The research by Payne and Saul reported in Chapter 9 used a survey to estimate the prevalence of angina symptoms in Sheffield. Their interest was in whether the need for coronary care services (indicated by angina symptoms) varied according to the affluence or poverty of the electoral ward in which people lived, and whether the availability of treatment varied likewise. Since their measurement of poverty or affluence was the poverty or affluence of wards, rather than of individuals, they needed a sample which represented the prevalence of angina accurately for each ward. There are 29 electoral wards in Sheffield. Angina is known to be both age- and gender-related. Older people and males are more likely to have symptoms. This means that for any particular ward a sample not representative of the ward for age and gender might give a misleading picture. Over-representing older males, for example, could give a higher angina figure for that ward because of the age and maleness of the sample, irrespective of whether there was a higher rate of angina in this ward compared with others for same age/same gender groups. Thus Payne and Saul needed a sample of people that was not only representative of each ward, but also representative of each age–gender group within each ward. To make matters more difficult, only a small percentage of people experience angina symptoms, so the sample had to be large enough to capture

Figure 10.3   Stratification by ward, age and gender in the Sheffield angina survey (see Chapter 9)

	Ward 1		Ward 2			Ward 29		Total (12,239)
	Male	Female	Male	Female		Male	Female	
18–34 years	Random sample	Random sample	Random sample	Random sample		Random sample	Random sample	3,738
35–54 years	Random sample	Random sample	Random sample	Random sample		Random sample	Random sample	3,837
55–94 years	Random sample	Random sample	Random sample	Random sample		Random sample	Random sample	4,664

a representative percentage of those few in each ward experiencing symptoms. Figure 10.3 shows the way their sample was stratified.

Thus the stratification divided the population into 174 categories (29 wards × 2 genders × 3 age groups) and a random sample was taken from within each category, using the health authority register as the sampling frame. When the survey was conducted these categories were to be divided again into those who had, and those who had not experienced angina symptoms. Hence the survey involves 348 unique categories of respondents. A key sample size issue here is about the size of a sample that would be adequately representative for the distribution of angina symptoms *across* the age profile *within* gender groups *within each* ward. Payne and Saul selected a sample of 16,750, and had returns of 12,240 (73 per cent). For each ward–age–gender group this gives an average sample size of 70 (each cell in Figure 10.3). Is 70 large enough to provide an accurate estimate of the prevalence of angina symptoms within these groups? Does a sample of 70 provide enough statistical power to distinguish real differences in angina prevalence between wards, from chance differences that might arise in the course of selecting the samples? An answer lies in the confidence intervals. These express the extent to which an estimate is likely to be wrong. The smaller the sample, the more likely the estimate is to be wrong.

Imagine three wards: one very affluent, one middling and one very poor and the figures for males 18–34 years old (Table 10.3).

In Table 10.3 the 'actual percentage' column shows what might have been the actual percentages derived from the survey at a sample size of 70 for each of the three ward–age groups. But as with all survey data, these are only estimates. The confidence limits show how big any error might be. Since these are the 95% confidence intervals they show where we can be 95 per cent sure what the true value will be. Thus for the 'middling' ward the 'actual figure' is 1.9 per cent, but this might

Table 10.3   95% confidence intervals at sample size of 70: angina symptoms males 18–34: three wards at different levels of deprivation[a]

	Sample size	Lower confidence limit	Actual percentage from survey	Upper confidence limit
Affluent ward	70	0*	0.95%	3.2%
Ward of middling affluence	70	0*	1.9%	5.1%
Very poor ward	70	0*	3.8%	8.3%

[a] Invented data based on Table 1 of Payne and Saul's study presented in Chapter 9.
* As calculated using the formula in Box 10.4, the lower confidence limits would be minus figures. But a minus percentage is impossible. In fact, zero is also impossible since in each ward *some* respondents were found who reported angina symptoms. This is an example of the way in which calculations that make good statistical sense are sometimes nonsensical in common-sense terms. It would be possible to calculate the minimum possible percentages and adjust the lower confidence intervals on that basis, but since these would be very near zero anyway there is not much point in doing so.

mean that the true value in the ward population for this age–gender group is anywhere from 0 to 5.1 per cent (though it is more likely to be closer to 1.9 per cent than to either extreme). Figure 10.4 displays the confidence intervals graphically. It shows how they overlap. So it looks possible that, despite the survey findings for the sample of different levels of angina symptoms in different wards, in fact the populations in all three wards have a similar percentage, at around 2 per cent, or any other percentage within the zone of overlap. This display illustrates a situation where we cannot see statistical significance 'at a glance' and would have to rely on statistical testing.

On this basis, had Payne and Saul only been studying three wards each with a sample of 70 for this age group of males, then their sample size was too small for comfort. But in fact they were studying 29 wards of varying affluence and deprivation and a wider age span. Hence, when all data for all poorer wards, all middling wards and all affluent wards are put together, it is highly likely that sampling errors will balance each other out. With a larger sample size thus created, the confidence intervals will be narrower and the estimates will be more precise,

Figure 10.4   Graphical display of 95% confidence intervals for data in Table 10.3

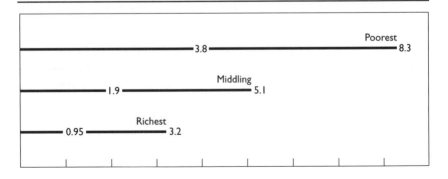

though now at the level of all males 18–94, in all poor, all affluent and all middling wards, respectively, in Sheffield. The confidence with which Payne and Saul could make claims about the prevalence of angina symptoms among males in *all poor wards together* will be much greater than the confidence with which they could make claims about the prevalence of angina symptoms among males in *any poor ward in particular*. Similarly, the confidence with which they could make claims about the prevalence of angina among all males aged 18–94 would be greater than the confidence with which they could make claims about differences in prevalence as between smaller age groups.

Payne and Saul actually cite their main results for all age groups, both genders, each ward. For this each ward has a sample size around 422. This is more than adequate for their purpose, which is to make comparisons of angina prevalence between wards. In general terms, 400 is a reasonable ball-park figure for the size of a sample needed in order to produce an accurate estimate of any dichotomous variable; that is any variable which can only take two values such as angina symptoms or no angina symptoms, the answer Yes or No, males and females. Accurate here means being 95 per cent certain that the value shown in the sample is accurate for the population with a confidence interval of 5 per cent. Thus, if the prevalence of angina symptoms found in a random sample of 400 was 4 per cent, then that would indicate a prevalence in the population of between 3.8 and 4.2 per cent (using the formula in Box 10.4) and we could be 95 per cent sure that the true value was between these limits. Note that adopting a confidence level of 95 per cent is not the same as aiming for plus or minus 5 per cent accuracy. A researcher may wish to be 95 per cent certain that an estimate is accurate plus or minus 10, 5, 3, 1 or any other per cent.

Table 10.4 shows that the ball-park figure of sample size 400 holds for samples drawn from populations of one million plus, however big they are. But with smaller populations smaller samples are possible.

Table 10.4 **Size of sample required for various population sizes in order to produce an estimate of a dichotomous variable in the population, 5 per cent confidence interval**

Population size	Sample size	Population size	Sample size
50	44	1,000	278
100	80	1,500	306
150	108	2,000	322
200	132	3,000	341
250	152	4,000	351
300	169	5,000	357
400	196	10,000	370
500	217	50,000	381
800	260	1,000,000+	384

Source: Krejcie and Morgan, 1970: cited in Bernard, 1994: 79

The figures given in Table 10.4 are rather 'tight' and some leeway should be allowed for non-response and unusable returns, and, if one of the values being investigated is small – as with angina symptoms – it is safer to err on the large size. One implication of Table 10.4 is that a sample size of 400 would be adequate for gaining an accurate estimate of the prevalence of angina symptoms in Sheffield as a whole with its population of 530,000 but that almost as large a sample would be needed to produce an accurate estimate for Sheffield's smallest ward, with a population of only 12,400. Moreover, while a probability sample of 400 could give a fairly accurate estimate of the prevalence of angina symptoms for Sheffield as a whole, it would not accurately show how the prevalence varied from ward to ward of the city. With a sample size this small it would not be very surprising if the people sampled from the poorer wards showed lower levels of prevalence than those sampled from the richer wards.

The important lesson from this example is that the total sample size is set by the size of the groups between which comparisons are to be made. Thus to compare the prevalence of angina symptoms between African Caribbeans in Sheffield and those of other ethnicities, a sub-sample of about 370 African Caribbeans would be needed: hence, the usual need for stratification by ethnicity when ethnic differences are of interest (see section 3).

Investigating variables which can take more than two values or attempting to achieve an accuracy greater than 5 per cent confidence intervals requires bigger samples than shown in Table 10.4. Electoral opinion polls, for example, usually use national samples of around 2,000 because there are more than two parties to vote for, and because they aim for an accuracy of plus or minus 3 per cent. The latter is because the difference in support for the leading parties is often less than 5 per cent. However, there are times when survey researchers do not need to aim for accuracy even at the plus or minus 5 per cent level. For example, in a survey designed to estimate the level of public support for a policy, the key information might be whether there was a majority for or against. In practical terms it would mean much the same if '76 per cent in favour' indicated any value between 83.6 and 68.4 per cent (plus or minus 10 per cent). Here, a smaller sample size than indicated in Table 10.4 would be adequate.

The remarks above apply to samples that are truly representative and where chance alone is likely to cause errors of estimation.

8 Under- and over-representation and their management

Having an incomplete sampling frame is one way in which samples fail to be representative (section 2). *Non-response* is the most important of the others. Among those selected to be representative of a population it will be impossible to contact some and some will refuse to co-operate. These excluded people are unlikely to be a representative sample of the sample. Subtracting an unrepresentative minority from a representative sample results in an unrepresentative sample. Cohen et al. (Chapter 8) illustrate the way in which deviations from representativeness can be checked by comparing the remaining sample with known characteristics of the population from which it is drawn. Thus, if the sample of people actually responding is on average older than the population, this is an indication that the sample of people who became respondents under-represents younger people.

The extent to which exclusion and non-response are a problem depends on a combination of four factors:

- How atypical the excludees/non-respondents are, in ways relevant to the survey.
- How great is their number.
- How large is the difference between groups in which the researcher is interested.
- How accurately the missing data can be estimated.

It is common to say that the results of surveys with non-response rates exceeding 25 per cent should be treated with suspicion. But this is slightly misleading. A larger non-response would be acceptable in a survey in which the researcher was interested in broad trends and where the non-respondents were not very atypical. By contrast, if a researcher were interested in, say, the differences between a majority population and a minority of people with disabilities, a very small non-response could invalidate the survey if disproportionate numbers of non-responders were from among the people with disabilities.

Sometimes *booster samples* are used to pre-empt or correct for initial exclusion and non-response, additional samples being taken and the results added into the main survey. The term usually implies that a different strategy for sampling is used for the booster(s) as compared with the main sample. If the strategy used for the main sample is likely to result in the under-representation of some groups then there is little point in using the same strategy in an attempt to remedy this. Adding together the results of what are, in effect, different surveys can lead to problems in statistical analysis.

Weighting is often used to manage initial exclusion and non-response. This is illustrated in Box 10.5 in terms of weighting for the under-or over-representation of age groups in a sample by comparison with the population. So long as the relevant percentages in the population are known, weighting can be done with regard to any demographic characteristic, for example, to redress the under-representation of people from a particular social class, household type and so on. For other uses of weighting, see Box 10.2.

Box 10.5   Weighting responses from a sample to manage a problem of under- or over-representation

Table 10.5 shows the percentage of males in each age group responding to a survey, compared with the percentage in the population. On each line, multiplying all the responses of the people in the sample by the 'age–sex weight' will produce a result as if there had been no under- or over-representation. These are age–*sex* weights since males make up only approximately half the totals and making these adjustments has implications for the weightings for females.

Table 10.5   Age–sex weightings to (re-)weight a sample to correct for under-representation in terms of age–sex groups

	A. Proportion in population	B. Proportion in sample	Age–sex weight To correct for under-representation multiply the sample proportion by A/B
16–19	3.8	3.4	1.12
20–24	5.9	5.0	1.18
25–29	6.6	5.6	1.18
30–34	6.0	6.0	1.00
35–39	5.3	5.3	1.00
40–44	5.3	4.9	1.08
45–49	5.2	5.2	1.00
50–54	4.2	4.4	0.96
55–59	4.0	4.3	0.93
60–64	3.8	4.0	0.95
All males 16–64	50.1%	48.1%	

Source: Based on Meltzer et al., 1995: Table A3.4. Office for National Statistics © Crown copyright 1995

There are problems in the kind of weighting shown in Table 10.5. For example, what is increased by 0.4 per cent in the first row will be the contribution of the responses of those males 16–19 who did respond to the survey. Males aged 16–19 will no longer be under-represented, but the responses of the kinds of males aged 16–19 who were originally under-represented may be even more under-represented now.

Weighting in this way also assumes that researchers have an accurate knowledge of the composition of the population against which to compare the sample. For survey work in general populations, the census is usually the most accurate source of such information, but census data become progressively more inaccurate in between census dates. In the study featured in Chapter 8, Cohen and his colleagues did not have up-to-date census data on the age composition of the Lothian region, and had instead to use estimates derived from various other surveys in order both to judge the age-representativeness of the Lothian sample and to re-weight the results in order to undo the effects of stratification in the original sampling design (section 3).

9 Case control (or case comparison) studies

A survey with a sample of adequate size drawn from the general population is often the only way of producing an accurate estimate of the frequency of a condition or circumstance in a population. If the condition is rare, a very large sample is required for this. For example, in 1998 it would have required a sample of millions accurately to estimate the frequency of new strain Creutzfeldt–Jakob disease (n-sCJD) since there had only been 35 known cases in the UK in the previous 18 years (National CJD Surveillance Unit, 1999). For many purposes it is enough to know that a condition is rare, without being able to put an exact figure on the frequency. However, when it comes to investigating the causes of a rare condition a largish sample of cases is needed. One way of managing this problem would be to use a stratified sample (section 3), taking a largish sample of cases, to compare with a random sample of 'non-cases'. However, with rare conditions, or conditions that are difficult to know about such as drug abuse or child abuse, there is no adequate sampling frame (section 2) to provide the starting point for the random sampling of cases. *Case control* (or *case comparison*) studies provide an alternative approach.

Here known cases are recruited to the survey. Usually these are cases known to services, for example, patients diagnosed with sporadic CJD (which includes n-sCJD) or children on an at-risk register. Then a sample of 'controls' is recruited to match the cases according to variables such as age, gender, socio-economic status, ethnicity and so on. Ideally matching should be for all characteristics that might be relevant, except the one for which causes are being investigated. But in practice matching has to be on characteristics that are easy to know about before detailed investigation begins. Matching may be done at the individual level using a *matched pairs* design, or it may be done group on group so that, although there are no individual matches between cases and controls, the two groups have similar profiles for age, gender, socio-economic status and so on (see Box 5.1 in Chapter 5). For example, a series of case control studies associated with the Confidential Inquiry into Stillbirths and Deaths in Infancy uses all known cases of sudden infant death in three NHS regions (1993–5) – 195 deaths – and 780 matched controls (Blair et al., 1996; Fleming et al., 1996). The controls in this case were selected from health visiting records. The logic of these studies is experimental (see Chapter 5). Those variables which are found equally associated with both the sudden infant death babies and with the living controls are unlikely to be among the causes of sudden infant death, and those variables which are associated more with the deaths than with the controls are possibly among the causative factors.

There are two problem areas for case control studies. The first concerns representativeness. Cases known to services are not necessarily representative of all cases. There is a risk that the cases recruited are a sample biased by *ascertainment bias*, meaning that those which are known about are different in significant ways from those which remain unknown. For example, offenders who have been arrested are unlikely to be a representative sample of all offenders. Similarly, problems can arise from the selection of the controls. For example, the earlier case control studies of n-sCJD used controls drawn from hospital populations. But in 1997 this was abandoned in favour of controls drawn from the general population because 'controls chosen from hospital patients may have medical histories which are not representative of the general population' (National CJD Surveillance Unit, 1999: 19). But the Unit point out that one of the costs of using controls drawn from the general population here is that fewer of them will have detailed medical histories, and more data will have to be collected directly by the researchers.

For these reasons, and simply because cases and, nearly always, controls will not have been chosen on probability principles, frequencies derived from case control studies cannot be generalised safely to wider populations.

The second problem area concerns the matching of cases and controls. The importance in experiments of creating matching comparison groups is discussed in detail in Chapter 5, section 3. Just as with experiments, faulty matching can lead to confounding and misleading results. For example, in the field of sudden infant death research, family smoking habits have been shown to be associated with sudden infant death: the more smoking, the greater the risk. However, some doubts have been expressed as to the adequacy of the matching of cases and controls for social class (Dwyer and Ponsonby, 1996). If the matching was imperfect such that the controls contained a smaller percentage of people from lower socio-economic groups than the cases, then some at least of the association found between smoking and sudden infant death may reflect the fact that people in lower socio-economic groups both smoke more, and that, for reasons not associated with smoking, their babies are more likely to experience sudden infant death.

10   Correlation, co-efficients, regression and scatterplots

In analysing the results of surveys or case control studies differences between groups are often of interest: for example, different percentages of different kinds of people expressing dissatisfaction with the NHS (Chapter 8), different rates of angina symptoms in different wards, or between different age groups (Chapter 9), or differences expressed in terms of odds ratios (Chapter 7, section 10.4). Such differences can be tested for their statistical significance in exactly the same ways as differences between groups in experimental research (see Chapter 7, sections 1 and 2) and all the remarks about kinds of data, and appropriate statistical tests in Chapters 6 and 7 apply equally to analysing surveys.

In survey work, however, correlations – measures of association – are just as important as differences. Correlation is the extent to which one thing varies with another. It is often called 'co-variance'. A good example of a correlation is given by the two ends of a see-saw. Since one end always goes up when the other end goes down there is a perfect *negative* (or *inverse*) correlation between the positions of the two ends. The movement of any two points on a roundabout show a perfect *positive* correlation. For every metre one point moves, the other will always make a corresponding movement; not necessarily a movement of a metre but always the same distance for every metre moved by the other point.

Correlations are usually expressed in terms of correlation co-efficients. Usually, but not always, these express a perfect positive correlation as 1, and a perfect negative (or inverse) correlation as -1. Zero designates no correlation at all. Seesaws and roundabouts apart, perfect correlations are rare, and 0.8 is usually a high positive correlation and -0.8 a high negative one.

Chapter 6 (sections 6 and 7) deals with the validation of research instruments which usually entails statistical correlation. Many such instruments are questionnaires and the questionnaires used in surveys are often validated in the same way for much the same criteria.

Another research tool used in surveys is the deprivation index, exemplified in this volume by the study by Payne and Saul (Chapter 9 exemplar), and described in more detail in Chapter 11, section 4. Deprivation indicators or indices are widely used in both research and social administration. They use easily obtainable population data of the kind which most people would agree indicates socio-economic deprivation; for example, percentage of people unemployed, percentage of single parent families, number of households without cars, and so on. Then from such indicators a score is produced for an area which is a good basis for predicting matters that are much more costly to find out about: for example, numbers of people suffering from depression, numbers of children who will suffer from glue-ear next year, and so on. Validation of a deprivation indicator means doing research to find out how well the unknown (and difficult to find out about) can be predicted from the known (and easy to find out about). The best deprivation indicators are the ones which show the highest

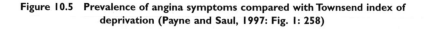

Figure 10.5   Prevalence of angina symptoms compared with Townsend index of deprivation (Payne and Saul, 1997: Fig. I: 258)

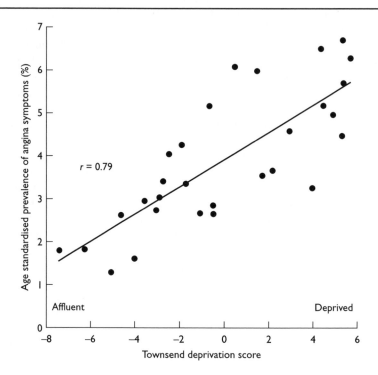

correlations between the deprivation score, and whatever else researchers were trying to predict.

Correlations are often displayed in terms of *scatterplots* or *scattergrams*. Figure 10.5 comes from the exemplar study by Payne and Saul in Chapter 9. Along the bottom of Figure 10.5 is a scale expressing the affluence or deprivation of areas according to the Townsend deprivation index. Zero is the middle score. Positive scores are an indication that an area is more deprived than average: negative more affluent than average. On the vertical axis there is a scale for measuring the proportion of people in an area experiencing angina symptoms. Each plot on the diagram represents a ward of Sheffield located according to its deprivation index score (horizontal axis) and the percentage of people in the ward experiencing symptoms (vertical axis). These latter are expressed after *age standardisation*. That is, after accounting for the fact that different wards have different age profiles. Age standardisation is dealt with in Chapter 11.

From eyeballing the distribution it is possible to see that the more deprived the area, the greater the percentage of people experiencing angina symptoms: or, to be precise, the greater the percentage of people in a sample of people from each area reporting that they experienced such symptoms in a survey conducted for that purpose.

The diagonal line drawn on the diagram is the *regression line*. If there were a perfect positive correlation between ward deprivation and reported angina symptoms all the plots on the diagram would lie on this line. It would be very surprising if they did, and the regression line represents the best estimate that can be made with these data about the relationship between angina and deprivation. One way of thinking about this is to think of how far this display improves our ability to predict the prevalence of angina symptoms from knowing the deprivation score (or vice versa if you prefer). If we didn't know the deprivation index then *for any area* the best bet is that it will have the same prevalence of angina as for *all areas*. This is about 4 per cent (with 95 per cent confidence limits of 3.7 to 4.4 per cent). This will under-estimate the rate for a highly deprived area, and over-estimate it for an affluent one. The regression line improves our ability to predict. Thus, with a Townsend score of 6, the regression line predicts an angina prevalence of about 5.5 per cent. Reading from Figure 10.5, the actual scores for wards with this, or a close degree of deprivation, are (approximately) 5.6, 6.1 and 6.5. The prediction is not perfect but it is nearer the mark than a prediction that these areas will have the average score for angina symptoms (4 per cent) and it improves the prediction in the right direction.

On scatterplots like this, plots clustering around a diagonal line sloping in the opposite direction would show negative (or inverse) correlation (see Figures 3 and 4 in Payne and Saul's study in Chapter 9), and plots showing no pattern at all would be showing no, or only a very weak correlation (see Figure 11.3 in Chapter 11).

Figure 10.5 also bears the legend '$r = 0.79$'. The r in this case is Pearson's product moment correlation co-efficient. As with other correlation co-efficients it expresses, in effect, the extent to which the observations cluster round the regression line. If they were all exactly on the regression line r would equal 1 (or minus 1). If there were no pattern at all r would equal zero. Since correlations can occur by chance, correlation co-efficients are also tested for their significance, although a score of 0.79 can usually be regarded as a 'high' correlation. In this case p was less than 0.001: there was less than one chance in 1,000 that this pattern of association was the result of chance factors (see Table 7.2 in Chapter 7 for the meaning of different values of p).

11   Correlations, causes and statistical control

Surveys – including case control studies (section 9) – can demonstrate correlations: what is associated with what. (For the expression of correlations, see section 10.) Causal links are often inferred from correlations. For example, being poor and dying earlier are correlated. One reasonable interpretation of this is that there is something about being poor which *causes* premature death. However, there is usually more than one interpretation of a correlation. For example, it is possible that the kinds of people who die earlier are also the kinds of people who are in poor health, and that it is being in bad health which both *causes* them to be poor and causes them to die earlier. In this case it is likely that both interpretations are valid; that there are two *directions of effect*. One may be more important than the other but a survey alone may not be able to establish the predominant direction of cause.

Payne and Saul in the Chapter 9 exemplar found that those with angina in the poorest wards of Sheffield were only about one-third as likely as those in the most affluent wards to receive angiography: there is a correlation between higher deprivation and lower rates of angiography. But what underlies this correlation? Is some aspect of poverty causing poorer people to receive angiography less often, or some aspect of affluence causing better off people to receive angiography more often? And, if either, or both, what exactly is, or are, the causal mechanism(s), and do they operate at the level of individual characteristics, or at the level of difference between services serving different parts of the city. These are not questions for which Payne and Saul's research design is capable of giving a final answer. This is partly because they did not collect the data to do so, but more importantly because surveys are not well designed to demonstrate causality. As noted in Chapter 5, only an experimental approach can do this, through setting up artificial situations in which variables are controlled, excluding all influences on what happens, except that which is of particular interest.

Survey researchers can, however, exert *statistical control* over variables. Age-standardising data provide a simple example. Two wards might show different levels of angina either because one ward has an older population than the other, or because it is more deprived than the other. To exclude the effect of age on differences in angina rates between wards all that is necessary is to compare the rates of angina between the wards, age group by age group, and, to exclude the effect of gender, to express the results for males separately from females. Age and gender will then have been *controlled* and any remaining differences in rates of angina between the two wards are available to be attributed to differences in deprivation. More elaborate techniques of age-standardisation are discussed in Chapter 11. This example shows how variables can be controlled statistically in analysing survey results, but it also shows a major problem with this. While the manoeuvre above will have eliminated the effects of age and gender on differences in angina rates between wards, any differences left will not solely be due to deprivation, but to deprivation plus other uncontrolled factors, or worse, due to other uncontrolled factors rather than to deprivation and affluence.

In discussing the reasons why people in more deprived wards are less likely to be treated with angiography Payne and Saul consider an alternative to a straightforward 'poverty' explanation: poorer people are more likely to smoke, and there is anecdotal evidence to suggest that doctors are less likely to allocate expensive coronary care procedures to smokers.

Payne and Saul exert statistical control over their data in order to see how well this explanation stands up.

> The angiography rate in those with angina identified through the survey was found to be 11% (13/116) in the 10 most affluent wards and 4% (9/216) in the 10 most deprived wards. National and local data suggest that about 83% of the affluent populations are likely to be non-smokers, but only 65% of deprived populations. Even if the smokers had been excluded from treatment (that is from the numerator) and if the denominator was adjusted to reflect the likely number of non-smokers, the angiography rate in affluent wards would still be twice that in deprived wards – that is 13% (13/(116 × 0.83)) v 6% (9/(216 × 0.65)), respectively. (Payne and Saul, 1997: 261; see Chapter 9)

As Payne and Saul note, it would have been better if their survey had collected data about whether people smoked or not, rather than relying on estimates. In the absence of evidence from their own sample they have to assume that *all* those receiving angiography were non-smokers. But that has the advantage of modelling what the situation would be if discrimination against smokers had the strongest possible effect. They also assume that the rate of smoking among people with angina symptoms would be the same as for those in populations of smokers and non-smokers of similar socio-economic status. This is unlikely, since coronary heart disease is itself correlated with smoking. But this will not alter the comparison being made so long as the correlation between smoking and coronary heart disease is of much the same strength irrespective of social class. If it is, any over- or under-estimate has the same effect on both groups being compared. Despite its speculative nature the analysis quoted above does illustrate the way in which a 'discrimination-against-smokers' explanation can be tested by controlling for smoking, that is, by comparing angiography rates just between *non-smokers* with angina symptoms from affluent areas and *non-smokers* with angina symptoms from deprived areas.

Notice that statistical control presents a version of a problem which may arise wherever comparisons are made in the search for important differences between groups. In experiments (Chapter 5) it is important to create comparison groups as similar to each other as possible prior to the intervention – otherwise any outcome differences may reflect prior differences between groups, rather than the effects of the different ways in which the groups were treated. In case control studies (section 9), imperfect matching of cases to controls may result in mismatches between the groups being mistaken for 'risk factors'. Similarly, sorting the data to exert statistical control may create groups which do not match for variables that should be controlled. For example, we might try to control for age by citing results in terms of age bands. But this still leaves it possible that in one 18–25 age group most of the subjects are between 18 and 20, and in another most are between 20 and 25. A difference shown between the groups may be due to this imperfect control of age.

Sample size limits the possibilities for exerting statistical control over survey results. This is because statistical control requires the respondents to be divided into sub-groups which will then be compared with each other. Payne and Saul started with a large sample, but for the analysis quoted above, they have deleted the results from nine wards of middling affluence, and from all the people without angina symptoms, divided the remainder into the richest 10 and the poorest 10 wards, then again into those receiving and those not receiving angiography, and then again into smokers and non-smokers. The result is that the differences between sub-groups they are comparing are very small (13/116 and 9/216). It would be impossible for them to take a further step and, for example, investigate gender differences in angiography rates between non-smokers according to ward affluence or deprivation. By this time the sample has run out of statistical power. Many surveys have smaller samples than this, and therefore much less capacity for testing the possible reasons for correlations.

Correlations from surveys can be useful even if the causal sequences which they reflect are unclear. For example, knowing that there is a correlation between socio-economic status and coronary disease is useful for planning services even if it is unclear as to the mechanism which links higher rates of coronary disease to higher rates of poverty. In many areas of practice the 'risk factors' identified result from correlations derived from surveys.

12   Contemporaneous and longitudinal surveys

Most surveys, including most case control studies, are *contemporaneous*: snap-shots of a state of affairs at a particular point in time, and therefore gather only *retrospective* data about events which happened in the past. Data that rely on people's memories must be regarded with less confidence than data about current matters. *Retrospective*, or *recall bias*, is not only a question of forgetting; it is a characteristic of human memory that people constantly revise their memories in the light of what has happened subsequently and in terms of the context in which they are asked the questions. For example, in the case control studies of sudden infant death (section 9) it is possible that since some people questioned have already heard that there are associations between sleeping posture and sudden infant death that they mis-remember what happened in a way that shows that they did what was right (Dwyer and Ponsonby, 1996). Again, mothers whose children have become delinquent may remember events in a child's past differently from those mothers whose children have not become delinquent, since they will have reconstructed their memories in a search for an explanation (West, 1969). This is to say nothing about the deliberate falsification of answers. Because data about what happened before and what happened afterwards all have to be collected at a single point in time, contemporaneous surveys are particularly weak designs for investigating causality and issues of effectiveness. Accurate service records can, of course, compensate for recall bias. Payne and Saul (Chapter 9), for example, check their respondents' answers about treatments received against medical records.

Longitudinal surveys (or prospective surveys) are able to produce more convincing evidence about what causes what by collecting data from people *before* the events of interest happen, and then following them up with one or more further studies later. Surveying at different points in time ameliorates *direction of effect* problems. A longitudinal survey, for example, can establish whether those who died prematurely were poor before they became ill, or got poor because of their illness (Goldblatt, 1990). Similarly, an evaluation study may take a longitudinal survey design, with a survey before the implementation of a policy, and a survey some time afterwards (Tudor Smith et al., 1998). Most longitudinal surveys are in fact a time series of snapshot surveys, perhaps just two, or perhaps more where the same *panel* of respondents is questioned on numerous occasions.

The terms *longitudinal surveys, prospective surveys* and *cohort studies* are often used as synonyms for each other. Usually all these terms imply that the same subjects are surveyed at different points in time, with the term *repeat survey* being used to refer to the same survey being conducted at different points in time with different subjects, as with the NHS Users' survey in Chapter 8. However, usage is imprecise in this field. 'Cohort study' is sometimes used more narrowly to refer to medical research where only a small range of factors are of interest and where a convenience sample rather than a probability sample is the starting point. A classic example is that by Doll and Hill begun in 1951 to investigate the link between smoking, lung cancer and coronary heart disease. This is illustrated in Box 10.6, which also explains the notions of *relative risk* and *attributable risk*.

Box 10.6   An example of a medical cohort study: relative risk and attributable risk

In 1951 Doll and Hill (1964) sent a questionnaire to all 59,600 doctors on the UK Medical Register asking about their smoking habits. Sixty-eight per cent returned questionnaires. From 1951 to 1961 the deaths of doctors and the causes of their death were monitored, mainly through the death registration process. There were 4,963 deaths. Some of the results are shown in Table 10.6.

Table 10.6   Deaths of doctors by smoking behaviour 1951–1961: some results from a cohort study

| | Deaths per 1,000 persons (doctors) per year | | | |
Cause of death	All doctors in survey	Non-smoking doctors	All cigarette smoking doctors	Doctors smoking more than 25 cigarettes a day
All causes	14.05	12.06	16.32	19.67
Lung cancer	0.65	0.07	1.20	2.23
Coronary heart disease	3.99	3.31	4.57	4.97

Source: Based on Unwin et al., 1997: 38

Two ways in which data like this are often expressed are in terms of *relative risk* and *attributable risk*.

Relative risk

$$\frac{\text{Rate in the group with the attribute or exposure}}{\text{Rate in the group without the attribute or exposure}}$$

For example: 1.20/1,000 doctors who smoked died per year of lung cancer in the 10-year period, and only 0.07/1,000 non-smoking doctors died of lung cancer

$$\frac{1.20}{0.07} = 17.1$$

meaning that those smoking were 17 times more likely to die of lung cancer than non-smokers.

Attributable risk   There are two versions of this: attributable risk (exposed) and attributable risk (population).

Attributable risk (exposed) is the rate among those with the attribute or exposure *minus* the rate among those without the attribute or not exposed. For example: 1.20/1,000 doctors who smoked died per year of lung cancer in the 10 year period, and only 0.07/1,000 non-smoking doctors died of lung cancer.

$1.20 - 0.07 = 1.13$ per 1,000 persons per year

meaning that out of the 1.20 deaths from lung cancer per 1,000, 1.13 can be attributed to smoking. This can be expressed as a proportion:

$$\frac{1.20 - 0.07}{1.20} \times 100 = 94 \text{ per cent}$$

94 per cent of deaths from lung cancer were due to smoking.

Attributable risk (population) is the rate in the population *minus* the rate in the group with the attribute or exposure. For example, deaths per 1,000 from lung cancer in the population were 0.65/1,000 and for smokers were 1.20/1,000. In this case, 'the population' is the sample of doctors responding to the questionnaire.

$$0.65 - 0.07 = 0.58 \text{ per 1,000 per year}$$

meaning that 0.58 deaths per year from lung cancer in this population were due to smoking. Expressed as a proportion:

$$\frac{0.58}{0.65} \times 100 = 89 \text{ per cent}$$

89 per cent of deaths from lung cancer in this population were due to smoking.

The same results might also be expressed in terms of other expressions of effect size (see chapter 7, sections 10.1–10.4).

Definitions and calculations based on Unwin et al., 1997: 38–40

As the material in Box 10.6 indicates, longitudinal studies some-times start with convenience samples, particularly those called cohort studies. In Doll and Hill's study this was all UK doctors, and in the so-called Whitehall study of mortality and morbidity (Marmot, 1995) the sample was taken from civil service employees. For longitudinal work there are some merits in starting with a sample of people who are likely to be easy to stay in touch with, rather than using probability sampling. This has the same effect as 'clustering' respondents (section 4). As with clustering *per se*, the cost of this convenience lies in the problems of generalising from a sample to a wider population. To generalise from the Doll and Hill study (Box 10.6) we have to make 68 per cent of all doctors stand as representative of all adults with regard to the influence of smoking on death rates. It is reasonable to assume that the research demonstrates an elevation of the risk of death for smokers everywhere – and other research has shown this. But it is not reasonable to assume that the extent to which the risk of death is elevated among doctors is the same as for other occupational groups. Thus it would not be safe to generalise the relative risk and attribut-able risk figures calculated in Box 10.6 from the sample of doctors to the population of all adults in Great Britain. The results of the Whitehall study (Marmot, 1995) show a continuous gradation of ill-health and premature death from the highest to the lower grades, but although the civil service covers a wide range of pay rates and work circumstances, it cannot be entirely representative of the social class spectrum of Great Britain.

Perhaps the best-known longitudinal surveys are the national birth cohort studies, which are so important in the knowledge base for practitioners in child health and child social work and education (Wadsworth, 1991,1996). These are studies through life of all or a large sample of the children born in a particular week in 1946 (5,362 children), 1958 (17,000 children) or 1970 (16,000 children). For the 1946 cohort the sample was fixed, but for the other two samples immigrant children with the same birth date have been identified and added in – an example of using booster samples (see section 8) However, in all the cohorts children from ethnic minority backgrounds remain under-represented in terms of today's population. The 1946 birth cohort study has been extended to cover the children of the original children (Wadsworth, 1996).

The sampling strategy for these studies might be regarded as a kind of systematic sampling (see Box 10.1), though with a single sampling interval, or as a form of clustering, by time rather than by place (see section 4). Systematic samples are as good as random samples so long as there is an arbitrary relationship between the sampling interval and the data collected. But there are important differences between children with summer birthdays and others, and hence no single week of birth will produce a sample of children representative of all children born that year for characteristics which depend on season of birth. This is a limitation of these studies, though for many purposes an unimportant one.

The longer a study goes on, the greater the opportunities to lose contact with respondents. However, in longitudinal surveys the problem of non-response is reduced somewhat by the fact that much data will have been collected about people before they disappear so that similarities and differences between those who get lost and those who don't can be specified, and the results interpreted accordingly, unlike the situation in a snapshot survey where it may be difficult to know about the characteristics of those people sampled, but not entering the survey. In fact these birth cohort studies have been very successful in retaining subjects. For example, in 1985 the birth cohort of 1958 was still scoring a 76 per cent response rate, and the loss includes people who died as well as those who lost contact for other reasons (Shepherd, 1985).

Longitudinal surveys conducted over a long time period also exaggerate another problem of generalisation; that of *generalising through time*. In March 2000 the children who entered the national birth cohort study in 1946 were 54 years old. The study does and will continue to provide an enormous amount of information on how circumstances in infancy and childhood in the 1940s relate to someone's life in their 50s at the turn of a new century. But how far will the findings also be true for someone born in the 1960s, or 1970s, or 1980s and in their 50s in 2010, 2020 or 2030 ? The circumstances of childhood in the 1940s are long gone. There can, of course, be time generalisation problems with any kinds of research as the research ages.

13   The ecological fallacy in interpreting survey results

To commit an ecological fallacy is to make unjustifiable assumptions about the behaviour or conditions of individuals on the basis of the characteristics of the areas they come from. Robinson (1950), who invented the term, gave as an example the possibly fallacious argument that unemployment causes high rates of crime, based on a survey finding that areas with high crime rates also have high rates of unemployment. Unless a survey has been specially designed to establish that it is unemployed people who commit the crimes, this would not be a safe interpretation of the survey results. For most of their study of the relationship between the need for coronary care services and the receipt of coronary care services, Payne and Saul (Chapter 9) take the electoral ward as their unit of analysis. They find both that people in poorer wards report more angina symptoms and that people in poorer wards are less likely to receive more advanced forms of coronary care. But since they did not collect information about the economic conditions of individuals their data *does not* actually show that it is poorer people in Sheffield who are most at risk of coronary heart disease and least likely to be treated for it. With their data it would remain possible – though very unlikely – that it is the richest people in the poorest wards who are at greatest risk, and the poorest people in the richest wards who receive most care. While their assumptions seem reasonable enough, there is a gap between ward-level data which they have collected and individual socio-economic conditions, about which they have no data and the gap has to be bridged by making assumptions. Since Payne and Saul were particularly interested in providing intelligence for planning services, and services have to be provided on a territorial basis, analysis at the level of the ward, rather than at the level of the individual seems justified. They address the problem of ecological validity in their article.

In terms of applying research results to practice, the ecological fallacy can sometimes lead to poor policy making. For example, in many rural areas poor people are in the minority and their deprivation gets lost in expressions of the socio-economic status of areas

(Abbott et al., 1992). Or again, the educational priority area pro-gramme of the 1960s was designed to improve educational achieve-ment. Additional resources were targeted to schools and educational welfare services in areas with high levels of socio-economic dis-advantage, since these were the *areas* with the lowest educational results. But the majority of under-achieving children, and the major-ity of poor children, actually did not, and do not, live in areas of high socio-economic disadvantage, but spread across all areas of the coun-try. Nor is the category 'under-achieving children' quite identical with the category 'deprived children' (Bernstein, 1970).

14 Questionnaires, reliability and meaningfulness

The main instrument used in surveys is the questionnaire. Usually the questions are posed to be answered by the people who are selected for the survey. Sometimes, however, the questions are actually answered by a practitioner or practitioner-researcher, who carries out a clinical examination or assessment on the people selected for the survey. This can lead to problems if different practitioners make judgements in different ways (see Chapter 6, section 5).

However questions are posed, the way they are posed will shape the answers given. In Chapter 8 Cohen and his colleagues illustrate this with regard to differences in response to what look like similar questions.

Most of the issues raised about research instruments in general in Chapter 6, apply equally to questionnaires, but in Part 4 of this book there is a set of critical appraisal questions to ask about surveys which includes questions to ask about questionnaires.

The results of a survey are a composite of comparisons and con-trasts. For this reason it is important that data about the same matters are collected in the same way from each respondent so that like can be added to like and contrasted with unlike. Put another way, survey researchers usually place a great emphasis on *reliability*. This follows from a long history of survey work which has developed a substantial research base showing that unless safeguards are used there is a strong danger that responses will reflect more about interviewers than about interviewees, or more about questionnaires than about those who fill them in (for example, Bradburn, 1983). *Social desirability bias* is a particularly important source of unreli-ability (Fielding, 1993: 147–50). While most respondents will probably want to show themselves in a good light, what responses they think will do this will depend on what cues they can pick up from the wording of the questions or the demeanour, persona or social status of the interviewer, or from the location of the interviews (Davies, 1997: Chapter 4). Interviews and interviewers may provide different cues as to social desirability to different types of respondents, and different respondents may read the same cues differently. By contrast with questionnaire studies the possibility for social desirability bias is much greater in loosely structured ('in-depth') interviews, where interviewers disclose far more of themselves and hence give more cues as to what would be a socially desirable performance by the interviewee, and where interviewees have much more opportunity to probe the views of their interviewer (see Chapter 16).

Unreliability undermines the credibility of comparisons made in analysing survey results. For example, different levels of dissatisfaction shown by the clientele of different agencies might turn out to be merely the result of their being questioned in different ways (see Chapter 8, for example). Apparent changes over time might be the result of a second survey asking questions in a different way from the first. Table 10.7 gives a synopsis of the main problems arising from unreliability of method in survey research and the main safeguards used to avoid them.

Table 10.7 also indicates one of the major trade-offs in research; here between reliability and meaningfulness. Following the policy suggested in the table to maximise reliability may mean, for example:

- asking people questions that may not be important or meaningful to them;
- asking some people questions that are important and meaningful to them, when the same questions will be less meaningful or important to others;
- not asking people, or some people, questions relevant to the survey topic which may be much more meaningful and important to them than the questions actually asked;
- forcing people to opt among responses which are pre-decided, when they might prefer to give a response which has not been provided for;
- offering some people the opportunity to give exactly the response they would like to give, but ruling this out for others;
- giving a performance as an interviewer which is congenial to some kinds of people, but not to others.

Qualitative research is often offered as an antidote to the problems listed above, though solving them usually means compromising reliability, representativeness and generalisability. Thus what a survey researcher might regard as poor practice because it is unreliable, a qualitative researcher might regard as good practice because it adjusts the collection of data to the particularities of each individual respondent, and therefore produces data which are meaningful to those who provide them (Oakley, 1981). Chapter 12 in this volume is by Mildred Blaxter, one of the main researchers involved in the large-scale *Health and Lifestyle Survey*. Here she contrasts the kind of data which

Table 10.7 Problems of reliability in surveys and some safeguards against them

Shortcomings in design	Problems of interpretation	Safeguards and remedies
Different questions might be asked of different respondents	If entirely different questions are asked of each respondent this will be many surveys each with a sample of one, and no sound generalisations will be possible. More usually, the result will be to reduce a larger, possibly representative sample to a number of smaller (probably unrepresentative) samples each consisting of a cluster of respondents asked the same or similar questions about the same topic(s)	Ask each respondent the same questions in the same ways. Brief each in the same way about the purpose of the survey
The same questions might be asked but in different ways of different respondents *Or* The interviewer might make different kinds of relationships with different respondents	Unless the differences are known precisely it will be impossible to decide whether differences in responses between respondents are due to differences between them, or to the different ways in which they were asked questions and/or the different relationships they struck up with the interviewer	Prepare each interviewer to follow a standard protocol for interviewing. If several interviewers are employed, analyse the results interviewer by interviewer to detect *interviewer effects*. Even if only one interviewer is used, analyse the results of, say, early as opposed to later interviews, interviews with males and interviews with females and so on, to look for interviewer effects
Interviewers with very different characteristics are employed	There will always be some *interviewer effect*, with results differing according to different interviewers – or even perhaps between interviews done at different times by the same interviewer	
Questions are open-ended and allow respondents to determine what are appropriate answers. There may be a good case for using open-ended questions but there will be problems of interpretation none the less	There will be acute difficulties of matching the answers of one respondent with those of another. Insofar as some people will give longer, fuller answers the results will over-represent the loquacious and under-represent the reticent	Preferably use closed/forced choice questions. If using open-ended questions do not assume representativeness for the distribution of answers
In epidemiological research, different diagnosticians might be using different decision-rules for making judgements	It will be difficult to decide how far the distribution of an illness or social problem shown in the survey reflects something real and how far it reflects different ways of defining or diagnosing problems	Use standardised protocols for assessment. Establish similarity or difference of judgement by subjecting at least a sample (of the sample) of judgements to inter-rater reliability testing (see Chapter 6, section 6)
Questions asked about past events are vulnerable to *recall bias*	It will not be clear whether differences between respondents are due to differences in the way in which they reconstruct their memories	Avoid asking questions about distant events. Find means to verify factual accounts

are produced by a questionnaire survey with the kind of data which are produced by informal, unstructured interviewing, which give an insight into how the people concerned themselves make sense of the topics about which they are asked questions.

15 Questions to ask about surveys

There is a checklist of critical appraisal questions about surveys in Part 4 of this volume. It deals mainly with questions to ask about whether a survey is valid in its own terms for the population the survey claims to represent. This may well be a population different from the practice population of the practitioner reader. It may be larger, in another place, or at another time. There are also questions to ask about how to extrapolate from a survey to a practice population. Two common purposes for extrapolation are:

- *Performance bench-marking*. For example, the NHS consumer satisfaction surveys reviewed by Cohen and his colleagues in Chapter 8 might be used to set norms for local performance. NHS Trusts might be surveyed separately to judge whether they were generating more or less satisfaction than the average for Scotland as a whole. Something like this is the purpose of the series of annual consumer surveys instituted by central government in 1998 (Department of Health, 1997). Insofar as 'performance' is only a small part of the cause of satisfaction ratings, Trusts would want to know how far the populations of their catchment areas were similar to or different from those of the national population surveyed, and especially in terms of those factors likely to influence satisfaction rates. For example, it is to be expected that the younger the population of a hospital catchment area, the lower the level of satisfaction which will be recorded in a satisfaction survey.
- *Epidemiological needs assessment*. Much survey work identifies the social distribution of illness, disability and social problems. This is useful information if it can be transferred from the population surveyed to another population about which service planning decisions are to be made.

Chapter 11 gives some details about extrapolating from an epidemiological survey.

16 Further reading on surveys and case control studies

On surveys

There is no shortage of good texts on survey methodology. A good introduction is Sapsford (1999). For survey methods in health care research in particular, see Bowling (1997, Chapters 12, 13 and 14), and in social work, see Alston and Bowles (1998, Chapters 5 and 6). For more technical information about sampling and questionnaire design, see Alreck and Settle (1995) or De Vauss (1995).

On case control studies

An excellent introduction to both case control and cohort studies is given by Mant and Jenkinson (1997).

References and further reading

Abbott, P., Bernie, J., Payne, G. and Sapsford, R. (1992) 'Health and material depriva-tion in Plymouth', in P. Abbott and R. Sapsford (eds), *Research into Practice: a Reader for Nurses and the Caring Professions*. Buckingham: Open University Press. pp. 129–55.

Alreck, P. and Settle, R. (1995) *The Survey Research Handbook*, 2nd edn. Burr Ridge: Irwin.

Alston, M. and Bowles, W. (1998) *Research for Social Workers: an Introduction to Methods*. London: Allen and Unwin.

Arber, S. (1993) 'Designing samples', in N. Gilbert (ed.), *Researching Social Life*. London: Sage. pp. 68–92.

Bernard, H. (1994) *Research Methods in Anthropology*, 2nd edn. London: Sage.

Bernstein, B. (1970) 'Education cannot compensate for society', *New Society*, 26th February, pp. 344–7.

Blair, P., Fleming, P., Bensley, D., Smith, I., Bacon, C., Taylor, E., Berry, J., Golding, J. and Tripp, J. (1996) Smoking and the sudden infant death syndrome: results from 1993–5 case-control study for confidential inquiry into stillbirths and deaths in infancy', *British Medical Journal*, 313: 195–8.

Bowling, A. (1997) *Research Methods in Health: Investigating Health and Health Services*. Buckingham: Open University Press.

Bradburn, N. (1983) 'Response effects', in J. Rossi, D. Wright and A. Anderson (eds), *Handbook of Survey Research*. New York: Academic Press. pp. 289–328.

Davies, J. (1997) *Drugspeak: the Analysis of Drug Discourse*. Amsterdam: Harwood Academic Publishers.

Department of Health (1997) *The New NHS: Modern, Dependable*. London: HMSO.

De Vauss, D. (1995) *Surveys in Social Research*, 4th edn. London: Allen and Unwin.

Doll, R. and Hill, A. (1964) 'Mortality in relation to smoking: ten years' observation of British doctors', *British Medical Journal*, 1: 1399–410; 1460–7.

Dwyer, T. and Ponsonby, A-L. (1996) 'Sudden infant death syndrome: after the "back to sleep" campaign', *British Medical Journal*, 313: 180–1.

Fielding, N. (1993) 'Qualitative interviewing', in N. Gilbert (ed.), *Researching Social Life*. London: Sage. pp. 135–53.

Fleming, P., Blair, P., Bacon, C., Bensley, D., Smith, I., Taylor, E., Berry, J., Golding, J. and Tripp, J. (1996) 'Environment of infants during sleep and risk of sudden infant death syndrome: results of 1993–5 case-control study for confidential inquiry into stillbirths and deaths in infancy', *British Medical Journal*, 313: 191–5.

Goldblatt, P. (ed.) (1990) *Longitudinal Study: Mortality and Social Organisation 1971–1981*. OPCS series LS no. 6. London: HMSO.

Layte, R. and Jenkinson, C. (1997) 'Social surveys', in C. Jenkinson (ed.), *Assessment and Evaluation of Health and Medical Care: a Methods Text*. Buckingham: Open University Press.

Kish, L. (1965) *Survey Sampling*. London: J. Wiley and Son.

Krejcie, R. and Morgan, D. (1970) 'Determining sample size for research activities', *Educational and Psychological Measurement*, 30: 607–10.

Mant, J. and Jenkinson, C. (1997) 'Case control and cohort studies', in C. Jenkinson (ed.), *Assessment and Evaluation of Health and Medical Care*. Buckingham: Open University Press. pp. 31–46.

Marmot, M. (1995) 'In sickness and in wealth: social causes of illness', *Medical Research Council News*, 65: 8–12.

Meltzer, H., Gill, B., Petticrew, M. and Hinds, K. (1995) *The Prevalence of Psychiatric Morbidity among Adults Living in Private Households: OPCS Surveys of Psychiatric Morbidity in Great Britain: Report 2*. London: HMSO.

National CJD Surveillance Unit (1999) *Creutzfeldt–Jakob Disease Surveillance in the UK: Seventh Annual Report*. Edinburgh: Western General Hospital.

Nazroo, J. (1997) *Ethnicity and Mental Health: Findings from a National Community Survey*. London: Policy Studies Institute.

Oakley, A. (1981) 'Interviewing women, a contradiction in terms', in H. Roberts, (ed.), *Doing Feminist Research*. London: Routledge and Kegan Paul. pp. 30–61.

Pett, M. (1997) *Nonparametric Statistics of Health Care Research: Statistics for Small Samples and Unusual Distributions*. London: Sage.

Robinson, W. (1950) 'Ecological correlations and the behaviour of individuals', *American Sociological Review*, 15: 351–7.

Sapsford, R. (1999) *Survey Research* London: Sage.

Shepherd, P. (1985) 'The National Child Development Study: an introduction to the background to the study and the methods of data collection'. London. *NCDS User Support Group Working Paper No 1*. Social Statistics Research Unit: City University.

Tudor Smith, C., Nutbeam, D., Moore, L. and Catford, J. (1998) 'Effects of Heartbeat Wales programme over five years on behavioural risks for cardio-vascular disease: quasi-experimental comparison of results from Wales and a matched reference area', *British Medical Journal*, 316: 818–22.

Unwin, N., Carr, S., Leeson, J. and Pless-Mulloli, T. (1997) *An Introductory Study Guide to Public Health and Epidemiology*. Buckingham: Open University Press.

Wadsworth, M. (1991) *The Imprint of Time: Childhood History and Adult Life*. Oxford: Oxford University Press.

Wadsworth, M. (1996) 'The survey that shocked the nation', *Medical Research Council News*, 69: 28–32.

West, D. (1969) *Present Conduct: Future Delinquency*. London: Heinemann Educational Books.

Wilson, P. and Elliot, D. (1987) 'An evaluation of the postcode address file and its use within OPCS', *Journal of the Royal Statistical Society: Series A*, 150 (3): 230–40.

Yin, R. (1994) *Case Study Research: Design and Methods*, 2nd edn. London: Sage.

CONTROLLING FOR AGE AND SOCIO-ECONOMIC CIRCUMSTANCES

Introduction — 1 Age standardisation — 2 Denominator problems in standardisation — 3 Standardised mortality ratios — 4 Deprivation indices — 5 Further reading on age standardisation and deprivation indices — References and further reading

Introduction

In 1971 in Bournemouth 1,223 males died. Is this a large or a small number of deaths? Obviously the answer depends on how many males there were to start with. Expressing deaths as *rates* allows for a sensible comparison to be made between areas with different sized populations, or the same area at two points in time where the population has increased or decreased. So in 1971 Bournemouth's male death *rate* was 18.7 per 1,000. The number of males in Bournemouth was 65,520 – the *population at risk*.

$(1,223/65,520) \times 1,000 = 18.666$
$= 18.7$ deaths per 1,000 of the population at risk.

With rates we can compare deaths in Bournemouth in 1971, 1981, 1991, 2001, discounting for changes in population size. But is this a high or a low rate? Simply comparing the male death rate for Bournemouth with the national average rate for 1971 suggests that it is on the high side, compared with that for England and Wales at 12.2/1,000.

However, death rates are predominantly influenced by the sex ratio and by the age profile of a population and by its socio-economic circumstances. So we can ask, 'Is this a high death rate *given* the age profile of the population of Bournemouth?' and 'Is this a high death rate given the socio-economic circumstances of Bournemouth?' or 'Is this a high death rate given the gender composition of the population?'. In each case the answer to the question would depend on the comparison being made: by comparison with England and Wales in 1971, by comparison with sixteenth-century London, by comparison with Calcutta today. And if the death rate in Bournemouth increased between 1971 and 1991 we would want to know how much of the increase was due to the population getting older, or getting poorer, or changing its sex ratio.

The first question might be translated as 'After controlling for age' or 'After discounting for the fact that different areas have different age profiles, is the male death rate in Bournemouth high?' And we could also ask the question 'Is the male death rate in Bournemouth high compared to the female death rate after discounting for the fact that females will on average be older than males?'

Answering these questions requires us to 'control for' different variables through some act of *standardisation*. What is usually just called a *death rate* might be better called an expression of 'deaths standardised for the size of the population at risk' since, in a rate, the size of the relevant population is standardised to 1,000 or 10,000 or some other convenient figure. A percentage is simply a rate out of 100. This chapter is about similar manoeuvres to standardise for age and socio-economic differences, and occasionally for gender and ethnicity. It is not only mortality which is influenced by age, gender, socio-economic circumstances and ethnicity. So also are patterns of illness, involvement in, and victimisation by crime, patterns of drug abuse and alcoholism, and so on (Benzeval et al., 1995; Gomm, 1996).

The reason for standardisation is to facilitate comparisons, but the comparisons might be in order to:

- Investigate causal relationships using standardisation to control variables: for example, estimating how much of the difference in crime between areas is due to differences in age profiles or differences in socio-economic conditions between areas. Chapter 8 uses age standardisation to discount the effect of age on responses to a survey in two areas with different age profiles. Age is, as it were, cleared out of the way so that other factors that might be causing the differences can be investigated.
- Predict the need for services in a local area. For example, estimating the number of cases of dementia likely in the next ten years may mean translating national figures in terms of a local age profile, since dementia is an age-related condition (Meltzer, 1992). Chapter 9 relates the need for coronary care services with degrees of socio-economic deprivation, and then judges the performance of services in meeting these needs. This current chapter also explains how deprivation measures are used to determine central government finance for local expenditure.
- Set local targets, or judge performance, in terms of what is feasible in a local area. For example, health improvement targets achievable in an affluent area may not be achievable in a poorer one or may require more resources to do so. The study in Chapter 9 implies

some performance targets which health services in Sheffield should adopt. Box 11.4 below in this chapter gives a further example.

1   Age standardisation

Researchers often give results in *age standardised* (or age weighted or age adjusted) terms. For example, a study by King and his colleagues (1994) gives the frequency of non-affective psychosis in different ethnic groups in Haringey (Table 11.1). As with many other conditions psychosis is age-related. The *incidence* – number of new cases – is highest in youthful populations, while the *prevalence* – number of all cases at a point in time – is highest in populations with larger percentages of older people. This apparently contradictory state of affairs happens with many chronic conditions because, while onset may occur in youth, giving youthful populations a high incidence rate, a large percentage of such people stay ill, raising the prevalence rate in older populations.

Differences in the *incidence* of psychosis between ethnic groups in Haringey might reflect the different age profiles of these population sub-groups, rather than anything else about differences in mental health. In order to compare like with like it is necessary to control for

Table 11.1   Incidence (number of new cases) of non-affective psychosis, including schizophrenia, in the catchment area of St Ann's Hospital, Haringey, 1991–2, from health service, social services, probation and prison contacts, by ethnic group

Ethnic group	Number of new cases 1991–2/ numbers in population at risk	Age standardised[a] incidence rate per 10,000 in local population (95% CI)[b]
White	24/121,438	2.0 (1.2 to 2.8)
Black		
Caribbean	15/14,973	8.9 (4.4 to 13.5)
Black African	8/9,381	8.7 (2.4 to 14.9)
Black other	4/2,994	12.0 (0 to 25.7)
Total 'Black'	27/27,348	8.7 (5.3 to 12.0)
Indian	3/6,326	4.5 (0 to 9.6)
Pakistani	2/1,065	15.3 (0 to 36.5)
Other 'Asian'	3/4,253	7.0 (0 to 15.0)
Total 'Asian'	8/11,644	6.9 (2.1 to 11.6)
Other	3/3,847	5.8 (0 to 12.3)
Total	62/167,984	3.6 (2.7 to 4.5)

[a] Recalculating the figures as if each ethnic group had exactly the same age profile as the age profile of the population of England and Wales.
[b] Where confidence intervals for percentages or rates give minus figures the lowest limit is expressed as 0 (see Chapter 10, Table 10.3).

Source: King et al., *British Medical Journal* 1994, 306: 1117, with permission from the BMJ Publishing Group

age differences. One way is only to compare the incidences between ethnic groups age group by age group. Another is to standardise for age, recalculating the figures to show what the differences between ethnic groups would be if each group had exactly the same age structure. For example, if in Haringey the percentage of black males aged 16–25 was twice that of the percentage of this sex–age group in the population of Haringey as a whole, then the figures could be re-calculated so that each new case of psychosis among black males aged 16–25 counted only half as much as each new case among males of this age group of other ethnicities.

In addition, as an inner urban area, Haringey will have a popula-tion which is on average younger than that of England and Wales. Hence findings on the incidence of psychosis here will not be repre-sentative for England and Wales as a whole. In order to deal with this kind of problem it is common to age standardise results from a local survey in terms of a *reference population*. One of the methods used is shown in Box 11.1.

Table 11.2 imagines a study of the prevalence of psychosis (columns A and C) in an area with a youthful population (column B), not unlike Haringey. Since psychotic illness is age-related the findings of this study do not provide a very good model for areas with different age profiles. Thus the calculations produce an estimate of the prevalence of psychotic illness (column E) for a reference population which has an age profile like that of the UK (column D). For example, the first row of the table shows that there are 15 cases of psychotic illness among the 3,400 people aged 16–19 years within the study population. That is a rate of 4.40 per 1,000 of this age group (column C). In the reference population, 7% are in this age group. The final column shows that, if the reference population had the same age prevalence rates as the index population, there would be 0.31 cases in this age group for every 1,000 people in the reference population as a whole. It may help you to think here of the reference population being divided into slices of 1,000, each slice with the same age profile. Adding the figures in column E gives an expected number of cases per 1,000 of the reference population of 5.38. Multiplying this figure by the number of thousands of people in the reference population would give the actual number of cases that could be expected in the reference population.

The reference population has a higher estimated rate of psychosis (5.38/1,000) than the study, or index area (4.75/1,000), because the reference population contains larger proportions of the age groups of higher risk of psychosis – more in the older age groups. (The series of government-sponsored, epidemiological needs reviews, standardise to a notional health authority which has an age structure as for England and Wales: for example, Stevens and Raftery, 1994).

Age standardisation is the most common form of standardisation. However, standardisation by social class, or for deprivation, and oc-

Box 11.1   A method for age standardisation

Age standardisation (or age adjustment or age weighting) expresses
frequencies from a survey of a local population (*index population*) in
terms of the population structure for a *reference* (or *standard*)
population, often the population of the UK, or one of its constituent
nations. The frequencies might be percentages of people giving
particular responses to a survey, death rates, rates of child abuse or, as
in the example below, rates of illness. The result is that differences in
age profile between the local area and the reference population are
discounted. In the language of experiments, age differences are
controlled (see chapter 5). If this is done ethnic group by ethnic group,
then differences in age profile between ethnic groups in a local area are
also controlled for and comparisons between groups can be made
having excluded the influence of age differences on differences in rates
(see Table 11.1).

Table 11.2   Age standardisation using the direct method

Age groups	A — Number of all cases of psychotic illness in study area (prevalence)	B — Population (%) in study area (index population) (100% = all 16–64)[a]	C — Prevalence rate per 1,000 in study area A/(B/1,000)	D — Percentage of population in age groups in reference area (100% = all 16–64)	E — (C × D)/100 = number of cases expected in each age group per 1,000 of reference population
16–19	15	3,400 (17%)	4.40	7%	0.31
20–24	20	3,800 (19%)	5.26	11%	0.58
25–29	18	3,600 (18%)	5.00	13%	0.65
30–34	6	2,000 (10%)	3.00	12%	0.36
35–39	6	1,600 (8%)	3.75	11%	0.41
40–44	4	1,600 (8%)	2.50	11%	0.27
45–49	4	1,400 (7%)	2.90	11%	0.32
50–55	6	1,000 (5%)	6.00	8%	0.48
55–59	8	800 (4%)	10.00	8%	0.80
60–64	6	400 (2%)	15.00	8%	1.20
All 16–64	93	19,600	4.75	100%	5.38

Age standardised prevalence rate for reference population as a whole =   **5.38/1,000**

[a] Percentages rounded. The percentages in column B are given here to show the profile of
the population. They are not necessary for the calculation.

Procedure

1   Take the number of cases for the first age group (A) in the index
    population and divide by the number in the age group (B) divided by
    1,000. That gives the age group prevalence rate for the index
    population (C).
2   Repeat for all other age groups. There is no need to calculate for the
    16–64 age group as a whole.

3   For the first age group multiply the age group prevalence rate (C) by the *percentage* of that age group in the reference population (D), i.e., in the first row of Table 11.2 4.4 (C) × 7% (D) or (4.4 × 7)/100 = 0.31 (E). That gives the number of cases to be expected for this age group per 1,000 of the reference population.

4   Repeat step 3 for all other age groups.

5   Add up all the expected cases in column E. This gives the standardised prevalence rate per 1,000 of the reference population for all age groups, 16–64.

6   (not shown on the table) Multiply the standardised prevalence rate by the number of thousands of people 16–64 in the reference population. If there are 6 million, for example, then multiply by 6,000; if there are 6,000, multiply by 6. This gives an estimate of the number of cases to be expected at any one time in this population.

For other ways of age standardisation, see Jones and Moon (1987), Unwin et al. (1997) or Marsh (1988).

casionally for ethnicity, are also done: sometimes all together. For example, even after age standardisation the imaginary study in Table 11.2 still doesn't necessarily provide a good model for other areas. With such a youthful population it probably refers to an inner urban area where it is to be expected that socio-economic deprivation and in-migration of people with mental health problems will push the rate of psychosis up (Giggs and Cooper, 1987). To compensate for this to some extent it would be possible also to standardise by social class; following the same procedures as in Table 11.2 with data for social class groups rather than age groups in columns A and B. However, if data about the social class of individuals are not available, a rather cruder form of standardising for socio-economic circumstances can be done using measures of the deprivation of the area in which they live (section 4), though this risks committing the ecological fallacy (see Chapter 10, section 13).

In order to apply findings cited in standardised (or reference area) form to another area, they have to be 'unstandardised' again to answer the questions, 'What would be the rates in a population with the same structure as the one I'm interested in?' or, 'How many actual cases should I expect to occur in my practice area?' Doing this is the reverse of the standardisation procedure in Box 11.1, and is shown in Box 11.2.

Taking Boxes 11.1 and 11.2 together gives the route shown in Figure 11.1.

Where the data were derived from a *national* survey, then, in effect, the national survey results serve as the results for a reference

Box 11.2   Extrapolating from age standardised (reference area) data to another practice area

Table 11.3 shows how to extrapolate age standardised figures to a local population in order to estimate the number of cases that would occur locally. This may be done to estimate local demand for service. It is often done to establish a benchmark against which the local situation is judged. An actual figure for the locality higher than the expected figure may indicate particular local health problems. If the actual figure is lower than expected this may indicate that local cases are escaping the notice of treatment services. The most common standardisation statistic used in this way is the standardised mortality ratio (SMR) (see section 3 in this chapter).

Table 11.3   Extrapolating from a reference area to a practice area to estimate the number of cases expected

	A	B	C	D
Age groups	Population (%)[a] in practice area (100% = all 16–64)	Prevalence rate in reference area[b]	(A × B)/1,000 = number of expected cases	Expected prevalence rate for practice area
16–19	800 (2%)	4.40	3.52	283 cases in a
20–24	1,600 (4%)	5.30	8.48	population of 39,200
25–29	2,000 (5%)	5.00	10.00	= a prevalence rate
30–34	2,800 (7%)	3.00	8.40	of 7.22 per 1,000
35–39	3,200 (8%)	3.75	12.00	
40–44	3,200 (8%)	2.50	8.00	
45–49	4,000 (10%)	2.90	11.60	283.20/(39,200/1,000)
50–55	7,200 (18%)	6.00	43.20	= 7.22
55–59	7,600 (19%)	10.00	76.00	
60–64	6,800 (17%)	15.00	102.00	
All 16–64	39,200	5.38	283.20	**7.22/1,000**

[a] Percentages rounded. The percentages are given here to show the age profile of the population. They are not necessary for the calculation.
[b] Note that the study area from Table 11.2 has been used here as the reference population.

Procedure

1 For the first age group multiply the number of people in the age group (A) in the practice area by the age group prevalence rate for the reference population (B) and divide by 1,000. That gives an estimate of the number of cases to be expected from this age group in the practice population (C).
2 Repeat for all other age groups.
3 Add together all the expected cases to produce the final figure for column C. That is the number of cases in all age groups 16–64 to be expected in the practice population. This is probably the most important figure for practical purposes.

4 Divide the total number of cases expected (the result of step 3 above), by the number of thousands of people there are in the population 16–64: if there are 39,200, then divide by 39.2. The result is the prevalence rate per 1,000 for the practice population.

You will notice that Table 11.3 assumes that the study which provided the index area data for Table 11.2 has been standardised to a reference population, as described earlier. For that reason, the age prevalence rates in column B of Table 11.3 are the same as those in column C of Table 11.2.

Because the practice area has an older population than the reference area, the overall estimate for prevalence in the practice area is higher, though the prevalence rates for each age group are the same. The calculation predicts that in the practice area there will be about 283 cases of psychosis per year among those 16–64 years old.

Figure 11.1 Standardising to a reference area, and extrapolating from a reference area to a practice area

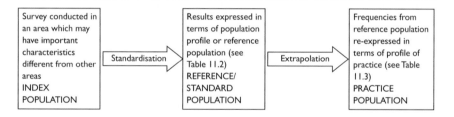

population. There is no reason why extrapolation should not be done direct from a research study area to a practice area elsewhere, using the same procedures as in Table 11.3 but with study area rates in column B. Data given in a reference format are only as good as the study from which they derived. For example, if the study area in Table 11.2 was the basis for the reference area data in Table 11.3, then the prevalences for those aged 55+ were calculated from rather rare cases in rather small populations. If they were in error, then the extrapolation in Table 11.3 will have exaggerated the error.

Remember also that these age standardising procedures only bring populations into line with each other in terms of age structure. There may be other ways in which populations differ which mean that applying the results from a study in one place to the situation in another can be misleading.

Extrapolations such as those in Box 11.2 are really only worthwhile for large practice populations (20,000 plus) and for fairly common conditions. For example, psychosis is a rare condition, and its most newsworthy form – schizophrenia – even rarer. It would not be sensible to carry out the extrapolation in Box 11.2 for a practice population smaller than 20,000. Given the association between psychosis and area poverty here, it would be wise to make allowance for differences in social deprivation or affluence as well.

2 Denominator problems in standardisation

Expressing deaths as rates, or age standardising a set of data, or calculating a standardised mortality ratio (section 3), all require some accurate knowledge about numbers of people in a population. The study by King et al. (Table 11.1) was a *case finding*, or a *clinical epidemiological study*. The researchers found the number of cases known to services and then expressed these as rates for the population as a whole. Thus, in order to produce an incidence rate of 8.9/10,000 for psychosis in Haringey for African Caribbean people, King and his colleagues not only had to discover how many new cases of psychosis there were in this group in 1991–2 (the *enumerator*) but also to know how many people there were in this category in total in 1991–2, in terms of which to express the number of cases as a rate per 10,000 of the population at risk (the *denominator*). This makes the accuracy of the calculation dependent on the accuracy of the population data from which the denominator is calculated.

Researching in 1991–2 King and his colleagues were fortunate since they were able to avail themselves of recent census data for Haringey. Even so, it is known that the census of 1991 particularly under-recorded numbers of young males in London, and perhaps especially young black males (London Research Centre, 1992). Given that the incidence of psychosis is highest from 16 to 25, this under-recording might be important. Census data are particularly inaccurate in Northern Ireland, even for census data which are up to date in their time (DHSS (NI), 1982).

Under-estimating the denominator figure for a rate will automatically increase the rate. This will have its greatest effect with regard to groups which are small in total. For example, in Table 11.1 if the population of African Caribbeans had been under-estimated by 10 per cent then the 'true' incidence of psychotic illness (before age standardisation) would be approximately 8.8 and not 10/10,000 (15 cases divided by 16.97 × 10 rather than 15 divided by 14.93 × 10). But an under-estimation of the much larger local population of white people by 10 per cent would only raise their rate before age standardisation from 1.8 to 1.98/10,000. Here a 10 per cent under-estimation of the denominator has almost a seven times larger effect on the prevalence for the smaller population as compared with the larger population.

During the 1980s research suggested that young black males were particularly prone to schizophrenia (for example, Cooper et al., 1987; McGovern and Cope, 1987). On the one hand this tended to feed racist stereotypes of 'big, black, dangerous and mad' killers on the rampage and, on the other, the notions that racism drove black people mad, or that political resistance against racism was being mistaken for mental illness (Fernando, 1988). However, much of this research was conducted without accurate denominator data, and it now seems likely that some at least of the higher rates of schizophrenia recorded were due to an under-estimation of the young black population. More recent research suggests only small differences in rates of psychosis (including schizophrenia) between black people and white at a national level, though this is not inconsistent with the possibility that locally there might be greater differences either way (Nazroo, 1997b).

As noted, the possibility for denominator errors to give misleading rates is greater the smaller the number of people in the relevant fraction of the population. In addition, the rarer the condition the greater the possibility for there to be errors in the enumerator. An *ascertainment bias* is a particularly common problem in clinical epidemiological studies, as in case control studies (see Chapter 10, section 9). The lesson here is always to treat with scepticism differences in rates as between small populations, or between a small and a large population, where there are any doubts about the representativeness of samples. Confidence interval calculations (Chapter 10, sections 6 and 7) will not show whether there are enumerator or denominator errors.

In the Haringey study (Table 11.1) the figures for the enumerators were taken from the survey – which attempted a 100 per cent count of all new cases – but the figures for the denominator were taken from census data. In the studies reviewed by Cohen et al., in the exemplar reading in Chapter 8, and for the angina symptoms survey of Payne and Saul in Chapter 9, figures for both the enumerators and the denominators were derived from the surveys, the total size of the sample being grossed up to stand as 100 per cent of the population, and the size of any sub-groups in the sample being grossed up to stand as 100 per cent of the sub-group in the population. But something of the same denominator problem remains. First, though researchers may aim to take (say) a 10 per cent sample from a population, they need data independent of the survey to tell them the size of the population and hence how many respondents equal 10 per cent. In stratified probability sampling (Chapter 10, section 3) accurate estimates of the actual numbers of people in sub-groups of the population are necessary. And the same data are needed in order to estimate the extent and shape of survey non-response (Chapter 10, section 8). Cohen and his colleagues (see Chapter 8) were faced with a situation where they wanted to square up the results of a survey which used one kind of random stratified sampling, with the results of another survey which used another kind of random stratified sampling. This is relatively easy, using procedures similar to those in Boxes 11.1 and 11.2, but the accuracy of the results depends on how representative the samples were. In turn, knowing how representative the samples were depends on having information about the size and structure of the population independent of the survey data. In the absence of accurate census data, Cohen et al. had to use hospital records and the results of two other surveys to estimate denominator figures.

3 Standardised mortality ratios

Standardised mortality ratios (SMR) are often used to compare death rates between sub-groups of a population. The term *ratio* is used, rather than rate, because 100 is set as a reference point and death rates for sub-groups are expressed as so many percentage points above or below 100. In reading such figures it is important to check what reference point is being used. The most common is an average for a whole population. Thus, if the average for the whole population is 100, and the figure for men is 110, that means that men have a death rate 10 per cent higher than the average for men plus women. However, the death rate for women might be taken as the reference point and calibrated at 100. Then if the figure for men was 110, that would mean that male death rate was 10 per cent greater than that for women. The principle of age standardisation was explained above. Box 11.3 shows how an age standardised mortality ratio is calculated.

As Box 11.3 shows, once age differences between populations are discounted, males in Bournemouth in 1971 had an SMR of 90, whereas England and Wales had, by definition, an SMR of 100. Hence Bournemouth had a 10 per cent lower (age standardised) death rate (SMR) than England and Wales.

The example in Box 11.3 is an SMR for deaths from all causes. But SMRs can be calculated for particular causes of death (see Figure 11.2). However, deaths per year, even for the most common causes, are rare in small populations, and hence vulnerable to large chance fluctuations. In their paper in Chapter 9, Payne and Saul use the SMRs for electoral wards for deaths from coronary heart disease in ages 35–64. To produce large enough figures they have to use deaths over a 5-year period. Standardised *morbidity* ratios are also possible, allowing for age standardised comparisons of rates of illness. Those for angina are cited in Chapter 9. The Bournemouth example above is calculated for the population of an area, but it might be calculated for a sub-group of a population: males, African Caribbean males, African

Box 11.3 Age standardised mortality ratio (SMR) calculations

Table 11.4 Calculating a standardised mortality ratio for Bournemouth, 1971

Age groups	A Male population: Bournemouth (000s)	B Male death rates for reference population[a] (deaths per 1,000)	C (A × B) Expected male deaths[b]	D Actual deaths for Bournemouth
Under 1	0.74	19.78	15	We don't need to
1–4	2.93	0.76	2	know the actual
5–14	8.38	0.40	3	number of deaths
15–24	8.83	0.92	8	for each age group
25–44	13.41	1.62	22	for this calculation
45–64	18.36	13.45	247	
65–74	8.23	51.82	426	
75+	4.64	137.42	638	
All ages	65.52		1,361	1,223

[a] The reference population here is England and Wales.
[b] If Bournemouth had the same death rates for each age group as the reference population (England and Wales).

Source: Based on Open University, 1975: 24

The SMR (males: Bournemouth: all ages: all causes)

$$= \frac{\text{Total actual male deaths}}{\text{Total expected male deaths}} \times 100$$

$$= \frac{1,223}{1,361} \times 100 = 89.86 = 90.00 = 10 \text{ per cent below average.}$$

Caribbean males living alone, and so on. The Bournemouth figures are also calculated for all adults, but often what is of interest is not death, which happens to everyone sooner or later, but premature death, which happens more often to men, compared with women, and poorer people compared to richer people. Usually this is expressed as death before the age of 60 or 65.

The two predominant factors setting the death rate for a population are age and social class. Gender is rarely important in making differences between areas, since most areas have similar ratios of males to females *within* each age group, but gender might be an important consideration in comparing death rates in two hospitals. Ethnicity seems rarely to be important in making a difference to the death rates of different areas once gender, age and socio-economic circumstances are accounted for (Smaje, 1995; Nazroo, 1997a). Thus, in making com-

Figure 11.2   Standardised mortality ratios for coronary heart disease (CHD) and social class, England and Wales 1979–80 and 1982–3 (Department of Health, 1995: 104; Office for National Statistics © Crown copyright 1995)

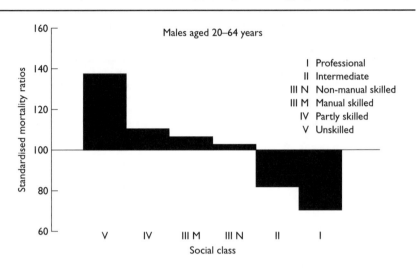

parisons between areas, once age is controlled through age standard-isation, what differences there are are largely caused by social class differences between populations. The death rate in Bournemouth, after age standardisation, is lower than the average SMR, reflecting mainly that Bournemouth has a more affluent social class profile than England and Wales as a whole.

SMRs are often used to show social class differences, as in Figure 11.2.

The data for calculating SMRs come ultimately from the process of death certification. Studies show that ascertaining cause of death in practice is a very unreliable process, insofar as different doctors will assign different causes of death to the same case (Bloor et al., 1987, 1989; Bloor, 1991, 1994). The SMR deaths from all causes can be regarded with more confidence than the SMR for deaths from particu-lar causes, and the more precise the diagnosis the less reliable the figures are likely to be. There is evidence also that particular doctors have their own favourite causes of death and that particular causes become and cease to be fashionable over a period of time (Bloor et al., 1987, 1989). SMRs for suicide are a particularly problematic matter since the ascertainment of suicide as the cause of death is itself so problematic. Differences in suicide rates between different areas, or occupational groups within a country may owe much to the idiosyn-crasies of particular coroners, and differences between countries may relate to differences in the medico-legal procedures of investigating and classifying 'unnatural' deaths (Atkinson et al., 1975).

In addition, death certification also provides the demographic data for an SMR. The sex and age of the deceased will most likely be accurately recorded, but recording the occupation of the deceased is less straightforward. It is on the basis of this that SMRs for social classes are calculated (Figure 11.2). For example, it has been shown that some 'notable' occupations are likely to be given as the last occupation of the deceased, even if this was not his or her last occupation. These include police officer, miner and fisherman. This means that occupations of these sorts – and the social classes to which they are allocated – will show death rates in the statistics higher than those in reality. Overall there is a tendency for those kinsfolk who register deaths to elevate the occupation of the deceased, thus leading to the production of statistics which under-record the link between low social class and age of death (Bloor et al., 1989). Social class SMRs for women are particularly quirky, since it may be a woman's own or her husband's occupation which is recorded on the death certificate (Moser and Goldblatt, 1985).

Ethnicity as such is not recorded at death and researchers have to make do with the recording of place of birth and nationality which are very poor guides to ethnicity (Nazroo, 1997a). Hence SMRs comparing people from different ethnic groups are difficult to produce from death certification data and have to be derived from specially mounted research projects.

4   Deprivation indices

SMRs for age groups 16–65 (or 20–60) are sometimes used as a *deprivation indicator* for an area since premature death correlates so closely with socio-economic conditions. The deprivation *index* of an area is a single score derived from combining scores for a number of deprivation indicators. The indicators are measures such as unemployment rates, percentages of unfit houses, percentages of households dependent on benefits, age-adjusted death rates and so on, all widely regarded as indicative of the poverty or affluence of a population. One of the simpler deprivation indices is the *Townsend index* which uses just four indicators: unemployment rates, car ownership, percentage of households owner-occupied and household overcrowding (Townsend et al., 1985). However many *indicators* are used, each produces a 'league table' of areas running from the most affluent to the most deprived. A deprivation *index* combines these into a single composite league table of affluence and deprivation (see Table 11.5).

Deprivation indices are very widely used in both research and in health and welfare administration. Differences in socio-economic conditions between areas are an important research topic in their own right (Noble et al., 1994). But, in addition, illness and social problems

Table 11.5 Deprivation indices and other deprivation indicators and socio-demographic indicators for areas of Barking and Havering: rates of death by selected causes, accident rates, selected morbidity rates and Health of the Nation Targets

| | Localities in | | | | | | |
| | Barking | | | Havering | | | |
Socio-demographic indicators	1st	2nd	3rd	4th	5th	6th	7th
Rank order for Jarman score, 1991 1st = most deprived	1st	2nd	3rd	4th	5th	6th	7th
Jarman score, 1991	39.1	16.3	15.5	6.9	-2.3	-4.2	-13.3
Jarman score, 1981	31.1	6.5	9.5	-2.5	-2.7	-4.2	-16.9
Townsend score, 1991	5.48	2.08	2.81	0.17	-2.12	-2.25	-4.19
Per cent population over 75, 1991	5.8	7.8	7.7	6.8	6.5	5.1	6.4
Per cent population over 85, 1991	1.2	1.6	1.5	1.1	1.4	0.9	1.5
Per cent non-white ethnic groups, 1991	16	4.6	4.3	2.3	3.5	4.1	2.6
Per cent households at >1 person per room, 1991	4.1	3.6	4.3	2.5	1.8	1.7	0.9
Per cent households owner-occupied, 1991	36.8	57.6	54.0	62.7	79.6	81.6	88.7
Per cent households in local authority/housing association tenure, 1991	57.7	37.9	42.8	33.0	14.4	14.7	5.5
Unemployment, 1991 (census definition)	10.3	7.0	7.3	6.4	5.4	5.4	3.9
Per cent households no car, 1991	51.1	39.6	41.6	32.7	26.0	25.6	20.2

Mortality rates (rates per 100,000 of relevant age group)	National Rates 1990	National targets 2000							
Ischaemic heart disease: ages 0–64, 1987–91	58.0	35.00	71.1	63.2	68.4	55.0	49.6	61.5	38.6
Ischaemic heart disease: ages 65–74	899.0	629.0	1078.2	973.9	1005.0	958.8	750.0	843.2	865.2
Stroke, ages 0–64, 1987–91	12.5	7.5	12.3	11.2	13.9	13.2	10.7	12.1	6.8
Stroke, ages 65–74, 1987–91	265.0	159.0	289.9	210.4	279.8	252.8	203.0	244.6	158.7
Lung cancer, ages 0–74 (males), 1987–91	60.0	42.0	72.0	85.5	78.2	78.3	50.6	62.3	39.9
Lung cancer, ages 0–74 (females), 1987–91	24.1	20.5	26.4	29.9	24.0	26.5	18.5	27.0	15.8
Suicide rate, all ages, 1987–91	11.1	9.4	12.3	12.0	8.7	11.7	7.9	10.2	8.2
Accident rate, ages under 15, 1987–91	6.7	4.5	6.5	3.9	11.5	7.1	6.2	9.8	6.5
Accident rate, ages 15–24, 1987–91	23.2	17.4	12.5	13.9	19.6	26.0	23.3	16.5	23.6
Accident rate, ages 65 and over, 1987–91	56.7	38.0	52.8	26.1	27.8	34.2	31.8	40.4	32.6
Cirrhosis males, ages 55–74, 1987–91	18.8	—	26.5	11.0	18.6	15.4	12.2	4.0	12.9
Infant mortality, 1983–92 (per 1,000 live births)	7.9	—	12.3	8.1	8.4	6.8	7.0	7.5	5.4
Hospital admissions per 100,000 of relevant age group									
Asthma, ages 0–14, 1991–3	593		498.6	700.7	458.9	777.5	534.5	550.1	557.9
Diabetes, ages 15–64	85.5		597.2	91.1	53.5	69.5	64.4	45.4	49.5
Dementia, ages 65+, 1991–3	544		567	418	404.7	624	376.4	373.5	416.3

Source: Based on Congdon, 1995: Tables 1 and 2: 1185–6

are so closely associated with an area's affluence or deprivation that knowing its rank order in a deprivation league table is a good basis for predicting the extent and kinds of illness and handicap likely in the area, its crime rate and so on. In turn this means that a deprivation index is also a proxy measure of the pressure on health and social services and of the need for services. The study by Payne and Saul in Chapter 9 is an example of this kind of usage.

Table 11.5 gives a picture of the way in which indices (in this case the Townsend and the Jarman-8) predict differences in mortality rates and hospital admissions. The localities in this table are not administrative territories, but areas composed such that each is fairly homogeneous in terms of its deprivation or affluence (Congdon, 1995). For some causes of death the indicators are good predictors. This can be seen to some extent without statistical analysis where rank order on the index is the same as rank order for rates of death from particular causes. For example, on Table 11.5 the rank order of areas for the Townsend index comes very close to accurately predicting the rank order of areas for ischaemic heart disease 0–64 and stroke 65–74, and the Jarman index is a fairly good predictor of these as well. Or again, locality 5 in Havering has a just below national average deprivation score. Comparing its death rates with those for England and Wales, shows that it has just below average death rates as well. For other conditions the predictive ability of these indices is less good, because differences between areas in terms of age or ethnicity complicate the picture. For example, Locality 1 in Barking has a massively higher rate of hospital admissions for diabetes than all the other areas, much higher than might be explained by differences in social deprivation, even though it is the most deprived locality in the table. Most ethnic minorities of colour have higher rates of diabetes than do white people and some difference remains even after controlling for the effects of social deprivation (Nazroo, 1997a). Table 11.5 also shows that Locality 1 in Barking has the highest percentage of minority ethnic people.

Deprivation indices are used in the following ways:

- Charting change in affluence or deprivation in an area between two points in time using the same index (for example Green, 1994; Phillimore et al., 1994).
- Charting the effects of government policy on poverty in terms of changes in index scores (Green, 1994; Phillimore et al., 1994).
- Investigating the relationship between deprivation and ill-health, or deprivation and social problems such as children at risk or crime (Townsend et al., 1985; Jarman et al., 1992; Abbott et al., 1992).
- Prioritising areas for expenditure in the local strategic planning of services (Congdon, 1995; see also Chapter 9 of this volume).

- Evaluating the availability of services between localities to judge whether those with greatest need are offered greatest provision (see Chapter 9).
- Weighting central government funding for local authorities, health authorities and primary health care to adjust it to differences of socio-economic circumstances (Judge and Mays, 1994; Senior, 1991).
- Setting or interpreting service performance indicators so that agency performance can be judged in terms of local socio-economic circumstances (see Box 11.4).

Studying deprivation at first hand would be prohibitively expensive for the purposes above, and for these purposes it is important to use a common scale of deprivation. This is especially so when fairness of treatment has to be demonstrated, as with the use of a deprivation index to weight the allocation of central government funding. Thus the data for such indicators are either drawn from bureaucratic data sets, such as welfare benefits data, or drawn from the 10-year censuses. The cheapness and availability of data for calculating a deprivation index are also important for applying research findings to another area. For example, many diseases show a close relationship with poverty (see Table 11.5 and Chapter 9). The results of a study demonstrating this which cites area deprivation indices can be extrapolated to another area with a similar deprivation index figure (making some adjustments for the age profile of the area as well – see section 1). Accuracy here cannot be guaranteed, but such extrapolation is more likely to be accurate than one from a study which makes vague comments about the 'poverty' of an area, to another area where people have different ideas about what 'poverty' means and different ways of measuring it. Extrapolation on this basis may be less easy with the Townsend index. This is because the scores on this index are calculated as deviations from the average for the overall area being studied, and standardised into so-called *z-scores* (Abbott et al., 1992). If the original study was about deprivation in the North East of England, then deprivation scores for the North East cannot be equated directly with scores for other areas of England. Typically, studies using Townsend scores cite their results for percentiles of the local area: for example, 'most deprived 10 per cent of wards', 'next most deprived 10 per cent of wards' and so on. Payne and Saul in Chapter 9, for example, contrast the poorest 30 per cent of wards with the most affluent 30 per cent of wards. What are the most deprived 30 per cent in one area, according to the Townsend index, may be more or less deprived than the most deprived 30 per cent in another. The index figures from most other deprivation indices, by contrast, mean the same wherever they are applied (Jarman, 1983).

For any practitioner in England, the index score for one of the major deprivation indices is readily available. This is the 1998 Index of Local Deprivation which is available for every local authority and local health authority in England based on 12 indicators, and available for every ward and census enumeration district for four indicators. (Department of the Environment, Transport and the Regions, 1998).

Different indices are used for different purposes. In research, the two most commonly used are the Townsend index, which features in Chapter 9, and the Jarman Under-Privileged Area (UPA) Score (see Table 11.5). The Jarman comes in two versions: the Jarman-8 and the Jarman-10, depending on how many separate indicators are combined for the final index figure (Jarman, 1983; Jarman et al., 1992). The Jarman-8 is also used by central government to calculate deprivation payments for GP practices in deprived areas (Senior, 1991). For adjusting health authority/board funding to socio-economic circum-stances yet a different index is used (Judge and Mays, 1994). And yet another, the Index of Local Deprivation, referred to above, is used to adjust the Standard Spending Assessment which determines central government funding for social services, housing and education in England. The other nations of the UK have various but similar kinds of deprivation-weighted funding.

The different indices have their own strengths and weaknesses. On the whole the Jarman index has proved to be both a sensitive predictor of disease patterns and to produce results which can be generalised from one area to another. Partly because of its simplicity, the Townsend index has been used most often to investigate geo-graphical patterns and temporal changes in inequality within an area. The indices chosen for administrative purposes are based on indica-tors which seem best to reflect the demand for services in a local area, different facets of deprivation having different implications for gen-eral practice, health authority expenditure and social work.

Different indices rank areas differently; compare the Jarman and the Townsend indices in Table 11.5 for example. This can have implica-tions worth tens of millions of pounds of income from central govern-ment. Unsurprisingly, the appropriateness, accuracy and fairness of the indices used for administrative purposes is a highly controversial matter. The controversy is heightened by the fact that so many components of these indices derive from census data which is collected only once in each 10-year period. There is a rural/urban dimension to controversy here. In rural areas poverty is often 'hidden' in small pockets in otherwise affluent areas and hence not reflected in the area's deprivation index figure (Abbott et al., 1992). While this is much less true of index figures for rural wards and enumeration districts, deprivation data at this smaller level are less available. What there is, is more dependent on census data and hence more likely to be out of date. But because it includes car ownership, the Townsend index is considered a more sensitive indicator of rural poverty.

Deprivation indices are predictors, either of the prevalence of diseases and social problems, or of the need for services in an area. What components go into a deprivation index and how different components are weighted to get the final score, has been arrived at by a long period of trial and error to see which particular combination best predicts differences between areas in terms of premature death, poverty-related disease, educational under-achievement, or crime rates. Hence they are validated by how accurately the index predicts – construct validity in terms of Chapter 6, section 7. For example, the Jarman index has been widely used in research on the need for mental health services. It seems to be a good predictor of the number of admissions to mental hospital at a district (though not at a ward) level. The higher the Jarman score, the higher the number of admissions (Jarman et al., 1992; Harrison et al., 1995). And again, the Jarman index has been validated as a predictor of GP workload: the higher the index score, the greater the pressure on GP surgeries (Senior, 1991).

The major problem in using deprivation indices comes from their reliance on census data. This means that their base data become increasingly out of date between census publication dates. This is particularly true of the Townsend index, which is entirely based on census data. There is a considerable degree of continuity in area poverty and affluence between censuses. The poorest areas in 1981 were usually the poorest areas in 1991 (Green, 1994). But inevitably there is much small-scale change in rank ordering and occasionally some more extensive changes. For example, with the expansion of higher education in the 1990s, some deprived inner urban areas have changed from housing poor families to housing students. The latter may not be affluent, but they certainly have different patterns of disease and social problems compared with the populations displaced.

Social fragmentation or *anomie indices* are similar to deprivation indices in using easily available data to predict problems or needs for services, but selected as a closer reflection of social exclusion or lack of community capacity; for example, numbers of single person households (Congdon, 1996), or non-participation in voting (Whitley et al., 1999). Such indices have been claimed to be better predictors of suicide than deprivation indices *per se*. It is almost certainly the case that each kind of illness, disability, social problem or service demand would be best predicted from its own custom-built deprivation or social fragmentation index. However, having separate indices for predicting separate problems would undermine the main functions of these indices which are:

- to serve as a general purpose predictor of the extent of need for services broadly defined;

Evaluating Research in Health and Social Care

- as a simple measure of inequality in order to demonstrate causal links between patterns of inequality and patterns of ill-health;
- as a basis for adjusting epidemiological data given for a reference area (see Section 2 above) to the socio-economic realities of a particular area. For example, while the national annual prevalence of psychosis might be 4/1,000 (Meltzer et al., 1995), it is likely to be twice if not three times this in an area with a high deprivation score (Harrison et al., 1995).

For reasons of expediency, the fewer the components of an index the better. Sometimes, as noted, the Standardised Mortality Ratio (SMR) is used as a single indicator index. For global comparisons infant mortality rates are often used as a single indicator index of national poverty and affluence, but infant deaths in the UK are now so rare that they are a poor discriminator of differences between areas within the UK, unless accumulated over a 10-year period. Kammerling and O'Connor (1993) have claimed that unemployment rates are almost as accurate predictors of mental health needs as the Jarman-8. For each index there comes a point where adding another component makes very little difference to the way areas are ranked. For example, the 1998 Index of Local Deprivation has no component taking account of the ethnic composition of populations. However, adding such a component makes very little difference to the rank ordering of areas by deprivation. Because people from minority ethnic backgrounds tend to be concentrated in poorer areas, other measures of area deprivation already put areas with large minority ethnic populations towards the top of the deprivation league table.

For planning purposes, deprivation indices and indicators are particularly powerful tools when incorporated into geographical information systems. These are software packages which allow for matters such as clients, diagnoses, accidents, burglaries and so on to be mapped to their location, usually to post code areas (Noble and Smith, 1994). The Office of Population, Censuses and Surveys is able to provide deprivation data for post codes which then map onto the enumeration districts of the census.

Insofar as deprivation indices are proxy measures of need for services, they are also useful for interpreting agency performance. This is the point of the study in Chapter 9. Box 11.4 provides another example.

Table 11.5 also provides some target figures: those derived from the Health of the Nation strategy. But these take no account of local differences in deprivation (nor do they take much account of age differences between areas). This raises a question of whether it is appropriate to set the same targets for improving health for different areas irrespective of their affluence or deprivation. As Table 11.5 shows, for many conditions the most affluent localities were already much closer to

Box 11.4   Comparing service expenditure with need using a deprivation index as a proxy measure of need

Figure 11.3 comes from an Audit Commission report on adult mental health services. It would have been prohibitively expensive for the Audit Commission to investigate the need for mental health services directly. Instead, they used the well-demonstrated high correlation between deprivation and need for mental health services in order to judge whether London health districts were allocating resources commensurate with need. The horizontal axis differentiates districts according to their score on the Jarman UPA index (high score = high deprivation). The vertical axis measures expenditure on mental health services *per head* of the population, thus standardising for different district population sizes. If the differences in district spend were commensurate with differences in district need then all the dots should cluster around a diagonal line running from bottom left to top right. There is actually very little relationship between need and spend. The same exercise might be done for spending on child protection services, drug and alcohol services and most other health services, insofar as in each case a deprivation index score differentiates areas in terms of need for services.

Figure 11.3   Expenditure on mental health services and need for mental health services: need estimated in terms of the Jarman-8 Underprivileged Area Index: London Health Districts (Audit Commission, 1994: 12 'Exhibit 6'; Crown copyright, reproduced with permission)

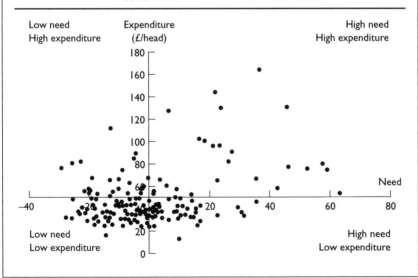

meeting the targets for AD 2000 than the poorer ones. In this case these are not the kinds of localities for which Health of the Nation targets are set, but the table does illustrate the fact that where a

Primary Care Group area has a population a large percentage of which has the characteristics like Localities 1, 2 and 3, it will find it much more difficult to meet the targets than one where more of the population is like those in Localities 6 and 7. Central government tends to take the line that because poorer areas receive more resources, this compensates them for their greater deprivation, and hence that standard national targets are appropriate for all authorities. Authorities way below target usually argue that additional resources do not compensate them enough, or that the extent of their deprivation has been under-estimated. The issue of how far it is reasonable to assume that service activity is able to overcome the effects of deprivation at given levels of expenditure is a matter for economic research of the cost-effectiveness kind (see Chapter 3).

Important questions to ask about studies using deprivation indices include the following:

- For what purpose is the index being used, and has it been validated for that purpose?

Some such studies will themselves be validation studies. Chapter 6 of this volume is relevant here.

- What are the component indicators of the index? How are they weighted to get the final score and how out of date are they?

And for the purpose of applying the results from a study in one place to a practice area:

- Are data available for calculating the score for the local area on the same index? If so, findings about the relationship between deprivation, disease, social problems or need for services elsewhere can be extrapolated to the local area.
- And if so, how accurate is the local index likely to be? Being based on out-of-date data is the major problem, but there are also difficulties of extrapolating from urban areas to rural ones and vice versa.

5 Further reading on age standardisation and deprivation indices

For age standardisation and SMRs, see Jones and Moon (1987: Chapter 2), or Unwin et al. (1997: 32–5) or Marsh (1988) (various chapters). For examples of the use of SMRs in relating ill health to social class, see Townsend, Davidson and Whitehead (1992). For deprivation indices a classic paper is Jarman (1983), which describes the development of the Jarman UPA index. Abbott et al. (1992), Phillimore et al. (1994) and Townsend et al. (1985, 1988) are all examples of the use of deprivation indices as research tools, as is Payne and Saul in Chapter 9 of this volume. Congdon's use of a social fragmentation index is also worth reading about (1996).

References and further reading

Abbott, P., Bernie, J., Payne, G. and Sapsford, R. (1992) 'Health and material deprivation in Plymouth', in P. Abbott and R. Sapsford (eds) *Research into Practice: a Reader for Nurses and the Caring Professions.* Buckingham: Open University Press. pp. 129–55.

Atkinson, M., Kessell, N. and Dalgaard, J. (1975) 'The comparability of suicide rates', *British Journal of Psychiatry*, 127: 427–56.

Audit Commission (1994) *Finding a Place: a Review of Adult Mental Health Services.* London: HMSO.

Benzeval, M., Judge, K. and Whitehead, M. (1995) *Tackling Inequalities in Health: an Agenda for Action.* London: King's Fund.

Bloor, M. (1991) 'A minor office: the variable and socially constructed character of death certification in a Scottish city', *Journal of Health and Social Behaviour*, 32: 273–87.

Bloor, M. (1994) 'On the conceptualisation of routine medical decision-making: death certification as an habitual activity', in M. Bloor and P. Taraborrelli (eds), *Qualitative Studies in Health and Medicine.* Aldershot: Avebury Ashgate Publishing. pp. 96–109.

Bloor, M., Robertson, C., and Samphier, M. (1989) 'Occupational status variations in disagreements on the diagnosis of causes of death', *Human Pathology*, 30: 144–8.

Bloor, M., Samphier, M., and Prior, L. (1987) 'Artefact explanations of inequalities in health: an assessment of the evidence', *Sociology of Health and Illness*, 9(3): 231–64.

Congdon, P. (1995) 'Localities for epidemiological monitoring and health policy', *Urban Studies*, 32 (7): 1175–98.

Congdon, P. (1996) 'Suicide and parasuicide in London: a small area study', *Urban Studies*, 33: 137–58.

Cooper, J., Goodhead, D., Craig, T., Harris, M., Howat, J. and Korer, J. (1987) 'The incidence of schizophrenia in Nottingham', *British Journal of Psychiatry*, 151: 619–26.

Department of the Environment, Transport and the Regions (1998) *Index of Local Deprivation.* London: DETR.

Department of Health (1993) *Health of the Nation: Key Area Handbook: Mental Illness.* London: Department of Health.

Department of Health (1995) *Variations in Health: What Can the Department of Health and the NHS Do? Report Produced by the Variations Sub-group of the Chief Medical Officer's Health of the Nation Working Group.* London: Department of Health.

Department of Health and Social Services (Northern Ireland) (1982) *Northern Ireland Census 1981.* Belfast: HMSO.

Fernando, S. (1988) *Race and Culture in Psychiatry.* London: Croom Helm.

Giggs, J. and Cooper, J. (1987) 'Ecological structure and the distribution of schizophrenia and affective psychoses in Nottingham', *British Journal of Psychiatry*, 151: 627–33.

Gomm, R. (1996) 'Mental health and inequality', in T. Heller, J. Reynolds, R. Gomm, R. Muston and S. Pattison (eds), *Mental Health Matters: A Reader.* Basingstoke: Macmillan. pp. 110–20.

Green, A. (1994) *The Geography of Poverty and Wealth: Evidence on the Changing Spatial Distribution and Segregation of Poverty and Wealth from the Census of Population 1991 and 1981.* Warwick: Institute for Employment Research.

194   *Evaluating Research in Health and Social Care*

Hall, J. and Dornan, M. (1990) 'Patient sociodemographic characteristics as predictors of satisfaction with medical care: a meta-analysis', *Social Science and Medicine*, 30: 811–18.

Harrison, J., Barrow, S. and Creed, F. (1995) 'Social deprivation and psychiatric admission rates among different diagnostic groups', *British Journal of Psychiatry*, 167: 456–62.

Jarman, D. (1983) 'Identification of underprivileged areas', *British Medical Journal*, 286: 1705–79.

Jarman, B., Hirsh, S., White, P. and Driscoll, R. (1992) 'Predicting psychiatric admission rates', *British Medical Journal*, 304: 1146–51.

Jones, K. and Moon, G. (1987) *Health, Disease and Society: an Introduction to Medical Geography*. London: Routledge and Kegan Paul.

Judge, K. and Mays, N. (1994) 'Allocating resources for health and social care in England', *British Medical Journal*, 308: 1363–6.

Kammerling, R., and O'Connor, S. (1993) 'Unemployment rate as a predictor of psychiatric admission', *British Medical Journal*, 307: 1536–9.

King, M., Coker, E., Leavey, G., Hoare, A. and Johnson-Sabine, E. (1994) 'Incidence of psychotic illness in London: comparison of ethnic groups', *British Medical Journal*, 306: 1115–19.

London Research Centre (1992) *Census Research Information Notes 92–93*. London: LRC.

Marsh, C. (1988) *Exploring Data: an Introduction to Data Analysis for Social Scientists*. Cambridge: Polity Press.

McGovern, D. and Cope, R. (1987) 'First admission rates for first and second generation Afro-Caribbeans', *Social Psychiatry*, 22, 139–49.

Meltzer, D. (1992) *Dementia: Epidemiology Based Needs Assessment: Report No. 5*. London: Department of Health.

Meltzer, D., Gill, B., Petticrew, M. and Hills, K. (1995) *The Prevalence of Psychiatric Disorders Among Adults Living in Private Households*. OPCS Surveys of Psychiatric Morbidity in Great Britain. Report No. 1. London: HMSO.

Moser, K. and Goldblatt, P. (1985) *Mortality of Women in the OPCS Longitudinal Study: Differentials by Own Occupation and Household and Housing Characteristics: Working Paper No. 26*. London: Social Statistics Research Unit, City University.

NHS Management Executive (1993) *Local Target Setting: a Discussion Paper*. London: Department of Health.

Nazroo, J. (1997a) *The Health of Britain's Ethnic Minorities*. London: Policy Studies Institute.

Nazroo, J. (1997b) *Ethnicity and Mental Health: Findings from a National Community Survey*. London: Policy Studies Institute.

Noble, P. and Smith, T. (1994) 'Children in need: using geographical information systems to inform strategic planning for social services provision', *Children and Society*, 8 (4): 360–76.

Noble, M., Smith, G., Avenall, D., Smith, T. and Sharland, E. (1994) *Changing Patterns of Income and Wealth in Oxford and Oldham*. Oxford: Department of Applied Social Studies and Social Research, University of Oxford.

Open University (1975) *Data Collection Procedures*. Milton Keynes: Open University Press.

Phillimore, P., Beattie, A. and Townsend, P. (1994) 'Widening inequality in health in Northern England 1981–91', *British Medical Journal*, 308: 1125–8.

Senior, M. (1991) 'Deprivation payments to GPs', *Environment and Planning*, 9: 79–94.

Smaje, C. (1995) *Health, 'Race' and Ethnicity: Making Sense of the Evidence*. London: King's Fund.

Stevens, A. and Raftery, J. (1994) *Health Care Needs Assessment: the Epidemiological Needs Reviews*. Oxford: Radcliffe Medical Press.

Townsend, P., Davidson, N. and Whitehead, M. (eds)(1992) *Inequalities in Health: the Black Report and the Health Divide*, new edition. Harmondsworth: Penguin Books.

Townsend, P., Phillimore, P. and Beattie, A. (1988) *Health and Deprivation: Inequality in the North*. Beckenham: Croom Helm.

Townsend, P., Simpson, P. and Tibbs, N. (1985) 'Inequalities in the City of Bristol: a preliminary review of the statistical evidence', *International Journal of Health Services*, 15: 637–43.

Unwin, N., Carr, S., Leeson, J. with Pless-Mulloli, T. (1997) *An Introductory Guide to Public Health and Epidemiology*. Buckingham: Open University Press.

Whitley, E., Gunnell, D., Dorling, D. and Davey Smith, G. (1999) 'Ecological study of social fragmentation, poverty and suicide', *British Medical Journal*, 319: 1034–7.

QUALITATIVE RESEARCH

CHAPTER 12

LOOSELY STRUCTURED INTERVIEWS: THE STORIES BEHIND THE STATISTICS

Blaxter, Mildred (1993) 'Why do the victims blame themselves?', from Radley, A. (ed.), *Worlds of Illness: Biographical and Cultural Perspectives on Health and Disease*. London: Routledge. pp. 124–42

EXEMPLAR

What you need to understand in order to understand the exemplar
What questionnaire researchers are trying to achieve by 'forcing' responses to questions – structuring the data prior to collection, and by adopting a standardised way of administering a survey. *See Chapter 10, section 14 and Chapter 16, section 1*
What problems the above give rise to and how loosely structured interviews are seen to solve them. *See Chapter 16, Section 2*
The meaning and procedures of the 'thematic analysis' of qualitative data. *See Chapter 16, section 2*
The kinds of generalisation which qualitative studies can produce. *See Chapter 16, section 8*
For any terms which are unfamiliar, try the index.

Introduction

With interviews that involve a questionnaire there is usually a pre-scribed order for asking the questions, and a prescribed wording for asking them, and only such matters as are already included in the questionnaire get recorded. This means that to a considerable extent the responses are already shaped before any respondent actually answers a question. For a loosely structured (or 'in-depth') interview the researcher will typically have a list of topics which the interview is supposed to cover, but latitude to ask about them in any way and in any order that seems appropriate, and the researcher will feel free to follow up previously unpredicted but interesting lines of enquiry. Such an open-ended approach then generates data which have to be organised after the interviews have been conducted.

The exemplar for this chapter provides a contrast between questionnaire research on the one hand and loosely structured interviewing on the other. The author, Mildred Blaxter, was one of the team involved in the large-scale Great Britain Health and Lifestyle questionnaire survey. With a large representative sample this was able to produce reliable generalisations about patterns of health-relevant beliefs and behaviours on the one hand, and patterns of morbidity and mortality on the other. However, while a questionnaire survey can gather data from a large and representative sample, it does this at the cost of only collecting small pieces of information from each respondent on each relevant topic. Typically, as in this case, most such data are in the form of yes/no/don't know or in the form of strong to weak agreements on a four- or five-point scale with statements provided in the questionnaire – a so-called Likert scale. Representative and reliable such responses might be, but what people mean by them can be puzzling. For every 'yes' and every 'no' to the same question there are almost certainly a variety of meanings. The loosely structured interview study reported by Blaxter investigates what respondents might mean by their responses on the Health and Lifestyle questionnaire to a question about whether people are personally responsible for their own state of health. The relevant page of the interviewer's instructions for asking questions is given as Figure 16.1 in Chapter 16. The exemplar also illustrates the thematic analysis of qualitative data (see Chapter 16, sections 2 and 6).

WHY DO THE VICTIMS BLAME THEMSELVES?

Mildred Blaxter

This investigation of what it means to say that 'the victims blame themselves' is presented as an example of the interaction of qualitative and quantitative methods. The question, raised by the inevitably superficial results of larger-scale surveys, is: Why do those who are most vulnerable to the environment seem to be most likely to stress self-blame for illness and self-responsibility for health? Can a biographical approach suggest some answers?

There are, of course, two perspectives on the determinants of illness, and especially the causes of social inequality in health: the idea that ill-health is primarily 'self-inflicted', and has behavioural causes, and the view that the major causes are structural and located in the environment. The extent to which people themselves subscribe to one view or the other is a topic which surveys often investigate, and though the alternatives are not necessarily mutually exclusive, the brief questions of surveys ('What is the cause of heart disease?', 'Do you think people are responsible for their own illnesses?'), perhaps with forced choice answers, tend to create dichotomies. One consistent finding is that although most people, of whatever social group, have learned very well the self-responsible lessons of health promotion, it is those who are most 'unequal' and most exposed to environmental risk who are least likely also to be aware of the structural perspective. Those who are in the lowest social classes, or have the least education, are most likely to confine their explanations to behavioural causes. The idea that the socially fortunate may be healthier is often flatly resisted.

The survey evidence

As evidence of this, a brief summary is offered of data deriving from the Health and Lifestyle Survey (Cox et al., 1987; Blaxter, 1990), a national sample survey, conducted by interviewers, of just over 9,000 respondents of all ages 18 and over. The design and analysis of the sections on beliefs and attitudes of this particular survey were strongly influenced by the experience of qualitative work. The relevant questions – about the causes of specific diseases, about the healthiness of the respondent's life and the perception of 'healthy' behaviour, about effects on health 'nowadays' for society in general, about the reasons for naming a 'healthy other person', and about attitudes to various health-related areas of life – were, deliberately, asked several times, in different contexts and in different ways, and almost always in open-ended format. Thus, the conclusions which follow are derived from the patterns of reply to many different questions throughout the survey schedule.

This method permitted the analysis to accommodate, in an imitation of qualitative methods, the sometimes contradictory and seemingly confused answers which any individual can produce on the complex subject of health. In particular, context was shown to be all-important. When the questions were about specific, named diseases, behavioural answers were overwhelmingly predominant: poor diet or lack of exercise could be the cause of almost any chronic disease. For ill-health in the abstract, considering 'what makes people unhealthy', voluntary behaviours were again primarily indicted, with little differentiation by social class or education. A surprising number of people asserted that more people smoked nowadays, compared with a generation ago, and illegal drugs received a perhaps undue emphasis. In the context of their own health and their own lives, rather fewer gave behavioural replies, as common sense might suggest: nevertheless, this was still the most popular form of answer: my life is unhealthy because I can't control my weight, because I smoke; it is healthy because I take exercise, because I watch my diet. [. . .]

It can be concluded, on the evidence of this one large-scale survey at least, that the lessons of public policy and health education – 'you are responsible for your health' – have been accepted, or at least that the population is aware of the 'correct' answers to give about the causes of health and ill-health. And, though it depends on the context in which the question is asked, it is those with higher incomes or better education who are also likely to be aware of the evidence of sociology and social epidemiology which stresses structural and environmental factors. [. . .]

The search for explanations

Why should this be so? There are possible explanations of a rather facile nature. It could be argued, for instance, that although this emphasis on the behavioural, as a taught response, has been generally very well learned, alternative or additional modes of explanation are more available to those who are better educated or more exposed to 'scientific' media presentations. The middle class are also more likely to belong to contemporary consumerist and environmentalist movements. It might also be suggested that these findings are no more than an artefact of method: the more articulate are more likely to give elaborate answers in the survey situation, and the less well educated or those without a ready vocabulary of abstract concepts are likely to seek the line of least resistance and give the easiest answers perceived to be the approved ones. Certainly, it was true in the Health and Lifestyle Survey that education of the respondent was, in general, clearly associated with the length of their open-ended replies or the number of different concepts that an individual expressed.

Are such explanations sufficient? If they are given time to express themselves in a situation less reminiscent of a 'test', is it true that those who are in the poorest social and economic circumstances are still least likely to place the blame for ill-health on their environment? And if it is, how do the disadvantaged, in fact, interpret the relationship between their health and the circumstances of their lives? To answer these questions, ideally, new and clearly focused research should be mounted. In the absence of this ideal, there is the possibility of an alternative strategy: to return to a re-analysis of the qualitative material which initially provided some of the themes guiding the analysis of the Health and Lifestyle Survey.

The qualitative data

The data referred to are long tape-recorded conversations with a group of 47 Scottish women of about 50 years old (Blaxter and Paterson, 1982). For other purposes of the study, they had been randomly selected from women who, at the time of their first childbearing 30 or so years before, were in social classes IV or V, and whose adult daughters lived in the same city and were still in the lowest social classes. Thus they belonged to families, neither geographically nor socially mobile, who were likely to have some generations of economic deprivation behind them: a group among whom the relationship between social circumstances and ideas about the cause of ill-health could be clearly tested. The data used here consist of inter-views, usually lasting for an hour and often much longer, in which the conversation was guided to cover the woman's health and health history, and her attitudes to illness, doctors and health services.

It must first be noted that the personal and family histories of the women demonstrated not only social deprivation in past generations, in their own child-hoods, and at the time of their childbearing (in the early 1950s), but also the very clear association of this deprivation with ill-health. As Herzlich and Pierret (1984) noted of their French respondents, 'the memory of the terrors of the past remained astonishingly vivid'. Diphtheria and scarlet fever had swept through families:

> Because I remember when I was taken away with scarlet fever. I mean, that night is as clear to me as though it happened last week. I wis only four, right enough, but I remember the hospital being packed wi' kids. My husband – there was him and his two brothers – the

three of them were taken out o' the house one night and my husband wasnae expected to come back. And after he did come back from the hospital he took it again. (G37)

Six of the 47 women had had TB, and several of their own children: one woman described how her son had caught TB from 'sharing a bed with a lodger, when he came home from sea – we didn't know he had it, you see'. A stark lack of adequate food, clothing and housing was described in the days before the Second World War:

> I always had sore throats, septic throats and that. Before I had diphtheria we stayed in an old house – my mother blamed that. We'd only one room and there was six o' us in one room, two beds in one room at that time. An' your sink was just on the stair an' outside was your toilet. (G3)

As young women in the 1950s their circumstances had been little better. Many husbands had been working away from home or otherwise absent, and almost all the women began married life either subletting crowded rooms from parents or other relatives, or renting crowded, damp slum property often without running water or inside sanitation. They represented themselves, at that time, as having little control over their fertility. Over half had conceived their first child before marriage, and twenty-nine of the forty-seven women had borne four or more children.

They were very conscious that part of the ill-health of the past had been due to an absence of medical services, and told many stories of not being able to afford or obtain care:

> When you had to pay for a doctor – well, to this day my mother still says that wa the reason I took rheumatic fever. Cos I took scarlet fever – and I was ill for a few days, and my mother took me to the dispensary. Now, I had to walk there, cos my mother didn't have the tramcar fare. With the result – I got my chill – we had to walk to the dispensary because it was free there, we couldn't afford to pull in a doctor. Cos my mother would have had the doctor in her house – well, at least twice a week, because she had eight of us. (G1)

[. . .] They were, however, very conscious that 'things had changed'. These family stories were usually told in the context of praise for the National Health Service, universally given credit (together with the 'medical advances' that had provided a cure for TB and, in their eyes, had been responsible for 'conquering' the childhood killers of the past) for major advances in health. One woman concluded by saying 'We hinna got that worry nowadays.'

Many of the women were of rural background. This acknowledgement of the effects of poverty produced some conflict with another strong and almost universal theme: the wish to present the days of their youth as in some sense 'healthier', with simple good food, fresh air and sensible living. This was an obvious appeal to a 'golden age' of the past, a response to all they disliked about modern life or all that irritated them about the way in which their grandchildren were brought up; in part, it represented the childhood memories of the rural as opposed to the urban, perhaps typical of a generation experiencing the period of rural depopulation. [. . .] At the same time, it would certainly be untrue to say that these women did not have a clear perception of the causes of their own specific, current chronic conditions lying in past circumstances. They seemed to be saying that their simple, healthy childhoods (leaving aside infectious disease, which was simply an ever-present but unavoidable danger, now removed by medical science) had provided them with a reserve of good health, better to withstand the attacks that later life circumstances might make. At the most difficult period of their lives, which most saw as their young married days, neglect of their own health had been inevitable. One woman was clear, for instance, about the cause of her long-term arthritis:

> Well, put it like this, when you've got young family you've got a lot of hard work. More so when you have five. It's nae easy work. And we'd nae washing machines, nae hot water, nae sink – well, we had a cold sink in the corner . . . there was a lot of hard work, there was stone floors. (G19)

Another had similar views about arthritis in her knees:

> Gaun aboot wi' auld shoes on – gaun aboot getting my feet soakin' – maybe, if I'd taken mair care o' mysel' earlier on. But wi' kids, no money for yoursel', you couldnae dae it. (G23)

Later, however, this same woman talked at length of the simple, austere upbringing of her own children, and explained how 'healthy' their childhoods had been by the same sort of reasoning that other women applied to their own childhoods:

> Well, my four was healthy. They was never pampered and wrapped up. They niver wore scarfs and hats in the winter time. They were jist out in a' weathers. And they jist ate a' thing that was going. And yet they were healthy.

To neglect their own health in the way they now admitted they had done meant that they were responsible, but on the other hand no one could have behaved differently:

> Three times in the city hospital with tuberculosis – I called it neglect. Well, I had pleurisy before my twins were born, and I cracked my ribs just before A. was born, and I had pleurisy, and I had naebody in, wi' six o' them, you know. And I had pleurisy, and there was naebody to look efter me, I just used to come an' get my poultice and heat it at the fire and put it back on. It was really neglect – my own – well, no my own fault, I had to look efter my bairns, you understand. (G7)

Many other women similarly struggled to reconcile a strong sense of self-responsibility with the conviction that all their health problems stemmed from childbearing and the difficult days of early motherhood. To present the process as one of self-sacrifice and 'good' motherhood was an obvious solution:

> When they were young, if I was ill, I couldn't afford to be ill and that was all there was to it. Because he was at sea and there was naebody. There wasn't anyone to watch the kids. If I was ill I still had to get up and work, you know – you couldn't be ill. (G25)

Immediate causes

This was all in the past, and things were different now. All the women felt themselves to be in at least 'comfortable' circumstances now. The privations of the 1950s were the bad old days, and now the NHS was available. In discussing their more recent illness, or the day-to-day fluctuations in their chronic conditions, the self-responsibility theme was paramount. A few complaints were ascribed to the environment, usually the weather or the immediate environment of their housing:

'dampness in these houses', 'the bedroom walls are running', 'there's something in this water'. Generally, these seemed to be expressions of dissatisfaction with their present house, in situations where they wanted to move and had perhaps got a 'doctor's line' in support of their application for different council housing. The women did not belong to more middle-class pure air or unadulterated food lobbies, and to complain about more general 'dangers of modern life' would have gone against their firm knowledge or conviction that living circumstances had improved. Nor did they perceive any dangers in over-medicalization, in any real way: many described how they 'didn't like pills' or criticized those who relied on them, but in fact they were observed to be very heavy users of prescriptions from their doctors. There were perhaps two exceptions to this trust of prescribed drugs: the contraceptive pill, and psychotropics. Both of these could be the cause of many problems. They were special, it seemed, because so intimately connected with the life events – marriage, childbearing, tragedies, growing older – which were the framework of their medical biographies.

Their working history – on the farms, or the cold, unpleasant work of fish processing when they were young, the hard work of hospitals, shops, and domestic service in later life – also represented both the hardships of their lives, and their strength in endurance. Work was also an important part of biography, and could be associated with the beginning of a variety of illnesses.

At a more superficial level, however, it was behavioural causes that were offered for almost every disease – certainly in the abstract, or in other people, but also for oneself. This seemed largely to be the recital of what they had been taught. Twenty-three of the forty-seven women suffered from chronic chest complaints, of this group twenty smoked, and all except one volunteered their smoking as a cause or at least a contributory factor. Lengthy reports were given of their interactions with doctors on the topic, in the course of which the women might express some degree of scepticism: 'If I did stop smoking I'd die of a heart attack overweight'; 'I've smoked since I was 14, so if there's anything going to happen it'll happen.' Nevertheless, at later points in the interview the association of smoking with bronchitis would always, and repeatedly, be ruefully acknowledged: 'that's smoking, of course', 'I'm breathless, I have to put it down to smoking'. Similar friction with doctors, spirited self-defences, but on the whole guilty agreement that it was their own fault, related to obesity. 'Blood pressure' was often the sufferer's own fault, for 'rushing around' or 'doing too much' and several other disease conditions were subject to discussion about 'what one had done' to get them: diabetes was described by more than one woman, for instance, as being caused by an over-fondness for sugar.

Health as biography

It thus seems that, if the women are considered as a group in this way, survey results are supported. Behaviour was the simplest 'public' answer to 'what is the cause of illness', the known 'expected' answer, and the one which they believed was medically authorized (Cornwell, 1984). To consider typical answers in this way, however, is largely to misrepresent the women's real thinking about cause. If, in a different manner of analysis, a single respondent's way of thinking is traced back and forwards throughout the hour or two of conversation, these answers are seen in context. In fact, nothing has one cause. Alternatives are tried out, rejected, associated with each other, traced from one period of life to another. Examples are given of different cases, and the different factors that might apply are reasoned out. An attempt is made to achieve that 'experiential coherence' (as distinct from abstract, theoretical coherence) which has been shown (e.g. Pinder, 1992) to be sought by those trying to interpret their own chronic disease. [. . .]

The women seek to answer the 'Why me? Why now?' questions in a way which, in Herzlich and Pierret's (1984) words, 'transcends the search for causes and becomes a quest for meaning'.

(*Editor's note*: The first example given by Blaxter is reprinted in Chapter 16, section 2.)

G19 – aged 43, five children

Major current problem is that she is waiting for a hysterectomy, 'I'm aye awfu' tired'. Ever since the fifth child (at 30) 'I've felt really tired and done.'	childbearing
Has also had bronchitis all her life. It 'comes back wi' the weather'. 'And of course I smoke.' It started with 'teething bronchitis' and runs through the family: 'My father had it, and my sister and myself, had it, and my daughter has it aff me, and her baby here, seven weeks old and it already has a whistle, so it must be taking it aff the mother.'	weather behaviour heredity
Returns to gynaecological problems. 'It's mental strain – and bringing up five kids is bound to leave something, I mean it's a' right for him [husband] – he gaed round the world when my kids was little, he cam home and put me pregnant and gaed awa' again!'	stress
Further talk of family history of chest problems, which leads to story of own mother's death from cancer.	heredity
Gynaecological problems: the state she is in is largely 'my ain fault' for not consulting earlier. 'It's jist anither phase of life. There's different things in life occurs, and you go on to anither phase of life. Me, I've come through all I've come through, it's only me I'm hurting now' (by neglect of health).	self-neglect life stage
Nevertheless 'healthy enough'. No reason to coddle self now. In comparison with days when children were young, life is easy. At that time she was almost overwhelmed with illness, but pulled herself through by her own efforts.	stress social circumstances
Returns to talk about mother. 'This is aye at the back o' my mind. Naebody kens until you're actually opened.'	some diseases unpredictable
Seems to retreat to talk again of bronchitis, which is more familiar and understandable: 'I mean, we're all made of an impression on our ancestors, arn't we? So if you've a weakness it must come out some way.'	heredity

One extended quotation is added from the respondent above, as an example of the lively, sophisticated and independent way in which the theme of stress and resentment as the cause of illness could be worked out. It also shows how, as Crawford (1984) noted, 'in the mind-over-matter formulation, one discipline is substituted for another': illness again becomes the sufferer's fault.

> When I wis bringin' up my kids, I was forever in at the doctor and I had like a chemist shop – I had tablets to mak' me sleep, I had tablets for heidaches, an' tablets for stomach aches, an' I just said tae mysel' tablets, tablets – I ta'en them a' an' I pit them in the bucket. I says, now they're nae helpin' me, I've got tae dae it mysel. So I got to work an' worked things oot mysel' . . . When I first got that heidaches, I thought I was goin' aff the heid. They put me to the [psychiatric hospital]. He [husband] says, 'You're a nut'. I says, 'Well, I'll be a nut, but I'll find out I am a nut, I'll ging to a psychiatrist.' A' they asked about was sex – well, it had nuthin' a'dee wi' sex. An' then it dawned on me fit it wis – the strain o' the kids were gettin' ower much for me an' I wis against him [husband] for aye bein' awa'! See? An' then, when things would crack up, I'd maybe smack them, for maybe little. I would sit doon an' greet – I shouldn't have hutten them. Ken? An' the heidaches would get worse an' worse – an' worse . . . Ken, gettin' tae ken things, has a lot to dee wi' it – ignorance is a lot tae dee wi' bad health. (G19)

Chains of cause

Several themes run throughout these accounts. First, there is the constant emphasis on life events, especially those identified with their female roles: childbearing, the care of elderly parents and their deaths, the menopause, widowhood, the deaths of children. Almost every chronic condition had its 'real' origins in one of these events. In particular, childbearing had been the crucial event: 'a woman's never the same after she's had children' was a popular aphorism.

These were all links in the chain of cause. A second notable feature of the accounts was the strain to connect, to present a health history as a chain of cause and effect, with each new problem arising from previous ones. There was a common concept of one disease 'going into' another, and many causes were sought in past injuries. A cough would 'go into' bronchitis, meningitis was caused by 'a knock', accidents many years before were blamed for arthritis. Accidents, like surgery, were assaults upon the body, unnatural breakings or openings which would leave it susceptible. Occasionally, disease might be seen as striking randomly: cancer is the most common example, though it must be noted that the reluctance to discuss cancer at length seemed also to be an expression of a taboo. Often the disease was not directly named, or the voice was dropped to a whisper. For most diseases, however, cause was not random. The women resisted the idea that one part of their body might have 'gone wrong' at one time, and another at another, without there being any connection. One thing must lead to another: there must be a logical biography.

These chains of cause stretched back through generations. Thus heredity and familial patterns were another pervasive theme in the talk of their own disease. In part, this was simply a natural human tendency towards 'pattern making', and, since families in the past had been large and certain diseases very prevalent, there was a high likelihood that if patterns were sought they could be found. Family weaknesses often lay in stomachs, or chests, or some other part of the body: 'They've all been bothered with their legs'. Alternatively, families could have some inherent strengths, resilience to certain types of condition. These discussions of family history, often very long, were commonly quite sophisticated, with the women working out in great detail exact degrees of relationship, the evidence of changes in environment (many older members of families had emigrated), or the different likelihoods of infection, direct inheritance, or 'susceptibility'. G37, for instance, explained:

> I think family traits have a habit o' – you know, cropping up. You might have a family that's prone to rheumatics. Rheumatics aren't infectious, but if it runs in a family, to me, you know, as it comes down the line, there's always going to be somebody that's sorta inclined to take that. In this climate . . .

This was set in the context of a recital of the lives and deaths of her own parents, siblings, and grandparents, and then of her husband's family. A digression considered the effects of voluntary lifestyles: her paternal grandfather died young, but he was a well-known drinker; on the other hand so did his father, 'and he was a very religious churchgoing man, he didn't smoke or drink'. The conclusion was:

> . . . families can be long-living families or short-living families. I think it must be something to do with the genes.

This fondness for familial 'explanations', as for connecting up the events of their lives, could be understood as a liking for continuity, a desire to give meaning to their lives. Their family histories, together with their own experiences, constituted their identity. Their present health status, including all the emerging problems of middle age, had to be accommodated into that identity.

Conclusion

In summary, it seems probable that if these women had been asked the brief direct questions of the Health and Lifestyle Survey, their answers would have been in accordance with the class patterns found. Illness was primarily one's own responsibility, not only at the superficial level of quickly offered survey responses, but also at a deeper level of claiming responsibility for one's own identity. They did not dwell on class inequalities because, though they were very conscious of the perils of the environment in the past, by contrast life seemed to be largely without such dangers now. They were perfectly capable of holding in equilibrium ideas which might seem opposed: the ultimate cause, in the story of the deprived past, of their current ill-health, but at the same time their own responsibility for 'who they were'; the inevitability of ill-health, given their biographies, but at the same time guilt if they were forced to 'give in' to illness. With this emphasis on selfhood and self-responsibility, and their knowledge of greatly improved general social circumstances, a rejection of ideas about (contemporary) 'inequality' was understandable.

Many such qualitative studies have shown that people reconstruct biomedical concepts, including those of aetiology, in the light of their own biographies. Perhaps sociologists and social epidemiologists may have to accept that their concepts, too, may have little reality at the level of individual perceptions.

References

Blaxter, M. (1985) 'Self-definition of health status and consulting rates in primary care', *Quarterly Journal of Social Affairs*, 1, 133–71.
Blaxter, M. (1990) *Health and Lifestyles*, London: Routledge.

Blaxter, M. and Paterson, E. (1982) *Mothers and Daughters*, London: Heinemann.

Calnan, M. (1987) *Health and Illness: The Lay Perspective*, London: Tavistock Publications.

Cornwell, J. (1984) *Hard-earned Lives: Accounts of Health and Illness from East London*, London: Tavistock Publications.

Cox, B.D., Blaxter, M. et al. (1987) *The Health and Lifestyle Survey. Preliminary Report*, London: Health Promotion Research Trust.

Crawford, R. (1984) 'A cultural account of "health": control, release and the social body', in J.B. McKinlay (ed.), *Issues in the Political Economy of Health Care*, London: Tavistock Publications.

Herzlich, C., and Pierret, J. (1984) *Illness and Self in Society*, Baltimore: Johns Hopkins University Press.

Pill, R. and Stott, N.C. (1985a) 'Prevention procedures and practices among working-class women: new data and fresh insights', *Social Science and Medicine*, 21: 975–83.

Pill, R. and Stott, N.C. (1985b) 'Choice or chance: further evidence on ideas of illness and responsibility for health', *Social Science and Medicine*, 20: 981–91.

Pill, R. and Stott, N.C. (1986) 'Looking after themselves: health protective behaviour among British working-class women', *Health Education Research*, 1: 111–19.

Pinder, R. (1992) 'Coherence and incoherence: doctors' and patients' perspectives on the diagnosis of Parkinson's Disease', *Sociology of Health and Illness*, 14: 1.

What you might do now

This study analysed qualitative data thematically, and assumed that what people said was evidence of their ways of making sense of their experiences. But there are other ways of analysing qualitative data, and different assumptions may be made as to what such data stand for. Read sections 5 and 6 of Chapter 16 and then reconsider Blaxter's data

⬆

Carry out a more systematic appraisal of the study using 'Questions to Ask about Qualitative Research' in Part 4 of this book

⬅ **What you might do now** ➡

⬇

Consolidate what you have learned about the relative strengths and weaknesses of questionnaire surveys on the one hand and loosely structured interview studies on the other by reading Chapters 10 and 16 and perhaps some of the further reading cited there

Use the Appendix to find some research of interest to you based on loosely structured interviews and appraise it using 'Questions to Ask about Qualitative Research' in Part 4 of this book

CHAPTER 13

NATURALISTIC OBSERVATION: MIDWIVES' ETHNIC STEREOTYPING OF THEIR PATIENTS

EXEMPLAR   Bowler, Isobel (1993) ' "They're not the same as us": midwives' stereotypes of South Asian descent maternity patients', *Sociology of Health and Illness*, 15 (2): 157–78

What you need to understand in order to understand the exemplar
What strengths a naturalistic observation study has over an interview study.   *See Chapter 16, Section 3*
The importance for readers of knowing what role the observer played in the setting observed; how it would make some things visible and not others.   *See Chapter 16, section 3*
The particular difficulty that observer researchers have in giving an account of their research to readers.   *See Chapter 16, section 7*
What it means to analyse data thematically.   *See Chapter 16, sections 2 and 6*
The issue of sympathetic bias in research.   *See Chapter 16, section 7*
The ethical issues of informing those studied of the uses to which the data will be put.   *See Chapter 16, section 3*
For any terms which are unfamiliar, try the index.

Introduction

The exemplar for this chapter is a report on a piece of non-participant observation research, though it included some pre-scheduled loosely structured interviews, and what Bowler calls 'natural interviews', by which she means that she asked questions and gained responses as and when opportunities arose in the course of the routine activities of the maternity unit she was studying. The major claim of any piece of naturalistic research is to give an account of how things normally happen, and that includes giving some attention to how the presence of an observer might have altered what there was to observe. It is not clear from the study as to how the people Bowler observed understood her research interests, and hence it is not clear how the presence of an observer might have influenced what was said and done. However, given that the final write-up is very unflattering to them, it seems unlikely that the midwives were fully aware of the picture Bowler was developing of them. Bowler states that nearly all of the data came from the natural interviews and from things said in the course of ordinary activities. These are both circumstances which, by comparison with a more formal interview, would make it more difficult for respondents to manage the impression they were giving to the researcher.

'THEY'RE NOT THE SAME AS US': MIDWIVES' STEREOTYPES OF SOUTH ASIAN DESCENT MATERNITY PATIENTS

Isobel Bowler

Abstract

The paper examines the stereotypes of South Asian descent women held by midwives in a British hospital. The data are drawn from a small-scale ethnographic study which investigated the women's maternity experiences. The midwives' stereotype contained four main themes: the difficulty of communicating with the women; the women's lack of compliance with care and abuse of the service; their tendency to 'make a fuss about nothing'; and their lack of 'normal maternal instinct'. The creation, perpetuation and effects of this negative stereotyping are examined in the light of the wider sociological research on patient typification. [. . .] Midwives used stereotypes to help them to make judgements about the kind of care different women want, need and deserve. It is therefore argued that stereotyping is a factor in the creation of the inequality in health experiences of black and minority ethnic patients.

Introduction

This paper presents findings from a small-scale ethnographic study of the delivery of maternity care to South Asian descent maternity patients. The stereotypes of these women held by health service staff (in particular midwives) are examined and set in the context of observational data. The South Asian descent women were generally referred to and regarded as 'Asian' women by midwives and other personnel. This term is also common in the literature (e.g. Rathwell, 1984: 123), but it masks heterogeneity in national, religious, and cultural background. However, because of the lack of differentiation by the midwives, their category of 'Asian' will be used in this paper.

The research was carried out in the maternity department of a teaching hospital in Britain in 1988. All the women received shared consultant directed care.[1] The hospital serves a city in southern England which has a South Asian descent population estimated[2] around 8 per cent, or 8,000 people. The largest group, about half of the Asian population, is of Pakistani descent. This group has a younger age structure and higher fertility rate than the British population as a whole (Coleman and Salt, 1992; Diamond and Clarke, 1989; C. Shaw, 1988). This results in a greater consumption of maternity services than would be expected from a consideration of numbers alone.

During fieldwork it became apparent that patient typification and labelling were common. The categorisation of clients as 'good', or more usually 'bad', is a routine feature of bureaucracies (Prottas, 1979) and medical settings are no exception (Kelly and May, 1982). In addition to individual patients being assigned a 'moral status', recognisable groups are likely to attract stereotypes. Midwives and other staff expressed stereotyped views of South Asian descent women which related to their customs and culture as well as their moral status as patients. The quotation in the title comes from an interview with a community midwife, and illustrates the common theme in the accounts: that 'they' are different from 'us'.

Midwives use stereotypes to help them pitch their interactions with women appropriately (Macintyre, 1978) and to make assumptions about the kind of care which different women want (Green et al., 1990). In the present study both of these observations held true. In addition, midwives used stereotypes to make assumptions about the kind of care different women deserve.

Midwives' views are contrasted with observational data which show that these were often contradicted by reality. However, midwives did not always recognise (or acknowledge) that individual women did not fit the stereotype. Even where midwives acknowledged a contradiction between experience and stereotype this did not necessarily cause them to question their view, but rather to treat the mismatch as the exception which proves the rule.

Green et al. (1990) and Macintyre (1978) report typifications of white women. Midwives in the present study also expressed stereotyped views of white mothers, although few data on this were collected. Examples given were of the 'thick' women from the large council estate and the educated NCT (National Childbirth Trust) middle class university women. Some of the aspects of the 'working class' stereotypes (e.g. low intelligence, lack of compliance) are present in the 'Asian' stereotypes. Indeed, the Asian women in the present study were all working class. However, this does not fully explain the extreme negative typification they suffered. The typifications go beyond class and echo the stereotypes of black and minority ethnic people common in wider society. The issue of racism (and anti-racism) is extremely complex (Gilroy, 1987) and beyond the scope of the present paper. Implicit throughout, however, is a recognition of the power relations between black women and white staff (Pearson, 1986).

Methods

The fieldwork with midwives[3] was carried out by the author alone over a three month period in the Summer of 1988. Access to the midwives and the maternity hospital was negotiated with the Director of Midwifery Services for the District Health Authority. The main method of data collection was observation, which was supported by data from interviews with twenty-five midwives.

The majority of the women observed were Moslem (of either Pakistani or Bangladeshi descent), but there were also Hindus and Christians. All were married and working class. Husbands were employed in local factories or on the buses; underemployed in family-run restaurants and shops; unemployed. Most of the women were recent migrants from rural areas; did not work outside the home and had limited contacts with non-Asian British people. Television, present in all the homes visited during fieldwork, was primarily used for the viewing of Hindi or Urdu videos. The use of medical services was therefore one of the few encounters they had with 'dominant' cultural values in British society.

The secondary method of data collection was interviews, primarily with the midwives, but also with a small number of other personnel, including hospital doctors and general practitioners, members of the local community health (CHC) and community relations (CRC) councils. The interviews were 'ethnographic' in character without a predetermined schedule but, instead, topics to be covered (Hammersley and Atkinson, 1983: 113). One of these topics was the midwives' attitudes to and perceptions of Asian women. Both directive and non-directive questions were used, although for the exploration of views about Asian women I favoured open-ended non-directive questions (Spradley, 1979). Questions used including the following: 'Would you say that there are different sorts/types of patients?' 'Are some women more difficult to care for?' 'Do some kinds of women have different needs?' There were two main types of interview. These may be characterised as *natural* and *formal* interviews.

The formal interviews with midwives were arranged in advance so that we would be able to talk at length. The *natural* interviews were interactions between myself and the midwives which occurred during observation, and in the context of general conversation. I took any opportunity to solicit accounts on the categories of interest, in particular views of black, and minority ethnic women. These occurred in the main with midwives I was shadowing when it was possible to introduce the topic with reference to individual Asian patients and/or particular events. Indeed it was often encounters with Asian women which would trigger expression of stereo-typed views. For example, in the case of a woman who had a low haemoglobin count and had not taken her iron medication I asked the midwife why she thought this was, whether it was a common problem, and so on.

Altogether ten formal interviews were conducted, which varied in length between 30 and 60 minutes, and fifteen *natural* interviews of significant length. Many of the comments about Asian women came, however, in shorter natural interviews, for example during a woman's labour or between patients in the antenatal clinic. In addition I recorded comments from midwives and other actors during observation which may be regarded as unsolicited accounts. Responses and other accounts were recorded longhand almost invariably as they occurred. During observation I always had a notebook in my hand and so this was not problematic. The majority of the data for this paper come from the natural interviews, and from unsolicited accounts.

The midwives' stereotypes of the women

The stereotypes of Asian women have four main themes: the difficulty of communication; the women's lack of compliance with care and abuse of the service; their tendency to 'make a fuss about nothing'; their lack of 'normal maternal instinct'.

Communication difficulties The level of competence in English among the Asian women observed was generally low. This resulted in the women being characterised as unresponsive, rude and unintelligent. It also helped to strengthen the stereotypes because it was difficult for women with little English to make a personal relationship with the midwives and therefore challenge the assumptions made about them.

One or two midwives had extreme opinions and felt the women's lack of English to be a 'moral' failing. They articulated the view common among white people in Britain that immigrants should be competent in English. For example, during observation on the labour ward a staff midwife commented with reference to a woman who had been in the city for eight years that 'It's disgusting not to speak English after so long in Britain.'

None of the midwives in the hospital was of Asian descent and the hospital did not employ interpreters or advocates. Some staff reported this as a problem, others felt that such facilities were not necessary since there were Asian men employed in the hospital who could interpret if necessary. However, during the period of the study, no one was ever used in such a way. An extreme attitude was expressed by a consultant. Asked if the hospital was considering employing interpreters he answered:

> Of course not. We haven't even got enough nurses. If you ask me they shouldn't be allowed into the country until they can pass an English exam.

Women who tried to speak English frequently offended the midwives. The main complaint was that the women did not say 'please' or 'thank you' and that they 'gave orders'. I know from my own attempts to learn Urdu that although the language has words equivalent to please and thank you, they are rarely used. In fact my Urdu teacher had to remind me frequently not to use them, pointing out that it was rather strange to use these words all the time 'like you English people do'. Instead in Urdu there is a polite form of the imperative with the 'please' built into the verb. The use of the imperative (fetch my baby, bring my lunch) without 'please' is indeed very rude in English, but was not so intended by the women.

Use of language indicates not only a person's attitudes towards those around them but also their intellectual abilities. The nature and content of speech (e.g. accent, vocabulary, grammar, syntax, dialect) are indicators employed to assess the other's competence. Black maternity patients in another study said that staff made them feel that they were 'too thick' to understand (Larbie, 1985: 19). In the present study some midwives described the Asian women as unintelligent. Commenting on their poor attendance at antenatal clinics (a part of the stereotype discussed below in the section on compliance with care) a clinic midwife remarked 'They're too stupid to remember when to come to the clinic.' One midwife remarked on Asian women's lack of intelligence in front of one, Asmat,[4] who was in labour. The midwife had asked for permission to give her a vaginal examination and gained no response. She said:

> Some Asian women are like blocks of wood, you know, thick [banging the side of her head]. Mind you others are delightful. It's impossible to know whether they've understood or not.

She used this as an example of how difficult it was to work with Asian women. Four other midwives told me that they found the women unrewarding to work with because they were unable to have a 'proper relationship' with them. Having a 'good relationship' with a mother was reported as an important part of a midwife's role.

The midwives were rarely motivated to take trouble with the women and to ensure that they understood. As a researcher I had far more time (and patience) to spend with individual women. For example with Asmat after the midwife had left I asked whether she had understood what had been said. She said that the midwives spoke too fast and were difficult to follow but she understood some of what they said. She had understood that the midwife thought that she was stupid. Many of the women in the sample said the same thing. They could understand a fairly simple conversation and would talk to me but not to the midwives.

Communication difficulties also stemmed from the use of colloquial language. It was common for staff to use culturally specific lay terms for symptoms and euphemisms for parts of the body which confused the Asian women. Terms such as 'waterworks', 'down there', 'the other end', 'tummy', and 'dizzy' are difficult even for those Asian women who are competent in English. Macintyre (1978) notes that in the antenatal clinic (and in other medical settings) staff modify their interactions with women according to the typifications made of them, based on such things as socioeconomic class, vocabulary and perceived intelligence. She argues that staff do this because they make the common sense assumption that standardised questions and vocabularies will not elicit standardised responses from patients in different categories. As she points out, the vocabulary used to those of low competence, social status and/or intelligence tends to be colloquial simplistic language. Ironically, these culturally specific terms were especially likely to be used with Asian women, who are of low status (by virtue of their ethnicity), were known to be of poor linguistic competence and perceived as being of low intelligence. This process can be seen in the following example.

I accompanied a community midwife on a home visit to a woman (Rubina). The midwife wanted to examine her to see if her fundus (i.e. uterus) had begun to contract back to its previous size. In order to do this examination properly (and to minimise discomfort) it is important that the woman's bladder is empty. Midwives therefore check with the woman first.

> *Midwife*: Do you need to go to the toilet – pass water?
> *Rubina*: Yes.
> *Midwife*: Or have you just been?
> *Rubina*: Yes.

Rubina looked confused and went out of the room, only to return immediately with an empty specimen bottle and an interrogative look on her face. The midwife waved it away crossly, told Rubina to lie on the sofa and began to feel her stomach.

While expansion of the question about 'going to the toilet' to include the phrase 'pass water?' in an interaction with an indigenous white English woman with limited vocabulary is probably better at eliciting a correct response than a question about 'urination', both versions may be equally incomprehensible to a woman who has English as a second language. [. . .]

Some of the misunderstandings between women and midwives can be attributed to differences in social and cultural background rather than the women's poor grasp of English. One area of confusion came over date of birth (DOB). Bureaucratic records of all kinds rely on DOB for classification and filing purposes (e.g. social security records, passports, driving licences) and hospital records are no exception. For Asian women DOB is particularly important since (as described below) there was often confusion over their names, which did not fit the Western surname/first name categories.

At their first antenatal clinic visit all women have to give their DOB. For the majority of women this question was expected, understood, and easy to answer. Some of the Asian women, however, did not know their birth date (age and birthdays do not have social significance in South Asia as they do in Europe), and were unaware of why it mattered. Some of the midwives took this as another example of poor linguistic competence. For those who realised that the women understood, but could not answer the question, this lack of knowledge of what in western society is an everyday fact, and part of personal identity, was mystifying. This reinforced the view that the women were stupid (so stupid that they don't even know when their birthday is). Some of the women had solved the problem. They knew (or estimated) the year in which they were born. Telling officials the year only did not satisfy the bureaucratic requirements. Therefore they gave their DOB as the first of January that year. One midwife, in all innocence, remarked how surprising it was that 'all these women' are born on the first of January.

Lack of compliance with care and service abuse   In interviews Asian women were described as non-compliant patients. Yet they were also (often simultaneously) characterised as service 'over-users' or even 'abusers'. Indeed in the midwives' accounts one often led to another. For example 'lack of compliance' with family planning advice led to increased fertility and therefore to 'over-use' and 'abuse' of the maternity service.

General examples of non-compliance given in interviews were that Asian women were poor attenders at antenatal clinics (cf. the clinic midwife's comment about women being 'too stupid' to know when to come, above) and did not go to parentcraft classes. Non-attendance could result from a variety of factors, including misunderstanding the date and time of the next appointment, and missing an appointment because of being called by the wrong name. Many of the Pakistani descent women gave the 'surname' Begum whereas Begum is a courtesy title, not unlike Mrs in English names (Henley, 1982). A woman called as 'Mrs Begum' would not immediately respond. This also contributed to the idea that the women were all alike: clinic midwives remarked that 'all these women have the same name'.

Another theme in the comments on non-compliance was that women had poor diets, suffered from anaemia and vitamin D deficiency and then failed to follow nutritional advice or take supplements. Few instances were actually observed in antenatal clinics. However, one community midwife shadowed was visiting an Asian woman daily to give her iron injections. The woman had previously been prescribed iron tablets but her haemoglobin count remained low. The midwife remarked:

> These women are very irritating. They don't take the tablets and then have to have injections. It takes time and its not nice for them . . . they hurt these jabs.

Midwives gave the women's fertility as an example of service abuse. Larbie cites examples of black women in hospital being told they have too many children (Larbie, 1985: 19). In the present study a staff midwife on the postnatal nursing ward remarked of an Asian patient, 'She's having her ninth baby. It's a disgrace. Talk about abuse of the service.' Midwives argued that Asian women were not motivated to use contraception. Discussing a woman on the postnatal ward a midwife remarked that her linguistic competence had disappeared when she had tried to talk to her about the topic. She told me that she had not pursued the point: 'She's not very interested in family planning is Mrs Begum.'

Several of the Asian women in the study had large families and women born in South Asia do have higher fertility than British born women (Diamond and Clarke, 1989). The only material in the hospital which was available in Asian languages was the information on Depo-Provera issued by the manufacturer. These were proudly shown to me by one of the consultants to demonstrate that he did take account of language problems.

Both midwives and doctors were ready to assume that Asian women have no interest in family planning. However, from the data collected in the separate sample of women[3] I found that this was not always the case. In her small scale study of Pathan women in Bradford, Currer (1983) found that of the 17 questioned at least nine were using a method of contraception. Nevertheless the assumption persists. The following example shows the stereotype being employed in the face of communication difficulties.

During postnatal home visits midwives discuss plans for future birth control with new mothers. The following exchange occurred in an Asian's woman's home 5 days after the delivery of her son. The community midwife asked the Asian woman (Saida) about her intended family planning practice. The following conversation ensued:

Midwife: Do you want any more children?
Saida: [confusion]
Midwife: You know, any more babies?
Saida: Four children
Midwife: More babies? Do you want to have five babies?
Saida: Not five babies, four babies.
Midwife: Well go and see Dr Smith in five weeks with your husband and discuss not having any more babies.

The midwife did not pursue the point any further. Saida appears to be answering the question of 'how many children do you have?' rather than 'how many children do you want?' Neither I nor the midwife could be certain either way. After we left the midwife told me that she tried her best with encouraging family planning but 'these women are just not interested'.

Not all the Asian women in the study were opposed to fertility control. In an antenatal clinic a consultation was observed between an obstetric senior house officer (SHO) and an Asian couple with one child of under one year and a second unwanted pregnancy. The referral letter from the woman's GP stated that she had been on the pill but had stopped taking it because of breakthrough bleeding. The GP pointed out in the referral letter that the pregnancy was the couple's fault: she had stressed that the husband must use a sheath and yet they had failed to comply with this advice. The SHO asked the husband about this and he said that he did not like the sheath. Both the doctor and midwife told me that they thought this couple were being unnecessarily difficult about the pregnancy. The SHO remarked, 'It's only her second baby. I thought these people liked large families.' The possibility of a termination was not discussed.

The second main issue which was cited in connection with 'service abuse' was circumcision, which was not provided on the NHS in the study hospital. One Asian couple observed had just had a second son. The first had been delivered in the hospital and circumcised, but they had not paid the bill for the operation. The ward sister told the father that this time he must pay in advance. He was not pleased, but paid up. A staff midwife told me that she was glad that they had been made to pay:

> These people will try anything. He tried to tell me that he didn't understand that he had to pay, but he knew full well. He was just trying it on.

A second midwife remarked:

> I'm sympathetic but I get fed up with the repeated abuse of the service by these people.

This unwillingness to pay was not common to all Asian couples. In another case, a paediatrician apologised to a father for the charge, and remarked that he thought it was discriminatory. The father disagreed and said that he was quite happy to pay:

> I am a guest in this country. This country has been very good to me, why shouldn't I pay if I want something different?

The debate became quite heated with the doctor and a midwife arguing with the father over whether or not he should have to pay. The paediatrician thought that circumcisions should be available in all health districts on the NHS. In addition to the fact that he thought that it was racist (because particular religious groups including Moslems have their sons circumcised) he had seen the results of circumcisions by traditional practitioners which had ended up in the accident and emergency department.

Associated with comments about service abuse, midwives reported that Asian women were demanding and complaining. During interviews with midwives on postnatal nursing wards a major complaint was that Asian women refused to be physically active after delivery of their babies and, a lesser complaint, did not do the recommended toning exercises. A quotation from one midwife which illustrates an extreme of this view is that the women just 'lie in bed all day and expect to be waited on hand and foot'. [. . .]

Making a fuss about nothing 'Making a fuss about nothing' was a phrase which recurred in interviews and was particularly applied to the intra- and postnatal behaviour of women. This view of black women has been reported in other studies. Larbie (1985: 22) found that black women were told by staff that they make too much noise when in pain or discomfort. Brent Community Health Council (1981: 13) reports the stereotype of black people having a low pain threshold and Rakusen (1981: 81) mentions this specifically with reference to Asian women. Homans and Satow (1982: 17) note that some health workers hold the belief that black patients are likely to 'make a fuss about nothing' and suggest that this will limit the health workers' willingness to try to communicate effectively with such patients.

In the present study Asian women were characterised as 'attention seeking'; making too much noise and 'unnecessary fuss' during labour (because of 'low pain thresholds') and constantly complaining of minor symptoms (particularly headaches) in the postnatal period. The issues of noise during labour and low pain thresholds were mentioned in interviews by all the midwives who worked on the labour ward. In response to a question about whether there were different sorts of patients who needed different sorts of treatment a typical response (from a labour ward midwife) was:

> Well, these Asian women you're interested in have very low pain thresholds. It can make it very difficult to care for them.

Six Asian and four white women's deliveries were observed. None of the Asian women made a great deal of noise or had pain control and yet one of the white women had pethidine and another an epidural for pain (although this latter case was a premature labour of an older and very frightened woman). It may be that this was partly observer effect. Two of the husbands of Asian women thanked me for being with their wives during labour because it had stopped them being frightened. One midwife noted that women who are frightened make noise:

> We perceive Asian women as whinging when they are just frightened. They just make more noise than we do.

This shows that it is possible to hold a stereotyped view without necessarily being unsympathetic to the stereotyped group.

Despite the fact that there was variation between women (and that non-Asian women also make a noise in labour) midwives saw making a noise in labour as the norm (although deviant behaviour) for Asian women. One woman (Shakila), expecting her eighth baby, had a long induced labour during which she vomited several times. On the postnatal ward she complained of a sore throat. The midwife said:

> I expect you were shouting a lot during labour. That's why your throat hurts.

I had been with the woman in labour and said that actually this was not the case. The midwife then went on to report a story to me which was the exception which proves the rule:

> I have a friend who's a Moslem. She's a GP's wife. She had a section and she had a lot of pain. But you know how much fuss they make. No one took very much notice. But I knew her so I knew that it really hurt. I made sure she got taken seriously.

This example provides circumstantial evidence that ethnicity is more important than class in the framing of typifications.

The noise Asian women were reported to make in labour was considered doubly inexcusable because they were perceived to have easier deliveries than Caucasian women. Some midwives cited this as a major (ethnic) difference. Others (and doctors I spoke to) pointed out that length of labour was primarily affected by parity (i.e. number of previous deliveries). Asian women have higher fertility and therefore make up a large proportion of the women of high parity delivered in maternity hospitals. For many of the midwives, however, ethnicity became the overriding factor. This is illustrated in the following example from my field notes. I was looking for an Asian woman on the antenatal nursing ward and a midwife told me that she had gone down to the labour ward. She was being induced and it was her first baby. Nevertheless the midwife remarked 'Oh, she'll be back in an hour, they're always quick.' In the event the woman had a slow and long labour. This example further demonstrates how a woman's ethnicity becomes her master status.

The midwife knew that it was an induction and a first baby, both factors which indicated a longer labour, and yet the woman's ethnicity was seen as the overriding factor.

On the postnatal ward the Asian women were unwilling to get up and therefore the midwives had to nurse them in bed. This made them unpopular. The following comments from a midwife were overheard in the ward coffee room:

> Mrs Kajoo is being difficult again. She wants me to bring her bottle [for the baby] but I'm not doing it. They're always ordering us around. Bring me my bottle indeed. [To a second midwife]. You're not to do it either.

Community midwives too cited examples of women 'making a fuss about nothing'. In the coffee room in the GPU two community midwives were discussing a woman who had been discharged from postnatal midwifery care. One midwife remarked to the other:

> I went to see Mrs Iqbal yesterday and finally got rid of her. She didn't want to be discharged . . . said she'd got a headache. These women they make such a fuss. In their own culture they get so much attention they have to invent it. I think it's pathetic.

Lack of normal maternal instinct   A theme running through accounts of Asian women given by midwives was that 'they're not the same as us'. In particular they were described as lacking normal maternal instinct and feelings. This was in part attributed to their large numbers of children and 'unhealthy' preference for sons.

In the everyday world in our society there is a concept of 'maternal instinct' which implies that humans (especially women) have instinctive drives towards reproduction. Macintyre (1976: 151–2) has pointed out that this and other aspects of 'normal' reproduction are socially constructed. However, she argues that although the majority of sociologists recognise the social construction of reproduction, most studies have defined 'normal' reproduction as occurring exclusively inside the statistically common nuclear family unit. The household formation (and different attitudes to marriage) of many Asian families (A. Shaw, 1988) puts them outside this Western normality. A more recent analysis of the psychological research into motherhood notes that the construction of 'normal' motherhood is based on white middle class behaviours (Phoenix and Woollett, 1991). Psychological studies have omitted black and working class mothers from studies of normal processes, but included them in studies of deviance. Phoenix and Woollett (1991) argue that the narrow focus of these studies has helped to maintain negative social constructions of black mothers (1991: 25). In addition, mothers from minority ethnic groups are themselves socially constructed as 'other' and hence by definition viewed as deviating from 'good/normal' mothering (1991: 17).

Thus constructions of normal reproduction and motherhood take no account of structural differences between mothers. Some of the Asian women's behaviours did not conform to the prevailing (Western) model of motherhood. For example, of the six South Asian women observed during labour, two reacted badly when the midwives delivered their baby onto their stomach, and three did not want to hold their newborn baby straight away. All those observed did not want to breastfeed immediately after delivery, and the majority of women in the study were likely to choose to bottle feed. Midwives were also upset by the preference for sons expressed by women (and related to the importance of male offspring in Islamic culture). Some of the women's behaviours could be interpreted positively in the light of dominant models: for example, none of the women in the sample worked outside the home, none smoked. However not one midwife mentioned this as a positive characteristic of Asian women although these issues were discussed with reference to mothers in general.

Models of childbirth and motherhood vary by culture. Many of the behaviours described above do not conflict with the South Asian Islamic models of motherhood described in Currer's (1983) study of Pathan women in Bradford. However, they caused midwives, with their different cultural perspective, to characterise women as lacking normal maternal instinct and feelings.[5]

Discussion

The examples above demonstrate how individual women's behaviours were interpreted within the stereotypes of 'Asian women' held by the midwives. This is not surprising since typifications of patients are common in medical settings. Menzies' (1960) classic paper on the defence against anxiety among nurses gives some indication of why this should be. She argues that depersonalisation and categorisation of patients (as, for example, bed numbers or illnesses) reduces the possibility of emotional attachment between carer and patient, and thus reduces anxiety and stress for the former. Green et al. (1990: 125) write that midwives on the labour ward commonly use stereotypes 'to make assumptions about what a particular woman is likely to want in labour and delivery'. In the present study midwives also used stereotypes to make judgements about the kind of care women deserved. When a woman speaks little English, stereotypes will be particularly likely to be employed in this way by the midwives.

The practice of typification described by Menzies leads to staff forming, transmitting and accepting stereotyped views of certain groups. For example the 'well-educated middle-class National Childbirth Trust type' or the 'uneducated working class woman' (Green et al., 1990), 'the demanding Jew' and the 'difficult Asian woman'. If an individual patient is easily categorised as a member of such a group she is more likely to suffer the effects of negative stereotyping. Black and minority ethnic women are particularly vulnerable to such typification because the colour of their skin makes it easy for staff to 'recognise them' and to assign them to a (negatively typified) group. 'Communication difficulties' were a major theme of the 'Asian' stereotype. The negative typifications were reinforced if women had poor English because midwives could more readily apply stereotypes to women with whom they could not communicate. Furthermore, women were unable to challenge the view that 'they're all the same'.

Communication difficulties: linguistic and cultural differences Communication difficulties occur at two levels: the linguistic and the cultural. As demonstrated in the examples above, language is a problem for some women. Their lack of English infuriated the midwives, and was one of the main 'problems with Asian women' mentioned by staff. More importantly, lack of English made the experience of hospital mystifying and often frightening for the women. However, language was not the sole cause of misunderstanding. Even women who spoke good English experienced culturally based communication difficulties.

Schutz (1976: 95) discusses the difficulty of the 'stranger', particularly (although not exclusively) an immigrant to a country, trying to interpret the cultural pattern of a social group which she or he approaches. He argues that the 'approached' (i.e. dominant) group has a system of knowledge, albeit 'incoherent, inconsistent and only partially clear', which allows anybody a reasonable chance of understanding and being understood. He describes this in terms of 'recipes' for interpreting the social world and expressing oneself within it. Garfinkel paraphrases this as 'common sense knowledge of social structures' (Garfinkel, 1967: 76). The stranger does not share the dominant recipes for communication. [. . .]

Applying these arguments to a medical setting, Hughes (1977) examines the way in which doctors in a casualty department use everyday knowledge to categorise patients: those needing immediate care; those who can wait; those who are deviant (drunk, down and out) and so on. He observed that overseas doctors had difficulty in typing patients and suggests that this may stem from their lack of 'conventional knowledge' (as opposed to medical expertise). It is possible to reverse this argument and to say that one reason why first generation black patients may become negatively typified is a result of the same phenomenon: they lack conventional 'common sense' knowledge about the system.

Ardener (1972, 1975, 1989) has discussed (with particular reference to the accounts of women rendered by (male) anthropologists in their monographs) how a subordinate group may become 'muted' in interactions with the dominant order. He argues not that they are dumb, but that when such groups become incorporated into dominant models and have to speak using dominant modes of expression then their meanings may become lost. They are muted because they are not listened to, or if listened to, not understood. Of course this argument can apply to all women using the maternity services: the dominant mode of expression is medical. However, black and minority ethnic women will be doubly muted because they will be dealing with two degrees of dominance: the white British and the male medical. [. . .]

Asian women as 'bad' patients   Stereotyping can be seen in the context of the research on patient typification (see Kelly and May, 1982 for a detailed review). The characteristics of Asian women included in the midwives' stereotypes echo the negatively typified characteristics cited in this literature. In addition, the women's ethnicity (which was never cited as a negative characteristic: no midwife told me that she didn't like black people) almost certainly plays a direct role in their typification as 'bad' patients.

Race, ethnicity and nationality have several effects. Patients who are not Caucasian, born outside Britain and who have poor command of English are likely to be unpopular. Several authors (Brown, 1966; Papper, 1970; Stockwell, 1972) cite these characteristics as leading to negative client assessment by health professionals. In addition, a patient's ethnicity makes her more likely to be classified as an undesirable patient because her knowledge and expectations of the medical services are different to those of indigenous patients. Goffman (1969: 366), in his analysis of the sick role, writes that the proper enactment of this role involves a characteristic etiquette, for example entailing (in Western culture) the belittling of discomfort, physical cooperation with carers and proper presentation of self. He notes that there are 'appreciable ethnic differences in the management of the sick role'.

There is evidence that patients become unpopular if they are perceived as constantly complaining (Armitage, 1980; Lorber, 1975; Stockwell, 1972); malingering; and receiving treatment under false pretences (Kelly and May, 1982). Those who fail to conform to the clinical regime are also regarded unfavourably (Basque and Merige, 1980; Gillis and Biesheuvel, 1988; Spitzer and Sobel, 1962).

A theme running through the data reported above is the role of communication difficulties which may be seen as a major factor in negative typification of Asian women. Because of these problems it can be more difficult and time consuming for midwives to care for them. Menzies (1960) leads us to expect that patients who cause a high level of anxiety or who cause staff to feel ineffective or angry (such as women who cannot communicate to staff that they are all right) may become negatively typified. This is supported by other studies (e.g. Gillis and Biesheuvel, 1988; Holderby and McNulty, 1979; Orlando, 1961; Schwartz, 1958; Ujhely, 1963). In addition, Kelly and May (1982) point out that some patients are defined as difficult because they hinder staff in their work. Finally, perceived patient intelligence has been shown to influence staff's evaluation of them (Gillis and Biesheuvel, 1988; MacGregor, 1960; Papper, 1970).

Accepting a rigid stereotyped view of Asian women may act as a defence against the anxiety generated in staff who cannot communicate with them. Stereotyping can allow staff to make assumptions about the care women need (or deserve). In the context of the present study, a midwife does not need to feel too anxious about the noise an Asian woman makes in labour because, according to the stereotyped view such women have 'a low pain threshold' and therefore do not need pain relief. In addition they 'make a fuss about nothing' and so do not deserve it either. Asian women's problems with English become part of the stereotype and so staff's willingness to try to communicate with them is reduced.

There is a second set of explanations for the prevalence of stereotyping associated with the different attitudes and behaviour (real or perceived) of the women. Several authors note that patients who are judged to be attention-seeking (Gillis and Biesheuvel, 1988; Jeffery, 1979; Lorber, 1975; MacGregor, 1960); demanding (Brown, 1966; Gillis and Biesheuvel, 1988; Jeffery, 1979; Papper, 1970; Schwartz, 1958); or who are thought to disrupt clinical routine unnecessarily (Lorber, 1975; Orlando, 1961) are negatively typified by staff. Those who are seen as manipulative (Armitage, 1980; Ujhely, 1963) are particularly unpopular. [. . .]

As Murcott emphasises, when typifying patients 'staff's concerns with getting through the day's work are of more immediate relevance than general moral concerns' (Murcott, 1981: 129). Second, and more subtly, women are unpopular if they prevent the midwives from fulfilling their role. This includes everything from carrying out their work well to feeling positive about themselves. Once a midwife has had several difficult encounters with women of Asian descent it is not surprising if, by virtue of their visibility, all Asian women become perceived by her as 'difficult patients'. In this way stereotypes form and are transmitted to other staff. [. . .] For black and minority ethnic women their moral status may (for some staff) be already compromised because they are black. Racist attitudes are not unknown among health service staff (Brent Community Health Council, 1981; Larbie, 1985; Phoenix, 1990). Midwives could employ a stereotype to allow them to practise discrimination based on ethnicity without having to admit that to themselves, or appearing to others to be racist.

The effect of stereotypes The data demonstrate the presence and construction of stereotypes of Asian women, but it is beyond the scope of the study to investigate fully their effect. The data strongly suggest that women are disadvantaged by the assumptions made about them by midwives. The two clearest cases concern family planning and pain control. In the examples of Mrs Begum and Saida neither midwife endeavoured to overcome language difficulties and talk about fertility control because they 'knew' that the women were not interested. Yet the example of the young couple with the unwanted pregnancy shows that this assumption should not be made. In that case it cannot be known whether termination would have been discussed with a similar white British couple.

None of the six Asian women observed during labour was offered pain control other than gas and air. Of the four white women observed two had intervention to control their pain. The sample is not matched and so no direct comparison is possible. The only indication is that in the case of Shakila, who suffered a long and painful labour, the registrar who saw her several hours after induction told me that pethidine could not be given because it was too close to the delivery. In the cases of the white women who had pain control this was at the suggestion of a midwife. The midwife looking after Shakila, who could have offered pethidine at an appropriate time, did not.

Stereotypes of Asian maternity patients, and black and ethnic minority patients generally, cannot be dissociated from the racist attitudes of many white people in Britain (one-third of the sample in the 1984 *British Social Attitudes* survey admitted to being racially prejudiced; Jowell and Airey, 1984). Space does not allow for a discussion of how the midwives' stereotypes reflect or feed into racist discourse but the following point can be made. Although it cannot be known whether the midwives were consciously or overtly racist *any* stereotype based on a racial or ethnic group is discriminatory, regardless of the stated attitudes of those holding the view.

Conclusion

This analysis has revealed several different ways in which stereotypes affect the interaction between staff and women, and how this interaction can reinforce the negative views of women. [. . .]

Individuals are typed according to a variety of criteria, cited in the literature review above. Macintyre (1978: 599) notes that staff revise their typification in the light of interactions with patients. It is difficult for women to assert their 'moral status' (and so get the typification revised) because language difficulties and cultural differences make it hard for them to make individual relationships with midwives.

There is evidence that ethnicity is a powerful criterion for typification, made stronger by its very visibility. Jeffery (1979: 90) shows how certain sorts of patients are unable to achieve entry into the legitimate career of sickness. The stereotypes emphasised the deviance of Asian women. If it is the women's ethnicity which causes them to be negatively typified then they are being disadvantaged because of ascribed ethnicity and not on the basis of individual action.

This analysis has implications for 'cultural awareness training' which can lead to static stereotyped views. It can encourage staff to make assumptions about ethnic difference based upon physical (racial) difference. If an Asian woman makes a noise in labour this is not because she is in pain but because Asian women in general have low pain thresholds and make fuss about nothing. There is therefore a difference in kind between stereotypes of black women and those of white women based on class. Race is a very hard boundary to cross. Stereotypes of Asian women can be applied purely on the basis of physical appearance and are therefore potentially racist.

A midwife in the present study asked me if I could recommend some information to help her understand her Asian patients. I suggested the booklets by Alix Henley (e.g. Henley, 1982, *Caring for Muslims and Their Families*). The midwife looked surprised

'I don't have time to read books,' she said, 'What we need is an A4 bit of paper with it all on so we can look things up when we need them.' This attitude to ethnicity is that all we need is some kind of cultural recipe book. Her reaction is similar to that of many health professionals to the complexities of other ethnicities: they're different to us (we need a map) but they're all the same (so one map will do).

Midwives were inclined to accept a view of 'Asian women' as a homogeneous group. In fact they were heterogeneous, not only in their cultural and religious background, but also in their relationships with staff. In other words the midwives held a rigid homogeneous view of these women, based on their physical appearance, in a way they did not for white British women. The behaviours and characteristics which led to negative typification of the women by midwives were not, therefore, common to all women of Asian descent. However characteristics of *some* women led to a stereotyped view which was attached to *all* women who were (or, more significantly, *looked* as if they were) of 'Asian' ethnic origin. As Phoenix (1990: 228) writes, 'The propensity to see black women as being "all the same" is not only inaccurate but also racially discriminatory in that it can mask individual black women's needs.'

Notes

1 Women are booked for care with a consultant obstetrician and delivered in the hospital labour ward. However, their routine antenatal checks are carried out by their GP and community midwife, i.e. the antenatal care is shared. This compares with GP directed care where all care is community based and the woman is delivered by community midwives in the General Practitioner Unit.
2 Estimated by the city council. The 1981 census did not collect data on ethnic origin, data from the 1991 census is not yet available.
3 This study is part of a wider project which also included a separate study of South Asian descent women who were recruited from an English language class and by snowball sampling. It is from this second study that the background information on the Asian women is derived.
4 Asmat is a pseudonym, as are all other names of respondents.
5 For a more detailed analysis of these issues see Currer (1983), Donovan (1986), Homans (1980)

References

Ardener, E. (1972) Belief and the problem of women. Reprinted in Ardener, S. (ed.) (1975) *Perceiving Women*. London: Dent.
Ardener, S. (1975) The problem of women revisited. In Ardener, S. (ed.) (1975) *Perceiving Women*. London: Dent.
Ardener, E. (1989) *The Voice of Prophecy* (edited by Malcolm Chapman). Oxford: Blackwell.
Armitage, S. (1980) Non-compliant recipients of health care. *Nursing Times Occasional Papers*, 76, 1.
Basque, L.O. and Merige, J. (1980) Nurses' experiences with dangerous behaviour: implications for training. *J. Continuing Education in Nursing*, 11, 47–51.
Brent Community Health Council (1981) *Black Women and the Maternity Services*. London: Brent Community Health Council.
Brown, E.L. (1966) Nursing and patient care. Reprinted in Davis, A. (ed.) (1978) *Relationships between Doctors and Patients*. Farnborough: Saxon House.
Coleman, D.A. and Salt, J. (1992) *The British Population*. Oxford: Oxford University Press.

Currer, C. (1983) *The Mental Health of Pathan Mothers in Bradford: A Case Study of Migrant Asian Women.* Coventry: University of Warwick.

Diamond, I. and Clarke, S (1989) Demographic patterns among Britain's ethnic groups. In Joshi, H. (ed.) (1989) *The Changing Population of Britain.* Oxford: Blackwell.

Donovan, J. (1986) *We Don't Buy Sickness It Just Comes.* Aldershot: Gower.

Garfinkel, H. (1967) *Studies in Ethnomethodology.* Englewood Cliffs, NJ: Prentice-Hall.

Gillis, L. (with Biesheuvel, S.) (1988) *Human Behaviour in Illness.* London: Faber & Faber.

Gilroy, P. (1987) *There Ain't No Black in the Union Jack.* London: Hutchinson.

Goffman, E. (1969) The insanity of place. *Psychiatry,* 32, 357–87. Reprinted in Black, N. et al. (eds) *Health and Disease: A Reader.* Milton Keynes: Open University Press.

Green, J. et al. (1990) Stereotypes of childbearing women: a look at some evidence. *Midwifery,* 6, 125–32.

Hammersley, M. and Atkinson, P. (1983) *Ethnography: Principles in Practice.* London: Tavistock.

Henley, A. (1982) *Caring for Muslims and their Families: Religious Aspects of Care.* Cambridge: National Extension College.

Holderby, R.A. and McNulty, E.G. (1979) Feeling feelings: how to make a rational response to emotional behaviour. *Nursing,* October, 39–43.

Homans, H. (1980) *Pregnant in Britain. A Sociological Approach.* Unpublished PhD thesis: University of Warwick.

Homans, H. and Satow, A. (1982) Can you hear me? Cultural variations in communication. *J. Community Nursing,* January pp. 16–18.

Hughes, D. (1977) Everyday medical knowledge in categorising patients. In Dingwall, R. et al. (eds), *Health Care and Health Knowledge.* London: Croom Helm.

Jeffery, R. (1979) Normal rubbish: deviant patients in casualty departments. *Sociology of Health and Illness,* 1, 90–107.

Jowell, R. and Airey, C. (1984) *British Social Attitudes.* London: Gower.

Kelly, M.P. and May, D. (1982) Good and bad patients: a review of the literature and a theoretical critique. *J. Advanced Nursing,* 7, 147–56.

Larbie, J. (1985) *Black Women and the Maternity Services.* London: Training in Health and Race.

Lorber, J. (1975) Good patients and problem patients: conformity and deviance in a general hospital. *J. Health and Social Behavior,* 16, 213–25.

MacGregor, F. (1960) *Social Science in Nursing: Applications for the Improvement of Patient Care.* New York: Russell Sage.

Macintyre, S. (1976) 'Who wants babies?' The social construction of 'Instincts'. In Leonard, D.L. and Allen, S. (eds), *Sexual Divisions and Society: Process and Change.* London: Tavistock.

Macintyre, S. (1978) Some notes on record taking, and making in an antenatal clinic. *Sociological Review,* 26, 595–611.

May, D. and Kelly, M.P. (1982) Chancers, pests and poor wee souls: problems of legitimation in psychiatric nursing. *Sociology of Health and Illness,* 4, 279–300.

Menzies, I.E.P. (1960) A case study in the functioning of social systems as a defence against anxiety. A report on a study of the nursing service of a general hospital. *Human Relations,* 13, 95–121.

Murcott, A. (1981) On the typifications of 'bad' patients. In Atkinson, P. and Heath, C. (eds) (1981) *Medical Work: Realities and Routines.* London: Gower.

Orlando, I. (1961) *The Dynamic Nurse–Patient Relationship: Function, Process and Principles.* New York: G.P. Putnam's Sons.

Papper, S. (1970) The undesirable patient. *J. Chronic Diseases,* 22, 777–9.

Pearson, M. (1986) The politics of ethnic minority health studies. In Rathwell, T. and Phillips, D. (eds), *Health, Race and Ethnicity.* Beckenham: Croom Helm.

Phoenix, A. (1990) Black women and the maternity services. In Garcia, J. et al. (eds), *The Politics of Maternity Care: Services for Childbearing Women in Twentieth-Century Britain.* Oxford: Clarendon Press.

Phoenix, A. and Woollett, A. (1991) Motherhood: social construction, politics and psychology. In Phoenix, A. et al. (eds), *Motherhood: Meanings, Practices and Ideologies.* London: Sage.

Prottas, J.M. (1979) *People-Processing.* Lexington MA, USA: Lexington Books.

Rakusen, J. (1981) Depo-Provera: the extent of the problem. A case study in the politics of birth control. In Roberts, H. (ed.), *Women, Health and Reproduction*. London: Routledge & Kegan Paul.

Rathwell, T. (1984) General Practice, ethnicity and health services delivery. *Social Science and Medicine*, 19, 123–30.

Schutz, Alfred (1976) The stranger: an essay in social psychology. In Schutz, A. *Collected Papers II. Studies in Social Theory* (edited by Arvid Brodersen). The Hague, Netherlands: Martinus Nijhoff.

Schwartz, D. (1958) Uncooperative patients? *Am. J. Nursing*, 58, 75–7.

Shaw, A. (1988) *A Pakistani Community in Britain*. Oxford: Basil Blackwell.

Shaw, C. (1988) Components of growth in the ethnic minority population. *Population Trends*, 52, 26–30.

Spradley, J.P. (1979) *The Ethnographic Interview*. New York: Holt, Rinehart & Winston.

Spitzer, S. and Sobel, R. (1962) Preferences for patients and patient behaviour. *Nursing Research*, 11, 233–5.

Stockwell, F. (1972) *The Unpopular Patient*. Royal College of Nursing Research project. Series 1 no 2. London: Royal College of Nursing.

Ujhely, G.B. (1963) *The Nurse and her Problem Patient*. New York: Springer Verlag.

What you might do now

You might like to consider further the different potentialities of interviewing and naturalistic observation. How far do you think that Bowler would have produced similar findings from a study relying on scheduled interviews as its main source of data? But what are the ethical implications of studying people when they cannot so easily determine the impression they are giving to the researcher?

Carry out a more systematic appraisal of the study using 'Questions to Ask about Qualitative Research' in Part 4 of this book

What you might do now

Think some more about the problems and possibilities of naturalistic observation by reading Chapter 16 and perhaps some of the further reading cited in that chapter

Use the appendix and find some research of interest to you based on naturalistic observation and appraise it using 'Questions to Ask about Qualitative Research' in Part 4 of this book

CHAPTER 14

UNDERSTANDING LANGUAGE IN CONTEXT: PROFESSIONAL UNCERTAINTY

EXEMPLAR Roger Gomm, 'Uncertain minds or uncertain times? Uncertainty in professional discourse' (written for this volume)

What you need to understand in order to understand the exemplar
What strengths a naturalistic observation study has over an interview study. *See Chapter 16, section 3*
The general idea of 'grounded theory', including the terms 'grounding', 'deriving theory from data', 'theoretical sampling' and 'constant comparison' and 'deviant case analysis'. *See Chapter 16, section 4*
'The linguistic turn in qualitative research'. *See Chapter 16, sections 5 and 6*
The exemplar does not describe how the data were analysed, but this was along the lines described in *Chapter 16, section 6*
For terms which are unfamiliar, try the index.

Introduction

The exemplar for this chapter has been written for two purposes. The first is to illustrate the use of a grounded theory approach to collecting and analysing data (Chapter 16, section 4). The second, and quite independent of the first, is to illustrate the kind of qualitative research which treats linguistic data as evidence of what people are doing with words when they utter them, rather than as evidence of 'beliefs', 'attitudes', 'interpretive frameworks', 'cognitive structures' or something similar, lying behind the words (Chapter 16, sections 5 and 6). The topic of the research is the assessment of health visitor students, but the paper is written to be relevant to a wide range of circumstances in which people utter expressions of uncertainty.

The paper concentrates more on telling the story of the research than on justifying its findings. To correct some of this shortfall readers may like to know that the data for the study were collected with the author as a participant observer, playing roles he would have played had he been engaged in research or not. At different times and in different places this meant doing research from the position of an internal examiner, external examiner, chair of an examination board, as a colleague to other participants and as a teacher of students. Data came from six colleges and were collected over an eight-year period. This may seem a very long time, but educational assessment consists of a cycle of events, each event of which is relatively short and happens only once a year. Data were collected from both the formal events of assessment, such as examination board meetings and viva voce examinations, and from interchanges in corridors and staff rooms. The author made no secret as to his research activities, but with the large number of people involved it is doubtful if all of them were aware of this, and, of those who were, most probably forgot this for long periods of time. The context was one in which doing research on one's ordinary activities was common and well understood. Some assessment events were audio-recorded, but most of the data were collected in the form of long-hand notes in order not to have to engage in protracted negotiations to gain permission to tape record, and not to disrupt events by so doing. During the more formal events the author concentrated on accurately recording short interchanges of talk chosen as relevant according to the way his theoretical framework was developing, noting who made them (recorded by role rather than by personal name) and when they were made in the context of the event. This could be done without disruption since most such events involved people taking notes. Immediately after an event he made diary notes on its more general features. Here agendas and other tabled papers provided useful *aide-mémoires*.

These are not ideal ways of recording data for studying the use of language in context but are less problematic when a researcher has a clear idea of the kind of data he or she is looking for and where events of the same kind happen over and over again. By the time someone has observed a hundred viva voce examinations, for example, they will have a pretty clear idea about their more usual features and of the kind of things to listen out for in the hundred and first. Given the danger of selecting data to fit a theory, it is particularly important to search for disconfirming instances and, as the exemplar makes clear, in this research much was learned about the usual from events that were exceptional: from deviant case analysis.

The research also involved the analysis of documents, such as student assessment work and reports on students, some recording of teaching events and a series of interviews with staff. The latter, however, added little to the research and are not referred to here.

UNCERTAIN MINDS OR UNCERTAIN TIMES? EXPRESSIONS OF UNCERTAINTY IN PROFESSIONAL DISCOURSE

Roger Gomm

Introduction

Uncertainty has been a long-standing theme in studies of professionalism and professional socialisation. At one level this idea has furnished an explanation for the existence of professional occupations as such. They are, it has been argued, the kinds of occupations which arise in society wherever there are important uncertainties: the unpredictabilities of life and death, of God's will, of engineering failure and so on. Such circumstances, it is claimed, either require highly skilled people to manage them on others' behalf (Parsons, 1950), or, alternatively, provide opportunities for charlatans to make a good living out of other people's uncertainties (Malinowski, 1935; Radin, 1935; Childe, 1959; Illich, 1977) and who are not averse to creating uncertainties to enhance their power (Friedson, 1975; Davis, 1960). Or again, on the more benign interpretation of professionalism, it has been argued that because people are made vulnerable by uncertainties, those occupationals who deal with them have to be bound by professional codes of conduct to prevent them from exploiting the vulnerable (Parsons, 1950), thus explaining a defining characteristic of a 'profession'. On a smaller scale the uncertainties allegedly inherent in professional practice have been cited to make sense of professional training as a process of learning to manage and otherwise cope with uncertainties (Fox, 1959, 1980 but see Atkinson, 1984), and, of course, the very idea that professionals make decisions in the face of extreme uncertainty, aggrandises such occupational groups; for only very special people could be expected to do so successfully.

The uncertainty featuring in this paper is the uncertainty expressed by staff involved in health visitor education in assessing students as to whether they should be recommended to receive a licence to practise, though it reached back into uncertainties as to whom should be given a place on the course in the first place (Gomm, 1986). As a researcher, I was struck by the fact that when staff were asked to offer an opinion about a student their responses often bordered on the incoherent:

> *Tutor 1*: Jane Marshall, do you think, I mean, will she/
> *Tutor 2*: Hhhh, mm well, you know with some of them, some of them like Jane, well, there are some where it is very difficult to tell.

Most student health visitors seemed to be 'like Jane', about whom it was 'difficult to tell'. Or at least they seemed to be like Jane some of the time, whereas on other occasions staff would issue detailed, definitive and sometimes apparently dogmatic judgements about students. Again, throughout a year-long course health visitor tutors and often other academic staff would issue doubts about whether this or that student would 'make a health visitor', or whether 'a lot of them would fail this year'. In fact, so few students ever failed that one would have thought that 'making a health visitor' was a forgone conclusion, not something to be uncertain about on such a grand scale.

Uncertainty manifested itself in numerous ways, but perhaps the quickest way to convey a sense of it is to say that often people behaved as if appearances were persistently misleading where students were concerned. Thus a student's performance in a viva examination could be a true reflection of that person, or due to the stress of the situation; what a student wrote in an essay might be a reflection of that student's ability, or perhaps evidence of a helpful spouse or a lucky find in the library; a student's expressions of enthusiasm might be evidence of that student's commitment to health visiting, or of an attempt to ingratiate themself with the tutor; apparent vocation might turn out to be an artefact of the peer group of which a student was a member; a poor performance now might be evidence of a 'slow starter', a good performance now of a someone who would peak too soon – and so on, such that every kind of evidence was treated as ambiguous. And staff had a fund of stories citing particular students who had seemed to be thus and thus, but turned out to be otherwise.

Uncertainty as a state of mind

Given the long-standing interest in uncertainty in studies of professional socialisation this uncertainty talk intrigued me. And so, of course, did the occasions when staff seemed certainly to know about their students. For me this raised questions about when, or how or why, staff claimed certain knowledge about their students, and when they did not. Initially I framed the problem in terms of uncertainty and certainty being 'states of mind'. Thus, when people spoke uncertainly I heard this as evidence that they didn't know about students, or that what they knew was complex and confusing and didn't lead them to any definite conclusion. This was a mistake, but I ask the reader to bear with me for a while.

Something which is often associated with a grounded theory approach (Strauss and Corbin, 1998) is a policy that the researcher should not import and impose inappropriate categories from elsewhere. Where possible, analysis should be in terms of the way in which the people studied themselves classify and categorise what they experience. Among the possibilities for explaining the distribution of certainty and uncertainty, one was that staff were certain about some kinds of student and uncertain about others. Here to ground the research in local understandings meant finding out what categories staff classified students into and what criteria they used to do so.

In an attempt to investigate this I used Kelly's repertory grid technique (Kelly, 1955; Norris, 1983). To elicit local categories of student this entailed interviewing staff by presenting them with the names of three students and asking what two of them had in common but where the third differed – and then asking about another three students and so on. Enthusiasts for the repertory grid claim that after ten or so rounds of the game, respondents run out of categories, and begin to cite the same criteria over again. Then the investigator has acquired a limited set of descriptors which are important in the way in which respondents structure their own experiences, and the researcher can use the same categories to structure the analysis of the data.

In other contexts I have used Kelly's technique successfully, as have other sociological researchers (Nash, 1976 for example). In this case it failed dismally. First, staff did not run out of descriptors to indicate similarities and differences between students. Second, different staff used different descriptors. There seemed to be no common culture with stock terms or ideas about students. One premature explanation I came up with for the widespread doubt was that it derived from staff having such rich and complex schemes for classifying students on so many multiple dimensions that it was unsurprising that they never came to any definite conclusion. But that threw no light on the occasions when judgements were made with no expressions of doubt at all.

The purpose for using the repertory grid technique was to provide a foundation for the process of constant comparison in terms of locally meaningful categories. Here this would have meant looking for examples, or creating them in interviews, of interesting permutations. For example: same staff member talking about students of the same local type: same staff member talking about students of different local types; different staff talking about students of the same local type; or more elaborate permutations such as different tutors talking about different students of the same local type, in terms of different assessment-relevant topics – for example, competence in communication skills or ability to make relationships.

In processual terms, doing constant comparison meant looking out for new data according to the comparison of the moment, or re-analysing data already collected. In fact, none of this led anywhere interesting, except perhaps some data about *when* staff made uncertain or certain judgements, as you will see.

Certainty as a commitment

The problem lay in conceptualising uncertainty as a state of mind. The solution came through taking the linguistic turn (Potter and Wetherell, 1994) and thinking about what people are doing with words when they make certain or uncertain utterances. What people do when they make certain utterances is to commit themselves to a position. Once committed to a position people are in jeopardy of being judged wrong, or incompetent, sometimes immoral, sometimes disputatious (Goffman, 1981: 142). This jeopardy is avoided by uncommitted speech. Uncertain utterances are one kind of uncommitted speech, but so also is 'for the sake of argument' speech, 'devil's advocate' speech and 'on the one hand, but then again on the other' speech or 'if I put this hat on' speech. And there were plenty of examples of these kinds of speech around. The subjects of the research were staff in their roles as assessors of students, employed allegedly for their particular skills in this regard. Every time assessors utter an assessment, they make themselves available for assessment by others as to their expertise in making judgements and as to their fair-mindedness.

Avoiding making definitive statements evades the problem of uttering a judgement with which others will disagree (Schiffrin, 1990) and in terms of which one might be judged adversely. But it also creates the risk of being seen to be confused, evasive and so on. However, in the culture of health visitor education it was a matter of common agreement that assessing health visitor students is a very difficult and complex task. More blame attached to expressing a certainty with which others disagreed than in avoiding making a definitive judgement – well, most of the time.

Certainty and uncertainty as states of play

Of course, sooner or later, usually later, definitive judgements had to be issued about students. Marks had to be assigned, reports written, distinctions, merits and credits awarded. For health visitor assessment to work, eventually uncertainty had to be put aside and certainty installed in its place. Having re-conceptualised uncertainty and doubt as speech acts the important issues became those of *when* certain and uncertain utterances were made, and *in whose hearing*. I came to think of these respectively as having to do with the *temporal* organisation of assessment, and the *social structure* of assessment events.

From this point, the theoretical sampling for constant comparison took a different slant. Previously it had been about types of staff, types of student and types of criteria for judging students. Now it was about different occasions in the sequence of assessment on the one hand, and different audiences for judgements about students on the other. Readers can imagine how this proceeded from the earlier discussion, but two examples will illustrate the importance of the temporal order of assessment and its social structure.

The first example concerns the marking of written papers. Students sat examinations which were then marked by an internal examiner – a member of staff at the institution to which the students were attached. The marks were regarded as provisional until scrutinised by an external examiner and then ratified by an examination board. Externals did sometimes query the marks. They usually did this with great delicacy, off-stage, informally with the examiner concerned. Encounters of this kind were often prefaced with long sequences of talk by the external about how difficult it was to mark students, about how he or she couldn't be sure but . . ., and responded to with agreements by the internal examiner. A shared agreement as to the inherent difficulty of assessing students constituted a facility through which agreement to change the marks could be reached without externals pulling rank on the one hand, or internals losing face on the other. Usually the marks were adjusted. However, when the marks were presented formally to the examination board they were almost never subject to any query. The idea that there might have been, or remain any doubt about them was nearly always banished from such occasions. Even on two occasions where an internal examiner had refused to amend marks in line with the externals' judgements, the externals made no comment about this in the examination board or in their reports.

A second example comes from the viva voce examinations to which students were subjected as the last act of assessment. Students were given viva voce examinations by an external and an internal examiner. Each student was then discussed. Examiners found it very difficult to begin these discussions. They typically began with sequences like this:

> *External:* Well, hmm I don't know, you know I always think its very difficult to get a rounded impression in a half-hour viva
> *Internal:* Yup, but I don't know about you but she hmm sort of kept her end up fairly well.

and then proceeded rather awkwardly towards a consensus as to why the student deserved to be granted a licence to practise. Or the interchanges might begin with a joke, the person taking the first turn with a joke angling the other into the position of being the first person to issue a judgement: though often the response was a joke capping the first. There was a great deal of humour at the beginning of these discussions.

It is worth remembering here that the number of students who were failed at viva was so small that uncertainties as to whether a student should pass or fail in a real sense were minimal. But, of course, for each examiner what was uncertain was the opinion of the other as to the particular strengths and weaknesses of the candidate. They played their cards close to their chests until each had disclosed enough to the other to allow for a prediction as to the kind of judgement to which both would agree. By contrast with these discussions marked by uncertainty, at the following examination board, both or one of the examiners would usually make very 'certain' statements about the quality of each student they had seen: judgements from which doubt was entirely banished. Though on several occasions examiners disagreed with each other in their post viva discussion, only on three occasions (out of 540 possibilities) was such a disagreement aired in the examination board.

In terms of its temporal organisation, the assessment system could be seen as a set of stages where uncertain utterances about students were preferred, followed by episodes where a definite judgement was made. After this, it was not only unusual, but could be objectionable, for someone to query the judgement by making remarks indicating that they were uncertain about the grounds for or the adequacy of the decision. After decisions ratified by the examination board, even in informal situations colleagues were inclined to censure each other for suggesting that such and such student shouldn't have gained a merit, or had 'pulled the wool over the examiners' eyes'. Informal settings allowed more latitude than the formal occasions of examination board meetings, but even here people were likely to signal the deviance of doubt by prefacing their own expressions of doubt with phrases such as: 'I know it's naughty of me to say so but . . .' In passing, it is perhaps worth noting that it took some effort for me not to lapse into the naive assumption that what people said in more informal and friendly settings was closer to what they 'really' believed, than what they said in the more formal and public situations. For one thing, how could it be known whether this were true or not, when all that can be heard are words and not beliefs? For another, there is no evidence available that we are less likely to adjust our speech to please our friends, than we are to do so for strangers or superiors.

The temporal organisation of assessment intertwined with its social structure. The most important point at which doubting became objectionable was *after* an external examiner had issued a definite and public judgement, or had nodded in agreement at a definitive judgement issued by someone else. External examiners' last words made it objectionable to raise doubts any further. Similarly, when staff issued judgements in a sequence that would end with the external's 'last words' they typically provisionalised and raised caveats and allowed room for the external to issue a contrary judgement: doubt before an external's last words – certainty afterwards.

When sociologists write of social structure they are usually referring to grand structures of social class, ethnicity, gender, age and such like. But in looking at the use of language in context the important social structure is the one that manifests itself through the way in which people take turns, by what topics can be raised by one kind of person and not by another, by who can interrupt whom, who can speak longest without interruption, and whose utterances close a topic off from further discussion. In health visitor assessment, external examiners had superior speaking rights compared with others, but there were other interesting features of the immediate social structure as well. For example, many of the important events of assessment were chaired meetings, where chairs managed the taking of turns and the length of turns taken. The most usual resource for this was subject expertise. Through the way in which the chair managed turn-taking the structure of the curriculum manifested itself as a social structure of speaking rights. Thus when the issue was a 'sociological' one, the chair nominated a sociologist to speak, when a 'health visiting one', a health visitor tutor. Doctors, though having a superior status outside the context of assessment, only had superior speaking rights with regard to 'medical' issues within it, and here still deferred to chairs in meetings and to externals even on medical topics, even though externals were not doctors. People would often signal their down-status position at a particular point in time, as in 'I know I'm not a psychologist, and this might be a silly question but . . .' as a preface to some comment querying the judgement of a psychology examiner. Subject experts would also disclaim the relevance of their own expertise:

> Sociologist: Sociologically speaking that is a bit dodgy, but this is an assessment for health visiting, so I'm not inclined to be precious about this.

Signalling a willingness to be overruled allowed externals free play to have 'the last word' without seriously contradicting anyone.

In the local social structure of health visitor assessment, gender, ethnic and age differences between staff seemed largely irrelevant. What was important was, on the one hand, who someone was in terms of the curriculum – which gave them primacy in issuing judgements about some topics and not others according to what was relevant at the time – and who someone was in the hierarchy running from externals downwards, externals having the right to make the final judgement about something, chairs of board exercising the right to determine who had a say about it at a particular point in time.

Deviant cases

This picture was pieced together through the process of constant comparison, constantly asking the question 'who says what about what or about whom to what audience and when in the sequences of assessment?' Valuable data came from unusual events. Deviant cases are particularly useful for testing grounded theory. It is often very difficult to see what rules of conduct people are following, until someone breaks the rules and this is signalled by an objection, a complaint, a raised eyebrow, or back-stage gossip. Thus my views on the importance of occasions for putting an end to doubt were greatly strengthened by observing people's reactions to one external who wouldn't commit herself to definitive views when recommending that students should pass. She said things such as:

> Given it's such an uncertain business, I suppose we had better say that is a pass, but I sometimes wonder.

This kind of utterance would have passed without notice outside the examination board meeting, but her performance in the examination board at a time when certainty was required eventually led to unpleasant scenes with the chair of the board, and a request by the college for her removal as an examiner.

Again there were examples of staff being given disciplinary interviews for arguing with the external, severe reactions to people who tried to revisit decisions already made and recorded, and an unpopular external who instead of havering about the quality of viva candidates immediately announced her views and imposed them on the internal examiner. Deviant cases then test a general hypothesis such that 'if such and such is the rule then there should be an observable reaction when someone breaks it'.

Generalisations

One of the generalisations which might be drawn from this study is an epistemological one to the effect that hearing people expressing uncertainty is not necessarily to be taken as evidence of their uncertainty of mind about the topic concerned. Indeed, I observed people moving from one context in which they disclaimed any clear idea about a student, quickly to another in which they issued judgements about the same student without caveat. More generally still, I would claim that hearing people say anything about anything is not necessarily a good guide to what they generally think, but may be a good guide to what they think is sayable in the current context.

The purpose of grounded theorising is to produce a theory from the data gathered in one place which will explicate situations in other settings. When the grounded theory takes a linguistic turn the generalisations are about what people accomplish with language in situations that arise quite commonly. One very broad generalisation along these lines is that uncertainty of utterance can facilitate consensus (Schiffrin, 1990). Serious dissensus only arises when people commit themselves to positions and invest themselves in a particular version of the truth. While people remain uncommitted by their speech acts there is room for the development of a consensus position without anyone 'backing down' or 'being overruled'. Externals, for example, almost never had to say anything publicly which could be regarded as 'overruling' other examiners, and a fiction that the views of all examiners were of equal weight could be maintained. Again, in diverse settings it is not uncommon to find situations where what the truth will be will emerge as a consensus, where there is some embarrassment or other penalty for individuals 'getting it wrong' but where no one can predict what the others will say. Uncertainty talk is characteristic of such situations. Silverman demonstrates this for interviewer talk following job interviews (1973), Myers (1991) for maintaining cohesion in scientific teams, and social psychology has provided much evidence of this, though usually expressed in terms of 'group pressure' following the tradition laid down by Asch (1940).

The research reported here also draws attention to organisational devices for producing 'certain' judgements and committing people to them. The legal system provides the premier example, where once a verdict has been reached it can result in severe penalties for people to behave as if the truth were otherwise (Atkinson and Drew, 1979). My own earlier study of the use of poison oracles to settle disputes in East Africa is another example (Gomm, 1974).

Among these devices is the time-tabling of doubt and certainty such that there comes a point when a definite judgement must be made and people committed to it, sometimes irrespective of the quality of the evidence on which the judgement is based. Indeed, social life as we know it would be impossible if all decisions had to wait until there was evidence which convinced all those party to the decision (Dennett, 1988). Another device is the allocation to some functionary of the right and the duty to 'have the last word': judge, referee, consultant, team leader, boss, external examiner. In the case of poison oracles, the 'last word' goes to the chicken, who dies or survives. The research which led to Glaser and Strauss developing grounded theory also had elements of this (1964). They were investigating the situation of patients who might, or might not have a terminal prognosis, who were trying to discover what their prognosis was. One of the factors impeding their search for information was the reluctance of nurses or junior doctors to answer patients' questions without knowing what the consultant had told or would tell the patient (see also McIntosh, 1978). In this regard investigating the distribution of utterances of certainty and uncertainty provides insight into the social production of truth: or rather, into the social production of what it is that all good members of the organisation should treat as true in the situation concerned, and who has the right to say what this is. Whether people believe this or not is something of a side-issue, because even if research could produce certain knowledge of what people believe, knowing this would be an inadequate basis for understanding what they do.

References

Asch, S. (1940) 'Studies in the principles of judgements and attitudes: II Determination of judgements by the group and by ego standards', *Journal of Social Psychology*, 12: 433–65.
Atkinson, J.M. and Drew, P. (1979) *Order in Court: the Organisation of Verbal Interaction in Judicial Settings*. Basingstoke: Macmillan.
Atkinson, P. (1984) 'Training for certainty', *Social Science and Medicine*, 19 (9): 949–56.
Childe, G. (1959) *It Happened in History*. Oxford: Oxford University Press.
Davis, F. (1960) 'Uncertainty in medical prognosis: clinical and functional', *American Journal of Sociology*, 66 (1): 41–7.
Dennett, D. (1988) 'The moral first-aid manual', in S. McMurrin (ed.), *Tanner Lectures on Human Values*, Vol. III. Salt Lake City: University of Utah Press. pp. 120–47.
Fox, R. (1959) *Experiment Perilous: Physicians and Patients Facing the Unknown*. Glencoe, IL: Free Press.
Fox, R. (1980) 'The evolution of medical uncertainty', *Milbank Memorial Fund Quarterly*, 58 (1): 1–49.
Friedson, E. (1975) *The Profession of Medicine: a Study of the Sociology of Applied Knowledge*. New York: Dodd, Mead and Company.
Glaser, B. and Strauss, A. (1964) *Awareness of Dying*. Chicago: Aldine.
Goffman, E. (1981) *Forms of Talk*. Philadelphia: University of Pennsylvania Press.
Gomm, R. (1974) 'East African poison oracles', *Cambridge Anthropologist*, 2(1): 7–15.
Gomm, R. (1986) 'Normal results: an ethnographic study of health visitor student assessments'. PhD thesis submitted to the Open University.
Illich, I. (1977) *The Disabling Professions*. London: Marion Boyars.
Kelly, G. (1955) *The Psychology of Personal Constructs*. New York: Norton.
Malinowski, B. (1935) *Coral Gardens and their Magic*, vol. 2: *The Language of Magic and Gardening*. London: George Allen and Unwin.
McIntosh, J. (1978) *Communication and Awareness in a Cancer Ward*. Beckenham: Croom Helm.
Myers, G. (1991) 'Politeness and certainty: the language of collaboration in an AI project', *Social Studies of Science*, 21 (1): 37–74.
Nash, R. (1976) *Classrooms Observed*. London: Routledge and Kegan Paul.

Norris, M. (1983) *A Beginner's Guide to Repertory Grid*. Guildford: University of Surrey, Department of Sociology.

Parsons, T. (1950) 'Illness and the role of the physician', *American Journal of Orthopsychiatry*, 21 (3): 425–60.

Potter, J. and Wetherell, M. (1994) 'Analyzing discourse', in A. Bryman and R. Burgess (eds), *Analyzing Qualitative Data*. London: Routledge. pp. 47–66.

Radin, P. (1935) *Men and Magic*. Glencoe, IL: Free Press.

Schiffrin, D. (1990) 'Management of a co-operative self during argument', in A. Grimshaw, (ed.), *Conflict Talk: Sociolinguistic Investigations of Arguments in Conversations*. Cambridge: Cambridge University Press. pp. 241–59.

Silverman, D. (1973) 'Interview talk: bringing off a research instrument', *Sociology*, 17 (1): 31–47.

Strauss, A. and Corbin, J. (1998) *The Basics of Qualitative Research: Techniques and Procedures for Developing Grounded Theory*, 2nd edn. London: Sage.

What you might do now

You might like to consider further the implications of treating linguistic data as evidence of what people are doing with language at the time they use it. You could do this by comparing this study with Bowler's study in Chapter 13. Bowler treats the words of midwives as evidence of what is in their minds–a stereotype, which shapes their actions. Would it make a great deal of difference if their utterances were taken as evidence of what they were doing with words when they said them?

Carry out a more systematic appraisal of the study using 'Questions to Ask about Qualitative Research' in Part 4 of this book

What you might do now

Think some more about the problems and possibilities of naturalistic observation by reading Chapter 16 and perhaps some of the further reading cited in that chapter

Use the Appendix to find some research of interest to you based on naturalistic observation and appraise it using 'Questions to ask about Qualitative Research' in Part 4 of this book

CHAPTER 15

ACTION RESEARCH: APPLIED QUALITATIVE METHODS IN THE FAMILY CENTRE

Winter, Celia (1996) 'Creating quality care for children in the family centre', *Educational Action Research*, 4 (1): 49–57

EXEMPLAR

What you need to understand in order to understand the exemplar
The general idea of 'action research'. *See Chapter 16, section 9*
Where claims are made about cause–effect relationships, the importance of having clear characterisations of the situation before and after the intervention. *See Chapter 5, section 10*
The difficulty of demonstrating cause–effect relationships convincingly without experimental control. *See Chapter 5, sections 1 and 3*
The importance of providing readers with information as to how the data were collected and analysed so that they can be evaluated. *See Chapter 16, section 7*
Insofar as the action research is presented as a model to follow, the importance of specifying very clearly exactly what actions were taken. *See Chapter 5, section 7*

Introduction

The major purpose of 'action research' is to effect some worthwhile change. In that sense its major objectives are those of practice rather than research. The research aspects of action research have to do with recording and analysing what happened in order to explain why, and perhaps to provide a clear model for others to follow in order to produce similar results. Thus it is possible for a piece of action research to be 'good practice' and 'poor research', or 'good research' and 'poor practice'. In the former case this would mean that something good happened, but for reasons which are far from clear, and in the latter case that something bad happened, but for reasons which are very clearly explained. From the point of view of *readers* of action research, its quality as research is much more important than its quality as practice, irrespective of whether the results of the actions taken were benign or not.

The exemplar study for this chapter is chosen from one genre of action research – *educational action research* (see Chapter 16, section 9), where most emphasis is placed on the value of what those involved in the research learn from doing it. The project also had the objective of improving the quality of services for children in a family centre. In both respects, claims are being made about changes and about causes and effects. Hence the kind of evidence required to make a convincing case involves some kind of 'baseline measurement' (how things were before, whether in terms of states of knowledge or quality of care) and some kind of 'outcome measurement' (how things were afterwards) and evidence that what was done was the cause of the changes recorded. There is no inherent reason why action research should not be quantitative. If n-of-1 experiments or single case evaluations (Chapter 5, section 13) are 'action research', then they are quantitative examples. But it happens that most researchers who describe themselves as action researchers record their work in terms of qualitative data. There are particular difficulties in using qualitative data to demonstrate cause–effect relationships, and particular difficulties in demonstrating cause–effect relationships where experimental control cannot be achieved (Chapter 5, Introduction and section 3; Chapter 10 section 11).

CREATING QUALITY CARE FOR CHILDREN IN THE FAMILY CENTRE

Celia Winter

Abstract

This paper is written on behalf of social work practitioners at the Wyrely Birch Family Centre, Birmingham, by Celia Winter, Project Leader. It is our first attempt at action research and tells how, as a team, we worked to consider the wishes of small children who come with their parents to a family centre. It covers a period of work over 6 months in 1992 which included evaluation and self-examination. It is the story beneath the external management view of the family centre as working to aims and objectives, tasks, roles, policies and purposes and shows how we tried to establish the centre as genuinely child focused without separating parents and children.

Much has been written about family centres and their impact on parents, but their impact on children has by comparison suffered neglect. For example, Kathy Cigno (1988), writing about 'Consumer views of a family centre drop-in', observes that they are something different from social work help for a range of adults and children but she does not interview any children. Similarly, Wendy MacFarlane (1989), in her paper 'Langleen Family Centre: a community social work approach to services for families', refers to children under the heading 'Bringing up children is problematic'. This adult perspective fails to recognise that children have an agenda in their own right. Jenus Qvertrup (1990) has commented in her *A Voice for Children in Statistical and Social Accounting: a Plea for Children's Right to be Heard* that information gained about families also comes from an adult perspective and therefore creates serious problems for those who want to give proper accounts of children's lives.

In our view, children have been lost from the family centre story. The following is an account of how, over a period of 6 months, my five colleagues and I set about creating quality care for children in a family centre.

The family centre is situated in the Wyrley Birch area of Kingstanding, Birmingham. It opened in September 1990 in a neighbourhood with few facilities, poor housing and people living with the effects of social isolation. The project is housed in a three-bedroomed maisonette, set amongst residential property and opposite the local shops. The model for the centre was developed based on ideas I had when I was a social worker based in an office going out to visit 'clients'. I used to wish there was somewhere to which I could refer my clients, somewhere where staff could give time to people and offer something to increase the self-esteem of parents. Here, local people can bring their children to a thrice weekly 'drop-in', they can seek advice if desired and we also provide individual work with families referred by the local Social Services Department, which results in our assisting and supporting families where child care and child protection is of concern. The emphasis is on voluntary participation. The centre also offers groups for parents such as cooking, swimming, discussion – all with a crèche facility – and also trips, outings and the 'drop-in'. This phrase is used to describe the facility open 3 days a week to parents and children under 5. People may 'drop-in' between 10 am and 3 pm for as little or as much time as they wish. Opportunity is given for socialising and for children to play. The Health Authority runs the baby clinic and a family planning clinic from the centre and staff from the Department of Social Security and local councillors run advice sessions.

We developed the centre within the almost taken-for-granted, perhaps typical, perspective of family centre workers, which assumes that in order to be successful one must engage the parents and offer an alternative way for social work. We assumed that we had an opportunity to have different, more positive and less threatening relationships with parents. We believed that we could offer the opportunity for parental participation in decision-making, experiencing choice and control, and for informal learning. These were things we had hitherto not found possible to offer within our local authority social work experience.

However, as a staff group we were interested to find after approximately 18 months that, through our evaluation of everyday life in the centre, we were all particularly concerned about the children and their situation in the daily life of the centre. Whatever our role within the centre, our encounter with children was held in common. We all had reason to give thought to addressing the same question – 'Where are the children in all of this?' In order to own the question, we agreed to consider how it linked to our experience. There was a tension for staff who were being placed between the demands of the parent and those of the child. We recognised that we were likely to be contributing to it because of our ambiguity about our responsibilities to parent and child interests. We were unclear about our expectations compared to staff in nurseries, schools or playgroups or even a health and welfare clinic which takes place in our building once a week. We recognised the need to work towards developing a policy towards children in the centre without invalidating the parents' experience gained from using the centre.

To pursue this policy task we had to disengage from our past thinking and perceptions. We had to criticise our assumption of the 'family' as user of the centre, as we could see that this failed to recognise the child as a person with rights. Children were being marginalised by being viewed as *visiting* the centre whilst it was being used by their parents. We concluded that our purpose in developing a policy was to give children the status of 'persons' within the centre, not that of 'somebody's child'. In order to be successful we had to bring about changes in adult behaviour and in the assumption that made children invisible or influential, as a 'bother to control' or 'objects of concern'. We thought our end result should produce guidelines accepted in the project to govern how children should be given rights to a quality experience of child care.

So, what had to be done? Our aim was to understand and to change a problematic situation. We chose our research methodology accordingly. A problem was emerging from the experience of staff in the family centre. We were experiencing an uncertainty in our work, the concrete meaning of which was not clear to us as a team. How were we to discover how to address a problematic situation in which we were all implicated?

In *Human Enquiry in Action*, Reason (1986) pointed to how we might regard ourselves as both the subjects and the objects of our research: how together we might inquire into the experiences we shared that we needed to understand more fully by systematic study of what happened in a situation we thought we knew well!

Prior to moving to the centre I, as Project Leader, had felt very strongly the need to research into the development issues of the project. I did not know exactly what method would be appropriate but was sure that a collection of statistical data would not be entirely satisfactory. As part of our practice, we had kept a daily diary within the centre and were already regularly reviewing and evaluating our activities and events. Therefore the idea of participatory research seemed the right method for the centre. It involved staff fully, enabled everyone to take an active and valuable role whilst enabling team building and a development of understanding between the group. We were as a group led by a consultant, who guided us throughout, as none of the staff had ever attempted action research or indeed any research before. Most of the children at the time of the research were under the age of 3.

The staff group is made up of six women, two of whom were formerly social workers. Practitioners reading this will be familiar with the experience of being jaded by the social work role, with its increased bureaucracy and lack of community involvement. This, as well as being seen in a negative light by clients, was a strong motivator for us wishing to work in a family centre. Other members of the team had worked with small children in nurseries and as childminders.

The development of the research took some time. Guided by our consultant, we did not arrive at our question immediately; rather we were led through a process of review and evaluation to the question, 'How can we create quality care for children in a family centre?' In order to begin becoming researchers we needed to share our own personal experiences. Each of us tried to articulate our own perspective on the children within the centre; how we felt towards them, how we thought about and perceived them, as well as how we behaved towards them in the centre. The change process therefore began with our personal learning. Sheila Harre-Augstein and Laurie Thomas write in *Learning Conversations* (1990): 'the group begins to understand that there is experiential and conversational evidence of learning about a situation and there is recorded behaviourial or performance evidence of learning'. In other words, if we were to resolve our problematic situation, we had to observe our process, record our observations, interpret the data and demonstrate that we were able to learn together.

These separate, personal reflections that began the research ensured that it became a collective learning process out of which we recognised that we needed to review our practice, look at our past experience with new eyes and consider change. During the research process, we saw the value in monitoring, recording and analysing practice and could see the development of the project team as a learning group.

After the initial period of sharing personal ideas and beliefs, we adopted the target of achieving a coherent picture of the quality of our practice through undertaking observations of the drop-in. We needed to know how it worked for the children. It was a difficult task as we found our attention being sought mainly by the parents. We collected data from amongst the everyday action, with no structured questions but by focusing our observations on the experience of the children as they arrived at the centre. Each member of staff undertook an exercise in tracking the arrival of the children and making notes on what they observed.

We all found the process of tracking interesting but difficult. Some children went about their business but others, familiar with our attention and interest, sought to engage us. Parents sought our attention and things would happen to distract us. As a team we spent time breaking down the situation, discussing and considering our personal perceptions and developing themes. One of the significant themes was the lack of continuity provided by the staff and this led us to recognise the need for certain 'ground rules' which would ensure a degree of overall continuity within the drop-in. This sounds quite a simple task but in fact proved to be quite time consuming. It necessitated self-examination and criticism of practice. Our consultant suggested how we might test the validity of our experiences to enable us to decide on necessary changes in practice. We did this by discussing the aspects of drop-in, the inconsistencies of what staff do at drop-in and what we would ideally like to achieve. The development of the research element of the work led us away from an awareness of the children themselves to a consideration of our own practice.

Another theme which affected the children was food. We became aware through the observation of the level of children's concentration spans, the amount of drinks and crisps being offered by parents and the interest shown by both parents and children at the staff's lunch-time activities. As a staff group, we are inclined to bring our potatoes to bake in the microwave, as well as beans, soup, etc., but initially, it was clear that the parents had neither thought about lunch for themselves nor for their children. This appeared to be due to lack of parenting skills, lack of knowledge about the culture of the centre and in some cases, lack of money. We found that we (the staff) were continually feeding little open mouths if we sat in the drop-in to eat. Some staff found this irritating. They felt the need for personal space but also felt concerned for the children – again, a self-awareness was highlighted by the research process. We encouraged the parents to bring lunch if they wanted to stay all day and indeed began to provide toast for the extremely hungry. We are pleased that this pattern of bringing lunch has now become established.

The reflection process and sense-making process encouraged by our consultant helped us to see that it would be important for two members of staff to be involved in drop-in – one for the parents and one for the children – even though sometimes the number of people in the building is very small. It sounds so obvious now as I write 3 years later, but by developing our idea together, it has become practice owned by us all. We do not make definite arrangements as to our role, other than a common understanding of the necessity for one of us to concentrate on the adults and one on the children. The children, as a result of these arrangements, have attention and focus from the adult who in turn encourages parents to value the pleasure their children gain from positive play.

The irritation felt by staff at the interest shown by others in their own food was recognised, as was the space needed by staff. Staff care and attention to our own needs was considered and measures to ensure this were incorporated into the Ground Rules. Our Ground Rules are outlined in the Appendix. Three years on, all these ground rules are an accepted part of life at the centre. They are the norm and it seems strange in retrospect that it took so long to develop.

Our next exercise was to consider the position of power held by the child within the relationship with the parent and the staff from the centre. We wanted to consider the impact of the centre on the children and whether they had any influence in their parents' decision to come to the centre. We tried to spot 'critical incidents' relating to the power held by the child with the relationship between parent and staff (see Figure 1).

We began to observe and reflect upon situations. For example: Polly aged 2 came to the drop-in with her mother just as we were leaving to go swimming. Mother was not prepared for swimming as she had visited the Housing Department. Polly insisted that she wanted to go swimming and in spite of her mother saying she had no costume, no time and no inclination, Polly won the day. They went home, fetched the costumes and both enjoyed swimming. They subsequently came swimming regularly. Jo, mother of Lance (aged 2), told us how Lance had pressurised her into coming to the centre. He shouted out the names of staff from the balcony as we arrived at the centre, which is situated beneath his flat. He took his coat, tried to put it on and made for the door. Jo knew exactly where he wanted

Figure I   Power in the parent–child–staff relationship

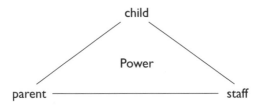

to go. She said he wouldn't let up until she agreed to come. Mark, aged 15 months, was struggling to get out of his pushchair on the opposite side of the road and pointing at the gate. His Mum said 'OK, OK, we'll go on the way back', which they did. These and other situations made us reflect upon how the children attach meanings of their own to being at the centre. Is it a place of safety, a place of peace or a place of stimulation? Is it somewhere they can recall which is local and almost within their reach where they can be assured of a welcome and recognition of themselves as people? We consider the power of children to influence their parents and all adults. Anna was not at all happy in the centre; although under 2 she made it very clear she did not want to come, and in spite of her mother's expressed desire to take part in a group, she ceased to do so. Anna won her point.

During both these processes, i.e. developing the ground rules of the drop-in and tracking and observing the children, the parents engaged themselves by questioning our interest in their children. We then included the parents in our observations and subsequently drew their attention to the pleasure of their children's actions: so often the 'magical moment' of a child's action and activity can be lost in the general 'hubbub' and chaos of everyday life.

These observations were especially interesting to us in view of our original perception that we had to 'hook' the parents to come to the centre, otherwise we would feel unnecessary and under-used. We could see that the children did have influence over their parents – clearly not a new idea, but it was interesting to us in relation to specific children who may have been perceived by adults as being appendages to their parents. It made us question what influence staff at the centre had on parents. We hoped that our positive child-aware approach was having a knock-on effect. Parents began to say, 'You are so good with them', which concerned us. We do not wish to be seen as more expert than the parents and we have continued to bring parents into our activities with the child where at all possible and appropriate.

In the wake of the drop-in research, we also reviewed the crèche. We run two groups each week for which we provide a crèche. Because of space, the groups are 'closed', enabling us to have an idea of numbers and personalities. Drawing upon our knowledge, we listed our 'ideal crèche' – the things we would like to do, the ages and number of children and the staff ratio. We then listed the 'reality' and compromised, creating as near to our ideal as we could under the circumstances. Plans were agreed regarding time, activities, staff, drinks, etc., and ground rules drawn up. These include a slot for parents and children to reunite and share their separate experiences at the end of a group.

Again with the benefit of hindsight, I believe that we are now more confident in ourselves as workers and as a team and that we should have invited parents to join with us at this stage, but we did not. At this stage, we believed that by providing a 'better facility', we would be creating quality care for children. We did not attempt to obtain the child's voice, merely our interpretation of the child's view based on our experience of child development theory.

The idea of doing some research running alongside the setting up of the centre developed into a learning process for staff. The fact that we had a 'reflective culture' already in place (i.e. we were accustomed to planning and evaluating our activities), meant that participative research fitted comfortably into the everyday work of staff. It began with a topic of common concern and developed into a task. The task led to reflection and agreed changes in working practice. This has enabled us to increase understanding of our role, and has given an example to parents of the importance of questioning how their children experience the world.

We have by no means finished. We are learning about the process of our learning and about how we can achieve change in a crucial area of our practice. We have developed as we have accumulated experience and awareness. We have become more accessible to children on their terms and are able to share this with their parents. Within the centre, negotiating ground rules and tracking and drawing attention to 'magical moments', has brought recognition of the child as an individual and has developed in the parents an acknowledgement and acceptance that their children do have rights.

In the light of our new knowledge and with the growth and development that 3 years' further experience affords us, both as individuals and as a team, we are currently using action research methods to develop a children's group in a refuge for women who have been victims of domestic violence. The work we did as described in this article has greatly enhanced our skills and I hope that a future article will show that development.

References

Cigno. K. (1988) Consumer views of a family centre drop-in, *British Journal of Social Work*, 18: 361–75.
Harre-Augstein, S. and Thomas, L. (1990) *Learning Conversations*. London: Routledge.
MacFarlane, W. (1989) *Langleen Family Centre: a Community Social Work Approach to Services for Families*. National Institute of Social Work.
Qvertrup, J. (1990) *A Voice for Children in Statistical and Social Accounting: a Plea for Children's Right to be Heard*. London: Thelma Press.
Reason, P. (ed.) (1986) *Human Enquiry in Action*. London: Sage.

Appendix

Ground Rules

1   *Role of organiser*

   Stage 1: **Organiser** welcomes, makes drinks, gets toys out. As the day progresses, organiser becomes **Facilitator**.
   Stage 2: **Facilitator** needs to communicate expectations, i.e. clearing centre by 3.15 pm, ensuring washing-up done.
   Stage 3: **Organiser** + team support for completing the day.

2   *Toilet*
Parent's responsibility.

3   *Child care*

- Care of children for short periods by arrangement, including other people's children.
- Users take responsibility for other people's children they are minding.

4   *Advice*
Advice by appointment but *publish opening times*.

5 *Safety*

- Bolt the garden gate.
- Use one garden only at a time.
- Delegate responsibility to parent or staff to supervise garden.

6 *Food*
Monday and Wednesday.

- Change staff at lunch-time or lunch-time cover.
- Respond to hungry child with toast – parent to prepare.
- Encourage parent to bring food for child and self.

Monitor feeding of children in Diary

- Care of self – own space.
- Care of children – hunger.
- Care of each other – celebrate food.
- Care of parents.

What you might do now

You might like to consider further the difficulties of demonstrating cause–effect relationships without clear baseline and outcome measures and without some kind of experimental control by comparing this study with the accounts of n-of-1 experiments and single case evalutions in Chapter 5, section 13

Carry out a more systematic appraisal of the study using 'Questions to Ask about Action Research' in Part 4 of this book

What you might do now

Think more generally about the investigation of 'effective practice' using various methods of research, dipping into Chapters 5, 10 and 16

Use the Appendix and find some action research of interest to you and appraise it using 'Questions to Ask about Action Research' in Part 4 of this book

CHAPTER 16

COLLECTING AND ANALYSING QUALITATIVE DATA

Introduction — 1 Forcing the answers in the Health and Lifestyle Survey — 2 Thematic analysis: structuring data after collecting them — 3 Loosely structured interviews contrasted with naturalistic observation — 4 Grounded theory research: structuring theory and data together — 5 The linguistic turn in qualitative research — 6 Thematic analysis and linguistic analysis compared — 7 The objectivity of qualitative research — 8 Generalisability and qualitative research — 9 Action research — 10 Further reading on qualitative research and action research — References and further reading

Introduction

This volume cannot hope to represent the huge and bewildering variety of kinds of research which are described as 'qualitative' by their protagonists (Denzin and Lincoln, 1998). Instead, three exemplar studies have been chosen to illustrate three methods of collecting data commonly used by self-styled qualitative researchers: in-depth or loosely structured interviewing (Chapter 12), non-participant observation research (Chapter 13) and participant observation research (Chapter 14). The latter refers to researchers becoming part of the setting they are studying and reporting on activities which would probably happen whether they were there or not. The term *ethnographic data* is often used as an alternative to qualitative data, when data have been collected through methods of naturalistic observation. But sometimes this term is used for qualitative data of any kind.

This part of the book also includes an exemplar of action research (Chapter 15). Action research is a term which is even more slippery than the term qualitative research. There is no inherent reason why action research should be reported in qualitative rather than quantitative terms. But, currently, most people who describe themselves as action researchers do not quantify much of their data. Hence the inclusion of this exemplar in this part of the book.

Patterns which show in data have always been put there by the activities of researchers in doing the research, analysing the data and writing it up. This is true whether the data are cast into numbers and manipulated statistically or whether they are expressed in verbal forms without attempts at quantification. To say that researchers create their data does not mean that what researchers claim are figments of their imagination. But it does mean that, in order to appraise the research, readers need to be able to reconstruct what was done by the researcher in order to judge whether the claims are credible or not. This chapter is primarily about the way in which the methods of qualitative research produce data.

1   Forcing the answers in the Health and Lifestyle Survey

The British Health and Lifestyle Survey (Cox et al., 1987; Blaxter, 1990; Cox et al., 1993) was a large-scale survey of people's health experience and health-related beliefs and behaviours, carried out in England, Wales and Scotland in 1984/5. There was a follow-up in 1991/2 so that changes over time could be measured. It was a questionnaire survey with a mixture of forced choice and open-ended questions. For some writers (Wright, 1997, for example) most of the data it produced would be regarded as *qualitative* since few of them reach the interval or ratio level (see Chapter 6, section 3). However, it is more usual to draw the line between any data which can be expressed numerically on one side, and call these 'quantitative', and data which are presented in the form of verbal descriptions ('qualitative') on the other. For survey research this line usually falls somewhere near the distinction between data which are produced from forced choice questions, and data which are produced from open-ended questions.

Figure 16.1 gives one of the pages from the interviewer's protocol for administering the Health and Lifestyle Survey. It is a good illustration of the *structuring of data prior to collection*. It has already been decided what relevant opinions people can have and whether, for the survey, they can hold these opinions in a binary way (*know/don't know* and if *know, yes* or *no*) as for Question 13, or with varying degrees of strength, as with the *rating scales* for Question 14. Apart from Question 13b, these questions are posed in such a way as to generate responses which are pre-classified and hence easy to count. With an initial sample size of over 9,000 and a follow-up of 5,352, handling responses in numerical terms is really all that is feasible. The results of the survey have to make statements, such as, for example, working class people hold a given opinion more strongly than middle class people, or that men say 'yes' to this question more frequently than women. And the aim is that such statements of

Figure 16.1 Interviewer's schedule for Questions 13 and 14 of the Health and Lifestyle Survey (Cox et al., 1987)

			Col./Code	Skip to:
13 a)	Do you think it is ever people's own fault if they get ill?		(358)	
		Yes	1	b)
		No	0	Q.14
		Don't know/not sure	8	
b)	IF 'YES' (CODE AT a) Why do you think it's their fault if they get ill? RECORD VERBATIM. DO <u>NOT</u> PROBE OR PROMPT			

							Col.
14	SHOW CARD B On this card are things people have said about health. I'd like you to say how far you agree with each statement. The answers you can give are shown on the top of the card. READ OUT EACH ITEM AND CODE						
	STATEMENT	Strongly agree	Agree	All depends (Don't Know)	Disagree	Strongly Disagree	
a)	It is sensible to do exactly what the doctors say	1	2	3	4	5	(359)
b)	To have good health is the most important thing in life	1	2	3	4	5	(360)
c)	Generally health is a matter of luck	1	2	3	4	5	(361)
d)	If you think too much about your health, you are more likely to be ill	1	2	3	4	5	(362)
e)	Suffering sometimes has a divine purpose	1	2	3	4	5	(363)
f)	I have to be very ill before I'll go to the doctor	1	2	3	4	5	(364)
g)	People like me don't really have time to think about their health	1	2	3	4	5	(365)
h)	The most important thing is the constitution (the health) you are born with	1	2	3	4	5	(366)

frequency, while derived from a sample, will be true also of the wider population (see Chapter 10, section 1).

The questions in Figure 16.1 were chosen in the light of what knowledge there was at the time about important ways in which people's beliefs about health do vary, and how variations in such beliefs correlate with both their health-related behaviour and their morbidity and mortality. Research using loosely structured interviews was an important preliminary to deciding on the questions for the questionnaire. The questions were pilot tested. With few exceptions, it was essential that the same questions were used in the follow up in order to measure changes over time reliably (see Chapter 10, section 14).

There are good reasons for using forced choice questions (Chapter 10, section 14) but the data they produce have obvious limitations. Responses to Question 13a on the Health and Lifestyle questionnaire would tell how many people of different kinds would say 'yes' when asked 'Do you think it is ever people's own fault if they get ill?' But 'yes/no/don't know' answers do not indicate what people mean by saying 'yes'. There is a very large number of different ways in which people might mean a 'yes' answer. Question 13b attempts to deal with this. But it immediately produces another problem. How are all the various answers to question 13b to be classified into a limited range of types about which some summary statements might be made? And with a very large sample some kind of summary statement will be necessary if the data from this question are to be used at all. Asking question 13b in itself, of course, puts some structure into the data collected. Note that there is no equivalent follow-up question for people who answered 'no' or 'don't know' to Question 13a – nor indeed are there any follow-up questions to people who answer 'strongly agree' to Question 14a, and so on. However, these other questions structure the answers *in advance* to a much greater extent than does the open-ended Question 13b: they are questions for which the responses are *pre-coded*. For Question 13b the data will have to be structured to a much greater extent *at the point of analysis*. A wide diversity of responses will have to be classified into a limited number of types, and the frequency of each type counted.

2 Thematic analysis: structuring data after collecting them

In the exemplar study for Chapter 12 Mildred Blaxter picks up a puzzle which was raised by answers to Question 13 on the protocol shown in Figure 16.1. As one of the members of the Health and Lifestyle team, she was intrigued by the finding that working class people were much more likely to blame ill-health on individual behaviour, than were people from other social classes. The puzzle came from comparing this with the substantial body of research (see Chapter 11, sections 3 and 4) showing that socio-economic deprivation is much more important than behaviour in delivering ill-health and premature mortality disproportionately to the working class. Hence her title '*Why do the victims blame themselves?*' The Health and Lifestyle responses to Question 13b gave some hints, but Blaxter investigated this further by re-analysing some loosely structured interviews which had been conducted as part of the Health and Lifestyle study.

The term 'unstructured interview' is quite commonly used in the literature but it is slightly misleading. Any kind of talk which is recognisable as 'an interview' has an 'interview structure' with one person playing the role of and talking as an interviewer and another person playing the role of and speaking as a respondent. What the term 'unstructured' (or 'in depth') usually implies is that the interviewer has some kind of checklist of topics he or she would like the interview to cover, but without specifying the order in which topics will be dealt with or the form of words in which questions will be posed. The term 'loosely structured' is a better term for this. The loosely structured interview will allow for interesting, but previously unpredicted lines of enquiry to be followed up, and for respondents to raise topics of interest to them.

Loosely structured interviews produce large quantities of data on which some structure has to be imposed. Box 16.1 contains an extract from Blaxter's study which shows part of the process of imposing a structure on data derived from a loosely structured interview. Note that the transcript only includes speech by the respondent, and sometimes in paraphrase. The implications of this are discussed in sections 5, 6 and 7.

The text in Box 16.1 shows extracts from one of Blaxter's interview transcripts coded in terms of *themes:* for example: 'life stage', 'stress, social circumstances' and so on. This is not very different in principle from the coding implied in the interviewer schedule in Figure 16.1: the coding there is shown in terms of code numbers. But for Blaxter coding is done at a different stage of the research process and respondents have had more opportunity to determine which codes will be used in analysing the data simply because they have played a more pro-active role in the interview than someone responding to a forced choice, fixed sequence questionnaire.

Where themes come from in qualitative research is sometimes a mystery. In some way or another they always come from the data, but since any set of data is capable of being analysed in terms of a very large number of themes, it is often difficult to know why a researcher has chosen one set of themes rather than another. However, the attempt is to find a limited set of ideas which are both relevant

Box 16.1   Coding data thematically

G14 – aged 54, 12 children

The main complaint chronic bronchitis: began with 'change of life at the time'. But also	life stage
began when husband, 'a war pensioner', could not work and she 'took on a really old house' with the idea of lodgers. 'And then I took ill. I had a' the work and a' thing, you see.'	stress, social circumstances
The bronchitis 'started off with flu, and developed from that.'	
Doctors told her it was smoking, and 'I stopped for nine months!' (But claims was better when she started again.)	(?) behaviour
Second, later, account of beginning of bronchitis: had a bout of pneumonia and neglected it, because she will never 'give in' to illness. 'Cos that was me, wi' pneumonia and bronchitis, walking down to the City hospital' (very long account of resisting hospitalization, on this and other occasions)	self-neglect
'I said, I'm nae gaun intae nae bed, I've a' these bairns at hame, I'm gaun back.' 'It's got to beat me first afore I'll call the doctor.'	life stage 'not giving in'
At about the same time she had a bad fall on ice in the street, 'Something gaed intae my leg'. Secondary trouble is still pains in the leg and and arms. 'It wis after that I first got the cold, and it went to my chest.'	effects of trauma
At present has laryngitis, but 'I'm blaming the weather.' 'And smoking disnae help.'	weather behaviour
The continued pain is perhaps 'just wear and tear on the spine'. Of course 'You couldnae expect onything else, wi' all that bairns.' She had two children after 40, which was 'too auld, maybe.'	natural ageing childbearing
Also has 'a kinda knot at the back o' my neck', which may be affecting the spine, but 'I think it's just a cyst maybe'.	
Also suffers from migraine. Considers whether it is perhaps associated with her neck? But 'I've had migraine since the last one was born.'	childbearing
Nevertheless describes self as healthy. 'The only recipe I say is nae to lie down wi' the least little thing that's wrang wi' ye. Sometimes, if ye ging awa' and do a little bit of washing or something, you forget a' aboot your pains.'	self-responsibility 'not giving in'

to the topic of the research and which, between them, constitute a common framework in terms of which the data deriving from different respondents can be described. In terms of contrasts and comparisons 'themes' have some similarity with the idea of 'variables' in quantitative research: where Maud said 'x' in terms of this theme, Geraldine said 'y'.

Thematic analysis of this kind can be done more or less rigorously. Sometimes qualitative researchers attempt to achieve inter-rater reliability (Chapter 6, section 6) in coding a passage of talk as being an example of a theme. This can be done by using a panel of judges to code a sample of transcripts and using an inter-rater reliability test to express their level of agreement (Armstrong et al., 1997). The process of data collection in qualitative research may not be very reliable when viewed in contrast to the use of a structured questionnaire (see Chapter 10, section 14), but there is no reason why the analysis of the data should not be highly reliable.

The analysis of qualitative data these days is often aided by one of the powerful software packages designed for this purpose, such as NUDIST or Ethnograph (Fielding and Lee, 1991; Richards and Richards, 1994). Occasionally the process is described as *content analysis*. This term is more frequently used for analysing printed or broadcast media, and sometimes suggests a numerical approach, but the principles are much the same (Silverman, 1993: Chapter 4).

Where data collection involves a questionnaire, many of the important decisions about what the data can mean have been made before the data are collected. Where loosely structured interviews are employed many of such decisions are delayed until after the interviews. Conducting loosely structured interviews may avoid the problem of imposing an inappropriate structure on the data, but the meaning of the data collected from one person will derive from making comparisons and contrasts with the data collected from all the people interviewed: something that can only be discovered after many interviews have been conducted. Interesting issues arising from interviews with some people may not have counterparts in the data from interviews with others. Perhaps this will reflect important differences between respondents, or merely the fact that what comes out of loosely structured interviews depends on the twists and turns of conversation. Where there is only one opportunity to collect data from each person this is a problem if the researcher does not know what is relevant until after all the interviews have been completed.

Sometimes researchers using loosely structured interviews will have an opportunity to do follow-up interviewing, and hence an opportunity to focus a second wave of interviews on the issues which have emerged as important from the analysis of the first wave.

Loosely structured interviews and questionnaire research are not necessarily alternatives to each other. They are very commonly combined in a single research programme. For example, the design of the Health and Lifestyle questionnaire (see Figure 16.1) was based on preliminary research involving loosely structured interviews which indicated the kinds of things which people believed to be relevant to their health. But because it is impracticable to conduct loosely structured interviews with large numbers of people it would have been unclear as to how far those interviewed were representative of the wider population. The questionnaire research with its large sample was ideally suited to accomplish representativeness, in the sense of being able to quantify how many people in the population would be likely to answer 'yes' to a particular question. But, as noted above, the survey could not provide detailed insight into the diverse meanings of 'yes', 'no' and so on. Some elucidation was available from the preliminary interviews, and this is the subject of Blaxter's study (Chapter 12), but had these data been unavailable it would have been possible to reverse the order of events: representative questionnaire survey first, followed by a programme of loosely structured interviews to find out what people might mean if they gave particular answers to the questionnaire.

3 Loosely structured interviews contrasted with naturalistic observation

The notion of validity which lies behind most qualitative research is rather different from that discussed in Chapter 6. There the discussion was in terms of the validity of research instruments. But from a qualitative researcher's point of view, instruments may get in the way of achieving *ecological* or *naturalistic* validity (Cicourel, 1982). As the term 'ecological' suggests, the analogy is often drawn between, on the one hand, the study of animal behaviour in zoos and laboratories where scientific validity may be great, but may only tell about what animals do in highly artificial situations, and, on the other, the study of animal behaviour, *naturalistically* in the field, where scientific validity may be lower, but ecological validity can be achieved. In health and social care research the strongest claims to ecological validity can be made by those who study events going on 'in their natural habitat' by observation or participant observation. None the less, the idea of ecological validity still guides those who prefer open-ended, loosely structured interviews to questionnaire research, and even to some extent, those who prefer open-ended questions on questionnaires over forced choice ones. The point they are making is that highly structured research methods may rip data out of their context, and the analysis put them together in ways that may be quite different from the understandings and experiences of the people from whom the data were derived. This leads to a policy of avoiding, as far as possible, imposing a structure *in advance* on what is being studied.

However, there must be serious doubts about the capacity of any interview to achieve ecological validity (Cicourel, 1982). Put crudely, what researchers learn by interviewing people is what people will tell researchers in interviews. This may or may not have any relationship to what they think, feel or do in other situations. Blaxter's study, for example, used loosely structured interviews to elicit ideas about health and illness. The responses took the form of stories – narratives – with plots in which one thing led to another, and characters – themselves and their kin – who had personality characteristics and motives and who responded to their circumstances in various ways. Blaxter was not interested in whether these stories were true in the sense of being historically accurate accounts of events as they had happened. She was interested in the stories as being illustrations of the ways in which these women, ordinarily, in everyday life, understood matters of health and illness. In this sense stories told to an interviewer during an interview have to stand for what would be going through a respondent's mind when, elsewhere, at another time, he or she was faced with some situation with health implications. Blaxter has no access to these other situations and there is no way of knowing whether the themes – see Box 16.1 – discovered in the interviews are constituents of the way in which respondents understood illness in the course of their everyday lives, or instead, just devices they use to put together stories to tell interviewers. It seems reasonable, however, to assume that there is some relationship between understanding and telling.

What happens in people's minds is never directly observable and there is always a problem of inferring what people *think* from what they say or do. This problem is doubled when the evidence for what people think *in one situation* is inferred from what they *say* in *another situation*, as is often the case in an interview. This is not necessarily a problem that respondents can help to resolve. In an interview a respondent will probably know what they think they think when they are in another situation. They will not necessarily be right about that and it is nearly always impossible to find evidence to judge whether they were right or wrong.

Putting a high premium on ecological validity favours researching situations at first hand by observing them happening, rather than at second hand, by hearsay via interviews, though using the two approaches in tandem is not uncommon (see Bowler's study in Chapter 13 for example). Various strategies of observation are possible, each of which has its strengths and weaknesses.

Participant observation research implies that the researcher is or becomes a member of whatever social situation is being studied. For example, if the research location is a hospital ward then the researcher combines the role of researcher with that of being a patient, a nurse, an ancillary worker or with some other role which is a constituent of the situation. There are various reasons for favouring *participant* over non-participant observation. One is to gain access to situations which might otherwise be inaccessible. Another is to minimise the effect of observation on whatever is happening, since people may behave differently when they are aware that they are being researched. Participation by the researcher in the ordinary activities of the setting serves to distract attention from the fact that research is going on. *Covert*, or secret participant observation will achieve this most completely, but there are strong ethical objections to spying on people (O'Connell Davidson and Layder, 1994: 214–17). It seems that if *overt* participant observation is conducted over the long term, people forget that they are being studied. There is an ethical argument for saying that they should be constantly reminded. But in practice it seems that few participant observers do this. While Bowler's research (Chapter 13) was not covert, it seems doubtful whether the midwives she studied had any clear idea as to how she would subsequently describe them.

There are problems with adopting a participant observation strategy. Someone, for example, who as a researcher plays the role of a nurse on a ward, will then always be communicated with as if a nurse, and will only have access to those situations where nurses can go. What he or she can observe will be limited and slanted by the role adopted. Again, once a role has been adopted researchers may become inhibited from asking the kinds of questions researchers need to ask, but people in their participant role would never ask (Pryce, 1979: 293). All this is particularly so with covert participant observation research where researchers are limited by the need not to 'blow their cover' (Patrick, 1973: 135).

There are, of course, roles which are inaccessible to participant observers. As an adult a researcher cannot adopt the role of a child; someone who is not a doctor cannot practise medicine for the purpose of research. Though Roth's famous study of a TB sanitorium was done from the viewpoint of a patient (1963), he did not contract his TB in order to carry out the research.

Again the tasks which come with the role may be inconsistent with observing, and particularly with recording observations. The issue of recording data is a particularly important one. Gomm, whose study features as Chapter 14, was fortunate in that most of the interesting action occurred in meetings where all participants were sitting at tables making notes from time to time. None the less, his data would have been better if these events had been audio-recorded. More usually there are difficulties in combining the role of the participant with the task of recording observations. Often participant observer researchers make records in retrospect and then there must be doubt as to the accuracy and completeness of these.

The merits of participant observation depend to some extent on the kinds of settings which are being studied. Those which are closed to outsiders may only be researchable by participant observation research, which explains why so many studies of criminal activities have been done using participant observation, covert in many cases. But there are many settings where it is quite normal to have participants standing around watching, asking questions and making notes: hospital wards are again an example. In settings like this, non-participant observation is unlikely to be disruptive of what usually happens and may give the researcher more freedom to concentrate on research tasks.

Readers of participant observation studies then need to know how the role adopted gave access to some scenes, settings and communications, disbarred the researcher from others, and how it constrained or facilitated the accurate recording of data.

Non-participant observation may also include the one-way mirrors which used to be common in psychological research, audio and video recording. There can be technical difficulties in using these methods, which include both the fixed viewpoint of the one-way mirror or the fly-on-the wall camera, and the difficulty of producing transcribable audio recordings of many people moving about in busy settings. None the less, records made in these forms constitute data which are relatively unanalysed and fix it in this state in such a way that it can be revisited again and again. By contrast the diary written by a participant observer at the end of a session of observation will contain data which are highly analysed in the sense that he or she will have only taken notice of what they thought was important, and will only have remembered and recorded some of that.

A major argument against non-participant observation and in favour of participant observation comes from the idea that a researcher can only explain what people do by sharing their experiences and coming to understand the world as they do. However, this is not an assumption which is shared by all researchers, and not all qualitative research is designed to capture the experience of those studied. Other researchers, by contrast, start from the position that people do not themselves know why they do what they do, and that therefore trying to understand the world as they understand it is not an important task for the researcher. This includes researchers who are interested not so much in what people *mean* by what they say, as in what people *do* by saying things (see Chapter 14).

Once the tapes had been transcribed and anonymised, I found that I was rarely able to tell which speaker had been me, and which had been someone else. Even if I could recognise myself I was able to give no better explanation for why I myself said something, than I could give for the utterance of someone else. Perhaps this was due to the kind of explanations I was seeking, which were not in terms of private beliefs and motivations, but rather in terms of public acts of speaking, of what was sayable, and how saying it produced a particular social structure. In such respects, insiders are likely to be in the very worst position to provide such explanations: what do goldfish know about water? (Gomm, 1986: 403)

This linguistic orientation to data is discussed in section 6 below.

4 Grounded theory research: structuring theory and data together

As Bryman and Burgess note (1994: 5–6), there are many studies claiming to use a grounded theory approach, but very few using the approach actually specified by Glaser and Strauss who coined the term (1967). Indeed, the exact nature of grounded theory has been a matter of some debate, even between Strauss and Glaser themselves. The account given of grounded theory below may well be contradicted by accounts in other books.

Many elements of grounded theory are used by people who do not use the term. The discussion below includes references to the work of Phil Strong and David Silverman, neither of whom claim to be 'grounded theorists'. While the exemplar for Chapter 14 was written for this book as an example of grounded theory, the original research on which it was based never used this term (Gomm, 1986). Whether what an author did was 'really' grounded theory, is much less important than what the author actually did in order to produce the study.

The term 'grounded' refers to the idea that theories should be derived from or 'grounded in' data, rather than data collected according to some theory formulated in advance. This relates to the research aim of achieving ecological validity (see section 3) and to the notion that theories formulated in advance impose an artificial structure on data which may give an erroneous picture of what happens naturally. The main elements of grounded theory are *theoretical* or *purposive* sampling and *constant comparison*, as will be discussed below.

Chapter 10 of this book deals with *representative sampling* where samples are selected to represent a population in a statistical sense, such that much the same frequencies of a phenomenon found in the sample will also be true of the population from which the sample was drawn. *Theoretical sampling* (Strauss and Corbin, 1998: Chapter 13) is also representative in a sense, but samples are selected to represent what is theoretically interesting, irrespective of how common or uncommon this might be. Thus Phil Strong in his studies of parent–doctor interaction in paediatric clinics opined that how the interaction proceeded depended on, among other things, doctors' notions of who was a proper adult to accompany a child to a clinic (Strong, 1979; Strong and Davis, 1978). While it was statistically rare for fathers, couples, grandparents, or older siblings to accompany a child, such rarities were none the less theoretically very interesting for showing how the features of the most usual consultation depended on it being the mother who accompanied the child. Hence grounded theory often involves *deviant case analysis*: looking at what rarely happens in order to illuminate what usually happens. In survey work, by contrast, the unusual is generally regarded as of lesser importance (Silverman, 1992).

Theoretical sampling operates alongside *constant comparison*. In the example of paediatric clinics this meant making comparisons between consultations involving mothers, fathers, couples, grand-parents, older siblings and so on to see how they differed. More generally, it means trying to find examples of all the different possible combinations of factors in order to find out what difference each factor makes.

Even *constant* comparison has to stop sometime and grounded theory exponents write about the end point as a state of *theoretical saturation*.

> the criterion for judging when to stop sampling the different groups pertinent to a category is the category's theoretical saturation. Saturation means that no additional data are being found whereby the sociologist can develop properties of the category. (Glaser and Strauss, 1967: 61)

In terms of Phil Strong's research, theoretical saturation would have been reached when studying additional consultations added no more to his explanation of why consultations proceed as they do. Obviously the more complex and elaborate a theory, the longer it takes to reach a point of theoretical saturation.

The final stage of grounded theory is the attempt to apply the theory to a much wider range of circumstances than those from which it was derived. Though only briefly, Gomm in Chapter 14 begins to generalise theoretical ideas about uncertain speech from findings on educational assessment, to hospital wards and terminal diagnoses, to job inter-viewing, to legal proceedings, to scientific project teams and to poison oracles in East Africa.

As a way of analysing data that have already been collected, theoret-ical sampling (within the data set) and constant comparison are not necessarily restricted to qualitative research. It is quite common for quantitative researchers to do this in analysing big data sets such as the General Household Survey or census data. Outside of grounded theory research the same procedures are often described simply as 'comparative method' (Ragin, 1987). What is more distinctive of qual-itative research is the use of a grounded theory approach as *a data gathering strategy*, starting with very little in the way of a theory, and then collecting data according to what becomes theoretically inter-esting as the theory develops. Here 'theoretical sampling' tends to mean the identification by the researcher of what to look out for and note down next, and what to re-look at in the field notes and think about again.

The method entailed continuous comparison of data and model throughout the research project. I began the research by developing a rough working framework based on the existing literature, conversations with colleagues and pilot interviews. I travelled back and forth between the emerging model and evidence throughout the data gathering and writing. In doing so, some elements suggested by the literature and prior intuitions could be grounded in evidence, while others could not. Other elements proposed at the outset or suggested by a subset of cases were retained but were modified considerably to conform to the evidence. (Sutton, 1987: 574)

It is interesting how similar this account of using a grounded theory approach seems to the kinds of 'discovery stories' told by researchers in the physical and natural sciences (Koestler, 1959). There is always a difference between the way research is done as a complex of intellectual and practical activities, and the way research is written up as a set of justifications for claims made by researchers: how researchers say they did the research is not necessarily how they actually did it (Knorr-Cetina, 1983). Looked at in this way it seems highly likely that something like a 'grounded theory approach' is common as a way of *doing research* in a wide variety of disciplines, but that as a way of *writing up* the research it is particularly popular with qualitative researchers in the social sciences (Atkinson, 1990).

5   The linguistic turn in qualitative research

Most of the data collected and analysed by qualitative researchers are linguistic: speech or writing. Most of the remainder are of other communicative acts: postures, gestures and other acts which convey some kind of meaning to others. There are two basic ways of orienting to such data. One way is to regard what people say, write or otherwise communicate as evidence of what is in their minds: of how they think, understand or feel in general. In this sense any utterance stands as a sample of some individual's, or of some category of individuals', cognitive and/or emotional processes. Thus in Chapter 12 Blaxter's interviews are presented as if producing samples of the way in which her respondents understand illness in the context of their lives, all the time, whether they are being interviewed or not. In Chapter 13 Bowler presents utterances by midwives as samples of speech indicative of their minds being inhabited by ethnic 'stereotypes' with the implication that racial prejudice is a persistent characteristic of these people. In both studies, some sample utterances by some people are used as the basis for making generalisations about how these same people, and others like them, usually think, make sense of their experience and act on their interpretations.

The *linguistic turn* (or a *rhetorical approach*) refers to a different way of approaching such data. Instead of regarding what people say as evidence of what people think or feel, utterances are understood in terms of what people are doing with language at the time, in the place where they use it. People do a large number of things with words, such as asking and answering questions, making polite refusals for not answering questions, issuing compliments or complaints, humouring the person they are speaking with, and so on. What they actually do with words depends on the context in which they are using them. From this point of view the data that derive from an interview are first and foremost evidence about how people – interviewers and interviewees – go about doing interviews. There is no safe generalisation from what someone says in an interview to what someone might say or think in another situation.

Linguistic orientations to qualitative data are diverse and have diverse origins. From linguistics comes the notion of *speech acts* which treats sayings as doings (Searle, 1969). Thus to say 'I'm feeling under the weather' may or may not be an accurate report by someone on their own feelings of health, but it is also a common way of doing a polite refusal, or casting a command for indulgence into a socially acceptable format. It might equally be one of a large number of other speech acts, such as jokes, insults, lies, excuses, answers to questions, commiserations and so on. In these terms what someone *meant* by an utterance is less important than what happened because they said it. Often the consequence of one speech act is another speech act.

From ethnomethodology comes the idea that all actions are *situated* and can only be understood in terms of what people are doing in the immediate situation (Heritage, 1984). *Conversation analysis* (CA) (Hutchby and Wooffitt, 1998) blends this with the idea of speech acts and involves a fine-grained analysis of speech data in terms of how this utterance here is to be understood as a consequence of some earlier one (see Section 6). Thus, for example, the explanation for 'an answer' is that it is a response to an earlier utterance which was heard as a 'question'. Or perhaps an utterance is to be explained as a refusal to answer a question which has not actually been asked, but which can be predicted from something said earlier, or from some other feature of the situation. Goffman's *dramaturgical* approach (1961a, 1963, 1967, 1971) has been influential in the sense that speakers are seen as performers, producing themselves as characters with identities that seem appropriate to them for whatever little playlet they think they are currently involved in. From this perspective it makes no sense to ask 'what is this person really like?' but only to ask how this person brings off an impression of themselves as being this kind of person.

Within the same field of studies, *narrative analysis* (Kohler Riessman, 1993) pays attention to the way people are always telling stories to show what led to what, with casts of characters with biographies, motivations, moral qualities and so on, and how people use storytelling to show what kinds of people they are and where they fit in the social structure (Dingwall, 1977). Though Blaxter's interviews (Chapter 12) elicited a large number of narratives from her interviewees, her study is not a thorough-going narrative analysis. She takes what her respondents say as evidence of how they understand their experience, rather than as a source of information as to how people construct plots, imbue characters with motives and use other story-telling devices in order to negotiate their relationships with other people.

The social structure of the immediate situation of *speech events* is also a matter of interest. In any situation some participants will have or claim more or different *speaking rights* than others. The right to ask questions, issue commands, raise new topics, interrupt or correct other speakers and so on are often asymetrically distributed. This is how we *hear* that one kind of person is more powerful than another (see Chapter 14). The social structure of a speech event is extremely important in shaping what is said and how it is said. Thus it is to be expected that what people say in a one-to-one interview will be different from what they say in a group interview such as a focus group. From this point of view there is little interest in whether people express themselves more honestly or authentically in individual interviews by comparison with the way they would express themselves in focus groups. For most topics there would be no way of deciding this matter. Rather, the interest is in the differences between people speaking in pairs and speaking in 'multi-party speech exchanges' where views as expressed are shaped by much more complicated processes of turn taking, topic raising, and so on (Myers and Macnaghten, 1999).

A close attention to the use of language in context has been especially enlightening in health and social care, where so much of the work is done through talking (for example, West and Frankel, 1991; Silverman et al., 1992).

6   Thematic analysis and linguistic analysis compared

Thematic analysis and linguistic analysis will often produce very different accounts of the same data, as illustrated by comparing Box 16.2 with Box 16.5. The interchange in Transcript 1 might be cited as evidence in support of the importance of two themes in an interview study of reactions to receiving a terminal diagnosis, as shown in Boxes 16.3 and 16.4.

Used in this way, feeling 'absolutely shattered' is being taken as an accurate report by Mrs Williams on how she felt at a moment 9 months previous to the interview, and her feelings taken as an equivalent to those of respondents who used the terms 'gob-smacked' and 'knocked sideways'. What she said in the interview about doctors is taken as evidence of her feelings of sympathy towards doctors.

Box 16.2 Transcript 1: Analysed thematically

Themes illustrated

Interviewer: And when you were first told about your diagnosis what did you, what did you, mm, what was your re—, your first reaction?

Mrs Williams: <u>Absolutely shattered</u>, I suppose [2 seconds silence]. Wouldn't anyone I mean [3 seconds silence] I mean I have <u>a lot of sympathy with them.</u> It;mmm. It mmm can't be easy for the doctors to errr, tell you that sort of thing and they do it as kind of gently as they can but it's, well it's not nice [laughs] sort of thing, and as I say it was rather shattering.

Theme 3: Reactions – disorientation

Theme 7: Feelings about doctors – sympathy

Box 16.3 Theme 3: Reactions to learning one's diagnosis

Many respondents reported acute feelings of disorientation on first learning their diagnosis:

'knocked sideways'
'gob-smacked'
'absolutely shattered'

were common descriptions . . .

Anger was also a common feeling experienced (see Theme 7 in Box. 16.4)

Box 16.4 Theme 7: Feelings about doctors

Anger at doctors was also a common feeling on first hearing the diagnosis . . . However, many respondents showed concern and sympathy for the doctors who had the unpleasant task of breaking the news to them, for example:

I mean I have a lot of sympathy with them. It can't be easy for the doctors to tell you that sort of thing

---

Either, both or neither might be true, but there is no way of verifying this. More importantly, to make what she says stand as evidence in this way, her words have been wrested from the context in which they

Box 16.5 Transcript 2: Analysed linguistically	Linguistic moves
1 *Interviewer*: And when you were first told about your diagnosis what did you, what did you, mm, what was your re—, your first reaction?	Question
2 *Mrs Williams*: Absolutely shattered, I suppose.	Answer
3 [2 seconds silence]	Silence [taken as negative evaluation of answer]
4 *Mrs Williams*: Wouldn't anyone I mean	Appeal as to adequacy of answer
5 [3 seconds silence]	Silence [taken as negative evaluation]
6 *Mrs Williams*: I mean I have a lot of sympathy with them. It;mmm. It mmm can't be easy for the doctors to errr, tell you that sort of thing and they do it as kind of gently as they can but it's, well it's not nice [laughs] sort of thing, and as I say it was rather shattering.	Repair of assumed complaint about doctors followed by restatement of answer given at 2 above

were uttered. The linguistic approach attempts to read her words in the immediate context of a speech exchange between an interviewer and an interviewee. It helps somewhat to re-organise the data and re-code it in linguistic terms, as in Transcript 2 (Box 16.5).

Mrs Williams is asked a question (1) and gives an answer (2). Her answer elicits no response from the interviewer: there is a 2 second silence (3). One of the important characteristics of conversations, including interviews, is that people take turns to speak (Sacks et al., 1974). Therefore participants are forever having to work out whose turn it is to speak. As in this example, this makes silences problematic for them, since the other person's silence can either be heard as a failure for them to take their turn, or as an indication that one hasn't finished one's own turn; that there is still something else to say. Among the things one might 'still have to say' is a correction of what one has already said. It is always more polite to give someone an opportunity to correct themselves, than to correct them, and silences leave a space for this (Levinson, 1983: 339–45). And as every school child knows, a silence following an answer to a question indicates that the answer has been incomplete, or deficient. In this case Mrs Williams' answer to a question is responded to by silence from the interviewer. Had this been an 'ordinary conversation' then one of the most predictable responses from the interviewer would have been some kind of commiseration or validation, such as 'I'm sure you were'. Of course there is a possibility that the answer Mrs Williams gave was one which was seeking for just that kind of validation, and had little to do with how she actually felt 9 months ago, but we cannot know this. In any event there is nothing in the way of validation from the interviewer and whatever response Mrs Williams expected, all she gets is a silence. Insofar as conversations are ruleful, it is a workable rule that the absence of a positive validation implies a negative evaluation. One of the most obvious interpretations of this silence available to Mrs Williams is that her answer (2) was incomplete or deficient. Mrs Williams responds as if this was so (4). She says 'wouldn't anyone I mean'. This might be heard as if Mrs Williams were saying 'for goodness sake, what do you expect people to feel when they are told they are dying? What other kind of answer could I possibly give?' But whatever she meant, it provokes the same response – silence (5). Two attempts to respond to a question, both followed by a silence can be taken by a respondent as a very strong message that the answer given was deficient.

Mrs William's next utterance (6) then expresses sympathy with doctors. What she says has the same effect as saying 'Though I was absolutely shattered, I don't blame the doctors for this.' One explanation for her saying this comes from assuming that she thinks she might have been heard to have complained about doctors when she said 'absolutely shattered'. This is to regard utterance (6) as an attempt to repair her earlier answers by disclaiming any imputation that the doctor who announced her terminal diagnosis was incompetent or unfeeling.

This reading of the data raises some questions as to whether Mrs Williams feels sympathetic towards doctors, or whether she expresses sympathy with them as a way of extricating herself from a sticky moment in an interview. The thematic and the linguistic readings are not incompatible with each other, but they are different.

The linguistic analysis of the data given above in Box 16.5, may or may not be an accurate reconstruction of how interviewer and interviewee produced what was said in the interview. However, it is a possible interpretation, and as such draws attention to the dangers of taking utterances out of the context in which they were made and citing them as evidence as to what the people concerned generally think or feel.

The distinction made above between thematic analysis and linguistic analysis should not be taken to suggest that there are just two ways of analysing qualitative data. Rather there is a wide variety of ways, some of which tend towards the thematic, and some towards the linguistic (Silverman, 1993; Miles and Huberman, 1994).

7 The objectivity of qualitative research

Quantitative research is, usually, highly accountable. Because of their emphasis on reliability and standardisation, quantitative researchers can specify precisely what they did to get the data they acquired. Figure 16.1 only says what the Health and Lifestyle interviewers were *supposed* to do, and not what they actually did. But increasingly survey research involves tape recording to check whether interviewers stuck to the brief, and various reliability checks (see Table 10.7 in Chapter 10). This high level of accountability means that readers can scrutinise the methods used and come to a conclusion as to whether they were appropriate, or how far the methods might have shaped the data in misleading ways. The exemplar reading for Chapter 8, concerning NHS consumer satisfaction surveys, is an exercise of this kind of scrutiny. In the absence of a full account being given, it is possible to *replicate* quantitative research to check it out. And as Chapter 4 suggests, experimental researchers who do not provide enough information do not get included in systematic reviews and their work is likely to be sidelined.

A long history of research with regard to interviews shows that even with forced choice questions the persona and behaviour of the interviewer has a considerable effect on the responses (Bradburn, 1983; Davies, 1997: 57–85). The bias is usually towards the social desirability of a response, respondents tending to answer in ways they imagine will show them in the best light. By contrast with questionnaire researchers, interviewers using loosely structured interviews disclose more about themselves and provide stronger clues as to what might be acceptable answers. It is not the shaping of responses by the situation of the interview which is the problem so much as its invisibility in much qualitative research. There are even more opportunities to create the conditions for this kind of bias in focus group research (Green and Hart, 1999).

A parallel tradition of research demonstrates the importance of researcher expectations in determining what the experimental researcher sees and how he or she interprets it (Rosenthal, 1966; Rosenthal and Rubin, 1978). If 'expectancy effects' are important in the highly controlled world of controlled experiments, how much more important must they be in the context of a participant observation study (Sadler, 1981). In experimental research the criteria that are used to define phenomena as being of particular kinds can be clearly specified and, in principle at least, the judgements can be verified. But qualitative researchers doing observation research have to make minute by minute interpretations of what kind of thing they are observing, often without themselves knowing quite how they are making these interpretations.

It is thus much more difficult to make data collection in qualitative research accountable than in quantitative research. Participant observation research and loosely structured interviews are unreplicable. Collecting the data can take a very long time, and it is part of the tradition that researchers adjust themselves to the circumstances of the research, and respond differently to different people rather than behave in a standardised way. This is a necessary requirement for achieving ecological validity (section 3). It would be virtually impossible for a participant observer researcher to give an account of everything he or she did that might have shaped the data collected over 6 months of observation. Qualitative researchers often provide *reflexive accounts*, discussing how their persona or their actions might have shaped the data (Grbich, 1999: 65–6), but these come nowhere near to matching the accountability of research reports in quantitative studies. Qualitative researchers who do interviews can, in principle, make themselves accountable by providing readers with transcripts of the interviews they do; the same is true with audio or video recordings of naturally occurring events. Then readers can judge how far the doing of the research shaped the resulting data. Researchers who receive funding from the Economic and Social Research Council now have to commit themselves to archiving their data for this purpose (Hammersley, 1997).

However, there are severe publishing constraints on conveying this information easily to readers. Note how Blaxter, for this reason presumably, does not present full transcripts: only edited highlights (see Box 16.1). For providing an objective account the crucial information that is missing is what the interviewer said in order to provoke the words said by the interviewee, as demonstrated in section 6 above. In the Blaxter and Bowler studies readers are given little insight into this and no insight into which data have been discarded, and hence no way of knowing how the researcher's behaviour shaped the data and whether this brings the results into question. Conversation analysts by contrast typically present long passages of transcripts including interviewer as well as interviewee talk, so that readers can make judgements of this kind (see section 6). Purists in the tradition of conversation analysis will sometimes refuse to draw on any data other than that which can be shared with readers in the form of a transcript (Anderson, 1979).

Bias in favour of, or against some types of people is a possibility in all kinds of research (Hammersley and Gomm, 2000), but there are particular possibilities for bias in qualitative research. Whether this is a problem depends very much on the assumptions made about the purpose of research. Some researchers, particularly those influenced by feminism, consider that the purpose of research is to advocate on behalf of groups who are misunderstood and oppressed; giving them 'a voice' they would not otherwise have (Mies, 1983, 1991; Stanley and

Wise, 1983). The genre of life-history research where researchers, in effect, 'ghost' the stories told by those researched is a case in point (Bornat, 1993). Mies recommends that researchers adopt a position of 'conscious partiality' (1983: 122). The idea that research should not be an activity restricted to researchers is currently popular. Writers such as Lather (1995) or Romm (1997) suggest that research should be a collaborative activity with the researcher 'empowering' others to produce their own accounts of the world. If this is the purpose of the research then taking on the partisan views of the group for whom the researcher advocates is not a problem for the researcher. But it remains one for the reader, who, with access to the same situations might have come to different conclusions and without such access may suspect that the data have been massaged for propaganda purposes (Hammersley, 2000; Hammersley and Gomm, 2000).

If the purpose of the research is to provide an account from multiple perspectives, and/or to explain why people do what they do, have the views they have, and what are the consequences of this, *sympathetic bias* of this kind is highly problematic (Becker, 1967). Dingwall suggests that an important criterion for judging qualitative research is whether:

> it displays its adherence to an ethic of fair dealing . . . does it convey as much understanding of its villains as its heroes? Are the privileged treated as having something serious to say, or simply dismissed as evil, corrupt or greedy without further inquiry? (Dingwall, 1992: 172)

8   Generalisability and qualitative research

For practical reasons qualitative researchers can only deal with small samples of people. There is a problem of *representativeness* here. However, it is important to be clear as to what the problem is. As noted in Chapter 10, section 1, representativeness is not an all or nothing matter. It depends on what it is that the researcher is trying to represent and its achievement is diversity-related. For some purposes a single individual can serve to represent the entire human race. Aliens who captured a single specimen of *Homo sapiens* could come up with some pretty accurate generalisations about some aspects of human anatomy and physiology, for example. Their problem would be that they wouldn't know what it was safe to generalise about! Anatomical and physiological homogeneity is what makes it less of a problem that experimental researchers in medicine often use convenience samples rather than samples that could be guaranteed to be representative (see Chapter 5, section 12), though the findings of the human genome project are suggesting that this is more problematic than was previously assumed. Blaxter's sample (Chapter 12) was of Scottish working class women in their 50s. It was necessarily a small sample. It would be unreasonable to assume that the way these women made sense of health and illness is representative of all working class people, male and female, or of all working class people who answered 'yes' to Question 13a (Figure 16.1), or of all working class *women* who answered 'yes' to this question. It is possible that their sense-making is representative of a majority of Scottish working class women aged 50 at the time of the interview; but the sample is still too small to be confident about this. For all these possible generalisations some evidence might be drawn from cross-checking with the Health and Lifestyle Survey data. Those surveys were, after all, designed to be representative and to yield valid generalisations.

The reason why generalisations of the kinds above would be doubtful is that particular beliefs about health and illness are likely to be highly diverse. None the less, there is an important generalisation which arises from Blaxter's study. This is along the lines that people's (all people's) beliefs and understandings of health and illness, whatever they are in particular, are in general woven into their understandings of life as a whole. The point of Blaxter's article is that picking off bits and pieces of their ideas with a forced choice questionnaire misses the way these ideas hang together into individually coherent systems of thought. Blaxter herself uses the term 'experiential coherence' (see Chapter 12).

Qualitative research has been quite successful in producing 'general' ideas which help to make sense of social, psychological and organisational processes. These include ideas such as 'total institution', 'moral career', 'deviancy amplification', 'stigma', 'suspicion awareness context', 'degradation ceremony', 'psychological survival' and such like, each of which draws attention to the similarities between phenomena which otherwise might appear quite different from each other. The first, for example, illuminates similarities between mental hospitals, prisons, military units, monasteries, cargo ships and boarding schools (Goffman, 1961b); the second draws attention to the way in which social affairs are organised to nudge people along more or less predictable trajectories as school children, patients, criminals, workers and so on, and how being at a certain stage of the 'career' determines the criteria by which someone's state and behaviour will be judged and interpreted by others (for example, Weir, 1977). The production of ideas with general currency is a rather different kind of 'generalisation' from that entailed in generalising from a representative sample to the population it represents. In a different way linguistic analysis has spawned a now large array of concepts which are generally applicable to the analysis of talk and writing (Hutchby and Wooffitt, 1998).

Robert Stake (Stake and Trumbull, 1982) coined the term *naturalistic generalisation* to refer to the everyday processes through which people learn things in one context and apply them in another. Along similar lines writers such as Stenhouse (1980), Donmoyer (1990) and others have suggested that the important function of qualitative research is to provide insights into other people's lives which can be learned from and then put to use in understanding ourselves and the other people we meet. In this regard qualitative research has similar functions to novels and plays, and its ability to develop empathy would be more important than its veracity. However, this is a dangerous argument for research. If producing common understanding is the most important aim, and if this can be produced through plays or novels, why bother to do research?

9   Action research

The term 'action research' is often applied so broadly as to include any kind of research which effects a change in situations and people (Hart and Bond, 1995). This includes experimental research such as RCTs (Chapters 1 and 2), n-of-1 experiments and single case evaluations (Chapter 5, section 13), as well as most evaluation research (Øvretveit, 1998). And sometimes the term is used so broadly as to include any kind of practice where practitioners take care to monitor the results of their actions. For this elasticity there are practical attractions. By labelling service provision as 'action research' it is possible to divert funds earmarked for research into service delivery. The reverse manoeuvre allows practitioners to present accounts of their practice for research degrees. However, the result is that, without further description, the term action research is now virtually meaningless. This problem notwithstanding, a somewhat arbitrary distinction can be made to distinguish three fields where the term action research is used, each of which does seem to have some internal coherence:

- **Action research in management studies.** When named as action research this is often associated with the work of Robert Rapoport in the USA (1970) and the Tavistock Institute in the UK (for example, Lievegoed, 1973). However, much the same kinds of activities go under the name of 'organisational development', 'team-building' and 'change management', and (in management education) 'action-learning'. Although the problems addressed are those defined by management, there is usually a strong emphasis on the importance of worker-involvement/participation. The primary objective of this kind of activity is to produce more effective and more humane organisations, often conceptualised as 'learning organisations' (Schön, 1975). This genre of action research is not exemplified in this book, but plenty of examples are to be found in management journals, especially those dealing with personnel management and with training (see also Argyris et al., 1985).
- **Community action research.** This is often a synonym for 'community development', and has been used as a means for building

more cohesive communities both in Third World countries and in deprived neighbourhoods in the UK and elsewhere in the developed world. To qualify for the appellation 'research', community development activities need to have an element of research conducted by members of the community themselves, usually in order to produce ammunition for a political campaign. Sonja Hunt describes aspects of anti-dampness campaigns in Scotland (Hunt, 1990, 1993), for example, and Greenwood and Levin (1998) provide a wide range of examples worldwide. A great deal of this kind of action research has been done by lay people, by-passes academia and, in the UK, is published in a propagandist way in the magazine *Community Action* or in ephemeral media such as community newsletters.

- **Educational action research.** Educational action research has its own journal of this title. The term 'educational' does not necessarily refer to action research in educational contexts – though these are the home-base of the genre. Rather it refers to a prioritisation of learning through the experience of conducting action research. There is a very strong emphasis on participatory research and on the empowerment of disadvantaged groups (Hart and Bond, 1995). It is this which is exemplified in this volume by Celia Winter's paper (Chapter 15) about action research in improving the quality of care for children in a family centre.

The distinction above has the advantage of pointing to three different kinds of outcome which are desired by action researchers – *apart from making a contribution to general, and generalisable, knowledge.* Though all would welcome each,

- the first prioritises improvements in the way an organisation functions;
- the second prioritises improvements in the quality of community life;
- and the third prioritises improvements in the knowledge and expertise of the people involved in the research, often particularly the knowledge and expertise of service user groups.

All these kinds of research are complex and procedures and results are heavily determined by the context in which research is conducted, which is often dynamic and politicised. Not only are any 'findings' unlikely to be generalisable to another context, but only in the broadest sense could the same methods reported in a piece of action research be applied by someone elsewhere. Reading such research should be regarded as something akin to reading a travelogue. It may tell the reader that there are some destinations which might be reached, and some routes which might be taken to get there, and provide some useful tips and warnings. But in significant respects someone else's journey will not be like the journey described and may not end up in the same place. Action research is more for doing than for reading about.

None the less, most self-styled action research does make claims about what actions led to what outcomes, and about what events meant to the people involved. In these regards it is open to appraisal in much the same way as other kinds of research. For example, if the claim is that the research activity improved the competence or knowledge of those involved, then what evidence is cited to support this claim, and how convincing is it? Or if the claim is that being engaged in the research improved community cohesion, how was this measured and what evidence is provided that this actually happened? A checklist of Questions to Ask about Action Research is provided in Part 4 of this book.

10   Further reading on qualitative research and action research

There is no shortage of texts on qualitative research, much of it featuring examples from health or social care settings. Jennifer Mason (1996) provides a sound introduction to planning qualitative research and collecting the data. David Silverman (1993) covers various styles of qualitative data analysis. Bryman and Burgess (1994) is an interesting collection of papers featuring different kinds of analysis of different kinds of qualitative data, and Hammersley (1990) is a critical reader's guide. For conversation analysis, Hutchby and Wooffitt (1998) is a comprehensive, and comprehensible, guide.

The term *grounded theory* is frequently used in the literature of qualitative research. For a manual on this methodology, see Strauss and Corbin (1998).

Hart and Bond (1995) provides an overview of action research with a strong slant towards the 'educational action research' variety (see section 9), while Greenwood and Levin (1998) deal more with community based action research. Though nowhere in their book do they use the term 'action research', Pawson and Tilley's *Realistic Evaluation* (1997) is none the less an excellent guide on how the quality and usefulness of action research might be judged. In many respects it is impossible to distinguish 'action research' from 'evaluation research'. Øvretveit's *Evaluating Health Interventions* (1998) catalogues virtually every known evaluation strategy.

References and further reading

Anderson, D. (1979) 'Talking with patients about their diet', in D. Anderson (ed.), *Health Education in Practice*. London: Croom Helm. pp. 177–94.

Argyris, C., Putman, R. and Smith, M. (1985) *Action Science: Concepts, Methods and Skills for Research and Intervention*. San Francisco: Jossey–Bass.

Armstrong, D., Gosling, A., Weinman, J. and Marteau, T. (1997) 'The place of inter-rater reliability in qualitative research: an empirical study', *Sociology*, 31 (3): 597–606.

Atkinson, P. (1990) *The Ethnographic Imagination: Textual Constructions of Reality*. London: Routledge.

Becker, H. (1967) 'Whose side are we on?', *Social Problems*, 14: 239–47.

Blaxter, M. (1990) *Health and Lifestyles*. London: Tavistock/Routledge.

Bornat, J. (1993) 'Oral history as a social movement: reminiscence and older people', in J. Johnson and R. Slater (eds), *Ageing and Later Life*. London: Sage. pp. 280–7.

Bradburn, N. (1983) 'Response effects', in P. Rossi, J. Wright and A. Anderson (eds), *Handbook of Survey Research*. New York: Academic Press. pp. 289–328.

Bryman, A. and Burgess, R. (eds) (1994) *Analyzing Qualitative Data*. London: Routledge.

Cicourel, A. (1982) 'Interviews, surveys and the problem of ecological validity', *American Sociologist*, 17 (1): 11–20.

Cox, B., Blaxter, M., Buckle, S.A., Golding, J., Gore, M., Huppert, F., Nickson, J., Roth, M., Stark, J., Wadsworth, M. and Whichelow, M. (1987) *The Health and Lifestyle Survey: preliminary report of a nationwide survey of the physical and mental health, attitudes and life style of a random sample of 9003 adults*. Bristol: Health Promotion Trust.

Cox, B., Huppert, F. and Whichelow, M. (eds) (1993) *The Health and Lifestyle Survey: Seven Years On*. Aldershot: Dartmouth Publishing.

Davies, J. (1997) *Drugspeak: the Analysis of Drug Discourse*. Amsterdam: Harwood Academic Publishers.

Denzin, N. and Lincoln, Y. (eds) (1998) *Strategies of Qualitative Inquiry*. London: Sage.

Dingwall, R. (1977) 'Atrocity stories and the professional relationship', *Sociology of Work and Occupations*, 4 (3): 371–96.

Dingwall, R. (1992) 'Don't mind him – he's from Barcelona: qualitative methods in health studies', in J. Daly, I. McDonald, and E. Willis, (eds), *Researching Health Care: Designs, Dilemmas, Disciplines*. London: Routledge. pp. 161–75.

Donmoyer, R. (1990) 'Generalizability and the single case study', in E. Eisner and A. Peshkin (eds), *Qualitative Inquiry in Education*. New York: Teachers' College Press.

Fielding, N. and Lee, R. (eds) (1991) *Using Computers in Qualitative Research*. London: Sage.

Glaser, B. and Strauss, A. (1967) *Discovery of Grounded Theory*. Chicago: Aldine.

Goffman, E. (1961a) *Encounters*. New York: Bobbs–Merrill.

Goffman, E. (1961b) *Asylums: Essays on the Social Situation of Mental Patients and Other Inmates*. New York: Anchor Books.

Goffman, E. (1963) *Behaviour in Public Places*. Harmondsworth: Penguin.

Goffman, E. (1967) *Interaction Ritual*. Harmondsworth: Penguin.

Goffman, E. (1971) *The Presentation of Self in Everyday Life*. Harmondsworth: Penguin.

Gomm, R. (1986) 'Normal results: an ethnographic study of health visitor student assessment'. Unpublished PhD thesis submitted to the Open University.

Gomm, R. and Hammersley, M. (eds) (2000) *Case Study Research*. London: Sage.

Grbich, C. (1999) *Qualitative Research in Health: an Introduction*. London: Sage.

Green, J. and Hart, L. (1999) 'The impact of context on data', in R. Barbour and J. Kitzinger (eds), *Developing Focus Group Research: Politics, Theory and Practice*. London: Sage. pp. 21–35.

Greenwood, D. and Levin, M. (1998) *Introduction to Action Research: Social Research for Social Change*. Thousand Oaks, CA: Sage.

Hammersley, M. (1990) *Reading Ethnographic Research: a Critical Guide*. London: Longman.

Hammersley, M. (1997) 'Qualitative data archiving: some reflections on its prospects and problems', *Sociology*, 31 (1): 131–42.

Hammersley, M. (2000) 'Taking sides in research: an assessment of the rationales for partisanship', in M. Hammersley (ed.), *Taking Sides in Social Research: Essays on Partisanship and Bias*. London: Routledge. pp. 16–34.

Hammersley, M. and Atkinson, P. (1983) *Ethnography: Principles in Practice*. London: Tavistock.

Hammersley, M. and Gomm, R. (2000) 'Bias in social research', in M. Hammersley (ed.), *Taking Sides in Social Research: Essays on Partisanship and Bias*. London: Routledge. pp. 151–66.

Hart, E. and Bond, M. (1995) *Action Research for Health and Social Care: a Guide to Practice*. Buckingham: Open University Press.

Heritage, M. (1984) *Garfinkel and Ethnomethodology*. Cambridge: Polity Press.

Hunt, S. (1990) 'Building alliances: professional and political issues in community participation: examples from a health and community development project', *Health Promotion International*, 5: 179–85.

Hunt, S. (1993) 'The relationship between research and policy; translating knowledge into action', in J. Davies and M. Kelly (eds), *Healthy Cities: Research and Practice*. London: Routledge. pp. 71–82.

Hutchby, I. and Wooffitt, R. (1998) *Conversation Analysis*. Cambridge: Polity Press.

Knorr-Cetina, K. (1983) 'The ethnographic study of scientific work: towards a constructivist interpretation of science', in K. Knorr-Cetina and M. Mulkay (eds), *Science Observed: Perspectives on the Social Study of Science*. London: Sage. pp. 115–40.

Koestler, A. (1959) *The Sleepwalkers*. London: Hutchinson.

Kohler Riessman, C. (1993) *Narrative Analysis: Qualitative Research Methods Series 30*. London: Sage.

Lather, P. (1995) 'The validity of angels', *Qualitative Inquiry*, 1: 275–89.

Levinson, S. (1983) *Pragmatics*. Cambridge: Cambridge University Press.

Lievegoed, B. (1973) *The Developing Organisation*. London: Tavistock.

Mason, J. (1996) *Qualitative Researching*. London: Sage.

Mies, M. (1983) 'Towards a methodology for feminist research', in G. Bowles and R. Klein (eds), *Theories of Women's Studies*. London: Routledge and Kegan Paul.

Mies, M. (1991) 'Women's research or feminist research. The debate surrounding feminist science and methodology', in M. Fonow and J. Cook (eds), *Beyond Methodology: Feminist Scholarship as Lived Research*. Bloomington, IN: Indiana University Press.

Miles, M. and Huberman, A. (1994) *Qualitative Data Analysis: an Expanded Sourcebook*. London: Sage.

Myers, G. and Macnaghten, P. (1999) 'Can focus groups be analysed as talk?', in R. Barbour and J. Kitzinger (eds), *Developing Focus Group Research: Politics, Theory and Practice*. London: Sage. pp. 173–85.

O'Connell Davidson, J. and Layder, D. (1994) *Methods, Sex and Madness*. London: Routledge.

Øvretveit, J. (1998) *Evaluating Health Interventions*. Buckingham: Open University Press.

Patrick, J. (1973) *A Glasgow Gang Observed*. London: Eyre Methuen.

Pawson, R. and Tilley, N. (1997) *Realistic Evaluation*. London: Sage.

Potter, J. and Wetherell, M. (1994) 'Analyzing discourse', in A. Bryman and R. Burgess (eds), *Analyzing Qualitative Data*. London: Routledge. pp. 47–66.

Pryce, K. (1979) *Endless Pressure*. Harmondsworth: Penguin.

Ragin, C. (1987) *The Comparative Method: Moving beyond Qualitative and Quantitative Strategies*. Berkeley: University of California Press.

Rapoport, R. (1970) 'Three dilemmas in action research', *Human Relations*, 23 (6): 499–513.

Richards, L. and Richards, T. (1994) 'From filing cabinet to computer', in A. Bryman and R. Burgess (eds), *Analyzing Qualitative Data*. London: Routledge. pp. 146–72.

Romm, N. (1997) 'Becoming more accountable: a comment on Hammersley and Gomm', *Sociological Research Online*, 2 (2).

Rosenthal, R. (1966) *Experimenter Effects in Behavioral Research*. New York: Appleton Century Crofts.

Rosenthal, R. and Rubin, R. (1978) 'Interpersonal expectancy effects: the first 345 studies', *Behavioural and Brain Sciences*, 3: 377–415.

Roth, J. (1963) *Timetables*. Indianapolis: Bobbs-Merrill.

Sacks, H., Schegloff, E. and Jefferson, G. (1974) 'A simplest systematics for the organisation of turn taking in conversation', *Language*, 50 (4): 696–735.

Sadler, D. (1981) 'Intuitive data processing as a potential source of bias in naturalistic evaluations', *Educational Evaluation and Policy Analysis*, July/August: 25–31.

Schön, D. (1975) 'Duetero-learning in organisations: learning for increased effectiveness', *Organisational Dynamics*, Summer: 2–6.

Searle, J. (1969) *Speech Acts*. Cambridge: Cambridge University Press.

Silverman, D. (1983) 'Interview talk: bringing off a research instrument', *Sociology*, 17 (1): 31–47.

Silverman, D. (1990) *Communication and Medical Practice: Social Relations in the Clinic*. London: Sage.

Silverman, D. (1992) 'Applying qualitative method to clinical care', in J. Daly, I. McDonald and E. Willis (eds), *Researching Health Care: Designs, Dilemmas, Disciplines*. London: Routledge. pp. 189–206.

Silverman, D., Bor, R., Miller, R. and Goldman, E. (1992) 'Advice-giving and advice reception in AIDS counselling', in P. Aggleton, P. Davies and G. Hart (eds), *AIDS: Rights, Risk and Reason*. London: Falmer Press.

Silverman, D. (1993) *Interpreting Qualitative Data: Methods for Analysing Talk, Text and Interaction*. London: Sage.

Stake, R. and Trumbull, D. (1982) 'Naturalistic generalisation', *Review Journal of Philosophy and Social Science*, 7: 1–12.

Stanley, L. and Wise, S. (1983) *Breaking Out: Feminist Consciousness and Feminist Research*. London: Routledge and Kegan Paul.

Stenhouse, L. (1980) 'The study of samples and the study of cases', *British Educational Research Journal*, 6 (1): 1–6.

Strauss, A. and Corbin, J. (1998) *Basics of Qualitative Research: Techniques and Procedures for Developing Grounded Theory*, 2nd edn. London: Sage.

Strong, P. (1979) *The Ceremonial Order of the Clinic: Parents, Doctors and Medical Bureaucracy*. London: Routledge and Kegan Paul.

Strong, P. and Davis, A. (1978) 'Who's who in paediatric encounters: morality, expertise and the generation of identity in medical settings', in A. Davis (ed.), *Relations between Doctors and Patients*. Farnborough: Saxon House.

Sutton, R. (1987) 'The process of organizational death: disbanding and reconnecting', *Administrative Science Quarterly*, 32: 570–89.

Weir, D. (1977) 'The moral career of the day patient' in A. Davis and G. Horobin (eds), *Medical Encounters: the Experience of Illness and Treatment*. London: Croom Helm. pp. 135–42.

West, C. and Frankel, R. (1991) 'Miscommunication in medicine', in N. Coupland, H. Giles and J. Wienmann (eds), *'Miscommunication' and Problematic Talk*. London: Sage. pp. 166–94.

Wright, D. (1997) *Understanding Statistics: an Introduction for the Social Sciences*. London: Sage.

PART 4

RESEARCH APPRAISAL QUESTIONS

This part of the book consists of seven sets of critical questions to ask about pieces of published research in order to judge the level of confidence with which their results can be accepted, and to judge whether there are any useful lessons for practice. Most published research includes several components. Sometimes these will be of the same methodological kind; two surveys perhaps. Then the questions in a checklist need to be asked, as appropriate, for each component. Sometimes a piece of research will include several different research strategies, and in that case you will need to use several checklists. Overall judgement will also depend on how well the various components work together to justify the conclusions proposed by the author.

The questions in the checklists had to be put in some order, but there is no correct order for appraising research. Rather, research appraisal is an iterative process. Often the implications of asking an earlier question do not become apparent until a later one is asked; sometimes the answer to an earlier question turns out to be irrelevant in the light of the answer to a later one. Considering each of the questions in a checklist is only half the task: it remains to consider all the answers, altogether; that usually suggests a second look at some of them. Nor should the questions be regarded as having an equal importance for each and every piece of research. What would be a fatal flaw in one piece of research is good enough for the purpose of another and vice versa.

It is very difficult to read research with an open mind. Most readers would either like or dislike the conclusions to be valid. If you would prefer the conclusions of a piece of research to be upheld, then be particularly rigorous in finding fault with it. And if you would prefer the conclusions to be invalid, try as hard as you can to find the merits in it.

QUESTIONS TO ASK ABOUT DATA COLLECTION INSTRUMENTS*

Questions

Comment

1 Has the instrument been validated at all?

The results of research which uses *ad hoc* methods or instruments which have not been trialled, tested, or validated must be treated with a lower level of confidence. The results may be correct, but readers will have less opportunity for making a considered judgement than where research involves validated instruments.

2 Validity (see Chapter 6, section 7)

Is the instrument valid – does it measure what it is supposed to measure?

Does the instrument merely (or even) have face validity, or has it been validated for content, criterion, or construct validity?

There are at least four notions of validity:

Face validity – the items appear to be relevant to the topic at hand.

Content validity – there is an adequate coverage of all relevant aspects of the phenomenon of interest.

Criterion validity – scores on the instrument will correlate with scores on some other instrument allegedly measuring the same thing.

Construct validity – the extent to which a score on an instrument measures what it is supposed to measure. Usually tested in terms of whether the instrument gives measures as predicted by theory which defines the entity in question.

3 Reliability (see Chapter 6, sections 5 and 6)

Is the instrument reliable – does it produce consistent results?

Test–retest reliability
The instrument will produce the same results when retested in the same population (assuming that what is being measured stays the same).

---

* If the instrument is a questionnaire used for survey purposes, see also 'Questions to Ask about Surveys'.

Has the instrument been validated for retest reliability
and, if appropriate for inter-
or intra-rater reliability?

Inter- and intra-rater reliability
The instrument produces the same results
when used by different people, or by the same
person on a different occasion. Usually measured by the Kappa coefficient: the higher the
κ, the greater the reliability (see Chapter 6,
section 6).

Internal consistency reliability
Items measuring a single attribute within an
instrument should demonstrate at least some
inter-correlation – usually measured with
Cronbach's alpha. The higher the alpha score,
the greater the internal consistency.

4 Discriminant validity

Is the instrument sensitive
(responsive) to the differences it is supposed to measure:
between people, or changes
over time?

If small differences are being looked for the
measuring instrument must be calibrated
finely. Beware floor and ceiling effects, where
change below a threshold or above a threshold
is not detected (see Chapter 6, section 4).

5 Robustness

Is the instrument insensitive to effects that are irrelevant to what is being
measured?

For example, would the measurement be affected by who was doing the measurement or
the place in which it was done?

6 Acceptability

Instruments need to be acceptable to both
those about whom data are being collected
and those who do the measuring: time taken,
comprehensibility, perceived relevance, cultural appropriateness and costs.

Non-response rates to particular questions
are sometimes used as a measure of acceptability (or 'feasibility').

7 Appropriateness to context and targets

Instruments designed for hospital use may
not be suitable for domiciliary use. Instruments designed for young people may not be
appropriate for older people.

Has the instrument been trialled, or better
validated, *in the setting for the clients* it is now
being used with?

8 Cross-cultural transferability

Is it cross-culturally transferable. Will it
translate?

9 Data level

Will the scores be sufficiently precise for the study? (see Chapter 6, sections 3 and 4)

If scores need to be continuous for statistical analysis, does the instrument provide these? If it only provides 'yes' and 'no' answers, is this adequate for the purposes of the study? Do the data produced take a normal distribution/can they be transformed into a normal distribution if it is necessary to use parametric statistics see Chapter 6, section 4, and Chapter 7, section 6; see notes on 'floor' and 'ceiling effects' in (**4** above)

QUESTIONS TO ASK ABOUT EXPERIMENTS

Questions and issues	Internal validity	External validity/
	You judge whether the experiment seemed true in its own terms (see Chapter 5, section 11)	**generalisability** You judge whether the same results could be achieved in practice and whether it would be worth trying to do so (see Chapter 5, section 12)
1 Was/were the question(s) to which the research was addressed clearly articulated? Can you see what this research is about?	Unless the study addresses clearly articulated questions it will be impossible to judge whether it has answered them satisfactorily.	Are the questions addressed relevant to decisions which might be made in practice?

2 Was this an experiment involving only one individual subject? If yes, this checklist is not appropriate. Read Chapter 5, section 13 instead.
If otherwise, go to **3**

3 From what population was the sample drawn?	These are questions of external validity – see right-hand column.	Only insofar as the sample was a representative one can the results be generalised to the population from which the subjects were drawn (on representative samples see Chapter 10). But the sample of subjects for the experiment is unlikely to be representative of the case mix in any practice. Do researchers provide enough information about subjects
Where data collection involved a survey technique, see 'Questions to Ask about Surveys'.		
What were the principles and processes for selecting *all* subjects for the experiment?		
Is it clear what wider population these subjects represent?		

for practitioners to be able to extrapolate the results to their own practices?

4 What was the unit of sampling?

Was it appropriate to the questions asked?

Alternatively ask, 'Was what happened to each subject independent of what happened to each other?' (subjects might be individuals, ulcers, clinics etc.) (see Chapter 5, section 4)

In experiments on individually delivered interventions the individual client is the appropriate unit of sampling. But where interventions are delivered at group or community level (e.g., group therapy), the outcomes for one will be influenced by the behaviour of all. A therapy group of six should then be regarded as a sample of 1, and sample size calculated accordingly (see **5** below).

Where the appropriate sampling unit is the individual there are no particular problems of application. But the results of group treatment trials are particularly problematic for application, since in order to reproduce the research results in practice a practitioner may need to reproduce the group dynamics which developed during the research.

5 What was the size of the sample?

Was it big enough to accommodate:

- all the relevant diversity among subjects, both within and between arms of the experiment
- any diversity of treatment within arms of the trial
- the diversity of outcomes on the chosen outcome measures

and to detect differences of the size of interest? (see Chapter 7, sections 7 and 8)

The more the relevant diversity among subjects, and between treatments within arms of a study, the more points of measurement on a measurement scale, the smaller the difference of interest and the rarer the event of interest the bigger the sample needs to be.

Statistical significance is reduced in small samples, perhaps giving spurious results – usually spuriously non-significant results.

If the sample was chosen to be representative of a wider population, a larger sample is likely to be more representative, but see **3** above.

A large sample has a better chance of including a wider range of the types of clients a practitioner might encounter in practice.

6 Was the sample divided into comparison groups selected to be rather similar but treated in different ways (an experimental/treatment group and a control/alternative treatment group)?

If yes, go to **8**
If no, go to **7**

7 Were there comparison groups selected to be different from each other according to some criteria, but otherwise similar, subjected to the same treatment to see whether it had different effects on different kinds of subjects?
[Note that this design may be nested within the structure described in **6** above: a factorial design (Box 5.1, Chapter 5). If so, go to **8**.]

Otherwise, if yes, go to **10**
If no, go to **11**

8 How were the comparison groups formed?

If by randomisation, go to **13**
If otherwise, go to **9**

9 This is probably a matched pairs, or a matched group/reference area design or groups have been formed by purposive sampling (see Box 5.1 in Chapter 5).

Is the way comparison groups were formed fully explained? Are you satisfied that the variables which should have been evened out between groups were actually evened out? Differences in outcomes for groups may be due to differences which were in the groups in the first place rather than due to differences of intervention.

Was a cross-check made to establish the equivalence of groups?

All other things being equal, experimental designs that do not create comparison groups by randomisation are a less secure basis for generalisation than those that do (Chapter 5, section 3). Properly conducted matched pairs designs are preferred to matched group/reference area designs.

Go to **14**

10 Was the purpose of the experiment to see how different kinds of people responded to *the same* intervention? If yes, check whether the sample seemed large enough to accommodate at least 10 and preferably more of each kind of person. The reason why the researcher didn't divide them into sub-groups in the first place will probably be because it was unknown at the outset as to which kinds of people would respond differently and the experiment was to find this out.

Go to **11**

11 Was the purpose of the experiment simply to see if there was a diversity of response to the same intervention, without being interested in who responded in what way? This is a common design for investigating practitioner decision-making, a group of practitioners being confronted with the same client/case notes/ diagnostic test results and asked to make a judgement about them. The results are usually analysed in terms of statistical correlations (see Chapter 6, section 6).

If yes, go to **16**
If no, go to **12**

12 This is probably a pre–post trial without controls (see Box 5.1 in Chapter 5).

A pre–post trial without controls, where what happened to one subject was not independent of what happened to another, is probably not worth reading (see **4** above).

Go to **17**

13 Randomisation
Was the sample divided into groups/ between arms by a truly random procedure? (see Chapter 5, section 3)

(Randomisation may be improved by stratification – see Chapter 5, section 3)

Go to **14**

14 Were the comparison groups checked for their similarity at the outset?

Were the characteristics of the subjects clearly described?

Did one of the groups have more extreme baseline scores than the other(s)?

Subjects (groups, communities etc.) are being compared with themselves before and after an intervention. Does the author make a convincing case that measurements posttrial were caused by the intervention and were not due to being involved in a research project (an experiment effect) or due simply to the passage of time?

Randomisation is used to ensure that each group is a representative sample of *all subjects in the trial* (not of the population from which the sample was drawn). Deficiencies in randomisation may produce treatment and control groups which are different in important ways from each other, the differences filtering through to create spurious differences on an outcome measure (see Figure 5.1, Chapter 5).

If the comparison groups are dissimilar, then these dissimilarities are likely to feed through to outcome differences creating spurious results. Groups with extreme scores at the outset set up the conditions for regression to the mean. If one group has more extreme scores than another this may feed through to outcome measurements

Unless the pre–post differences are very large and/or the same differences have been demonstrated in other studies, it is speculative to generalise from the results of pre–post trials (without controls).

In routine practice practitioners do not select clients for particular treatments at random. Their selection criteria may produce results which are different from those reported in a randomised study even if they 'do the same'. However, since there are no controls in practice, this may not be apparent.

Unless practitioners are told about the subjects, practitioners will not know how like or unlike they were compared to the clients they deal with.

Go to **15**

15 Did the design include planned 'crossover'? Were the same subjects subjected to a sequence of treatments? (see Box 5.1, Chapter 5 and Chapter 5, section 13)

to give spurious differences in 'improvement' or 'deterioration' (see Chapter 5, section 6).

With cross-over were the subjects and the experimenter blind to the treatments being given? Was it certain that carry-over effects were not confounding the results? With random and blind assignment of treatments and proper management of carry-over effects this is a very powerful research design.

For n-of-1 experiments and single case evaluations (Chapter 5, section 13) generalisation is not the main purpose, though these designs do demonstrate the diversity of response to the same treatment. For group trials generalisation will depend on the similarity of the practice case mix with that of the subjects researched.

Go to **16**

16 Drop out and unplanned cross-overs

Were the characteristics of any unplanned cross-overs, and any subjects lost to the experiment recorded? Were the effects of lost subjects on the results estimated?

Did the loss of subjects from any group make the groups no longer similar?

If differences in outcome were actually produced by differential drop out then the results cannot be generalised.

Are the results expressed in terms of 'intention to treat'? (Chapter 5, section 8)

[Intention to treat] In the final analysis were results for those who were switched from one arm of the trial to another, and for those withdrawn counted as results for the arm to which they were originally allocated?

Results in terms of intention to treat may be closer to what happens in practice.

Go to **17**

17 **Subject reactivity** (see Chapter 5, section 5)

What were the subjects' understandings of the experiment: how might these have influenced the results?

Where subject interpretations and understandings influence the results of only one arm of the trial this may create spurious outcome differences.

If, as usually happens, all subjects know they are involved in an experiment this may affect outcomes for *all* arms of the trial. Where such effects implicate all subjects this may

Were the subjects blinded as to the intervention they received? Were they successfully blinded?

Were Hawthorne/experiment effects likely – changes due to the fact of being researched, rather than to the intervention itself? (Chapter 5, section 12)

Go to **18**

Reactivity is a particular problem where the judgements of subjects are used as the basis for outcome measures.

invalidate the generalisability of the results.

In routine practice clients should know what treatment they are being given. In this respect they differ from a blinded group. Clients in the know may be expected to respond differently from blinded subjects.

18 Subject compliance

Did the experiment depend on subjects doing what they were supposed to do?

If so, what means were taken to judge whether subjects had been compliant?

Go to **19**

Hidden non-compliance may give misleading results.

In routine practice non-compliance is common. Trials that enforce compliance successfully may give misleading results for practice where compliance cannot be enforced.

19 Practitioner/researcher judgements
(see Chapter 5, section 5)

Were practitioners/researchers blinded as to the interventions received by subjects? If so, were they successfully blinded? If not, how might their knowledge of group membership have altered their behaviour towards subjects, perhaps confounding the results?

If practitioner judgements were used in making baseline or outcome measures, what

Blinding practitioners/researchers is sometimes impossible and sometimes ineffective. Is there any reason to suppose that the practitioners in the research treated members of different groups differently over and above the planned difference in intervention? Is there any reason to suppose that researchers did things to produce results they preferred? Is there any evidence of 'conflict of interest'?

Different practitioners may not make judge-

In routine practice, practitioners know what treatments they are giving to clients. They will rightly do all that they think is necessary to produce benign outcomes, including all kinds of things not featured in the research. Hence the results in practice may differ from the results of an experiment where practitioners were blinded and tied to following the research protocols.

devices were used to ensure that their judgements were reliable? (see Chapter 6, section 6)

Go to **20**

ments in the same way. The effect of this may filter through as spurious outcome differences if different practitioners furnished data for different groups.

20 Specification of intervention (s)

Was what was done to each group of subjects clearly specified?

Unless what was done to/for subjects in *all* groups is clearly specified it will be impossible for readers to judge the results of the experiment as being the results of different treatments being given to otherwise similar groups, or as the result of the same treatment being given to groups with different characteristics. It will also be impossible to replicate the experiment, or to compare its results with those of others.

Unless practitioners know precisely what was done in the research they cannot successfully replicate this in their own practice. And would it be possible for practitioners to deliver the same intervention in practice: issues of resources, expertise and so on?

Go to **21**

21 Standardisation of intervention

Was what was done to/ for each subject within an arm of the experiment similar to what was done for each other in the same arm?

Where there is considerable heterogeneity of treatment within an arm of a trial, this is not really one arm but many arms and results should really be analysed in as many categories as there were differences in treatment. This requires a larger sample size (see Chapter 5, section 9 and Chapter 7, section 7).

Most routine practice entails customising interventions to the particularities of each client. The more this is true, the more difficult it is to investigate the effectiveness of such treatments, since investigations of effectiveness require reasonable sized groups of similar people treated much the same as each other.

Go to **22**

22 Observations and measures

What baseline, interim and outcome measures were made? Was the same kind of data collected for each subject? Is there missing data?

Would the observations and measures used in the research be feasible for someone in routine practice – if not, it will be difficult for practitioners to know whether they can do, or

Were the instruments used appropriate for the research question?

Had the instruments used been validated for use in a similar way?

Did the instruments used generate data in a form appropriate for the statistical analysis conducted?

Insofar as practitioner judgements were involved were they reliable judges? (see **19** above).

If the study was aimed at measuring effectiveness, what criteria of effectiveness were used? Might other definitions of effectiveness have been more appropriate? Go to **23**.

See 'Questions to Ask about Data Collection Instruments'.

could achieve the same results in practice.

Are the researchers' ideas about effectiveness the same as those of practitioners and/or of their clients?

23 Duration

Was the period of the study long enough to ensure that all important differences and similarities of outcome would show themselves?

If the duration of the study is too short then:

- some important 'side-effects' might not show
- short-term, but temporary advantages may be mistaken for long-term and permanent gains
- some long-term benefits of intervention (or non-intervention) might not show.

For what duration of care is the practitioner responsible? Can practitioners track their clients for longer, or shorter than the period of the experiment?

Go to **24**.

24 Statistical analysis

Were all the subjects accounted for in the analysis?

If a large proportion of subjects are missing from the analysis then it is unlikely that the comparison groups are similar any more (although there are ways of estimating the effects of missing data).

Were the tests used appropriate for the data produced and the questions posed?	This is a question for which reference to a statistics textbook may be necessary, but see Chapter 6, sections 3 and 4; Chapter 7, sections 6, 7 and 8. If tests of association/correlation were used, see Chapter 6, section 6, and Chapter 10, section 11.
Were the differences statistically significant?	See Chapter 7, sections 1 to 4.
Were confidence intervals calculated/was there enough information given for readers to calculate CIs?	See Chapter 7, sections 4, 5 and 9.

Go to **25**

25 Effect sizes

An effect size which is statistically insignificant should be ignored. But a statistically significant effect may still be too small to be important in practical terms (see Chapter 7, section 10 *passim*).

Is any statistically significant difference shown also of practical significance? For example, is it big enough to convince a practitioner that it would be worth the cost and effort of changing practice?

Go to **26**

26 What works for whom?

Does the study describe what happened to sub-groups within each arm of the experiment? For example, those in a control group whose condition improved as much as those in a treatment group, or those in a treatment group whose condition deteriorated more than those in the control group. This is desirable, but sample size which is adequate for showing statistically significant differences between two arms of a trial may well be too small to show statistically significant differences between sub-groups within an arm of a trial. Beware of small trials making claims about sub-groups.

Does the study identify sub-groups affected differently by the intervention / non-intervention in a way that could be used to guide practitioners' decisions as to whom to treat by what means: indications and contraindications, or 'risk factors'?

Go to **27**

27 Conclusions

Were the conclusions answers to the questions asked initially?

Did the conclusions follow logically from the evidence presented and the analysis conducted?

Beware of research that asks one question and concludes with an answer to another. The research was probably not designed to answer the second question!

Were conclusions stated in practice-relevant terms? For example, in terms of 'numbers needed to treat' (Chapter 7, section 10.5).

Did the conclusions drawn about the applic-

Is the conclusion restricted to what the evidence will support?

Go to **28**

ability of the research take account of the realities of practice and the diversity of practice circumstances?

28 Other research

Did the authors place their research in the context of other research? (see also Questions to Ask about Systematic Reviews and Meta-analyses)

Go to **29**

Does the study confirm findings from other studies, or run against them? Better evidence is needed to make a convincing case which runs against the grain.

All other things being equal, similar results from several studies are a safer basis for practice than results from a single study.

29 Ethical considerations

What evidence is there that the study was conducted in an ethical way: look for the way subjects were screened for entry to the experiment, the gaining of informed consent, measures to prevent harm and ensure confidentiality. Is there reference to approval by an ethics committee?

Go to **30**

Unethical research may none the less be internally valid.

Would it be ethical to apply the results of this research in practice?

30 Was the experiment the basis for a cost-effectiveness analysis? If so, see Questions to Ask about Cost-effectiveness Studies.

QUESTIONS TO ASK ABOUT SYSTEMATIC REVIEWS AND META-ANALYSES

Questions about the relevance of the review

Comments

1 Does the review relate *at all* to the questions for which you want an answer?

Read the abstract or the introduction to the review to avoid wasting time on a review which won't answer your questions.

2 Does it provide evidence in relation to the outcomes you are interested in?

Do a quick check as to what outcomes feature in the review. Are they of the kind which you could relate to your own practice?

3 Does it provide evidence that would be relevant to the practices/kinds of practitioner/kinds of agency in which you are interested?

Is this a topic where local socio-economic conditions, institutional arrangements or practice arrangements are likely to affect outcomes and if so how similar are your circumstances to the circumstances of the studies reviewed?

4 Does it provide evidence relevant to the kinds of clients you are interested in?

Are the clients in the studies reviewed sufficiently like the clients you are interested in?

5 If you are interested in cost-effectiveness, does the review provide the kinds of cost data which you can relate to cost data from your own circumstances?

See Chapter 3 of this volume and 'Questions to Ask about Cost-effectiveness Studies'

Questions about the quality of the review

Comments

6 Is this a systematic review emanating from an authoritative source, and itself peer-reviewed?

Most systematic reviews are published in peer reviewed journals or via one of the agencies specialising in systematic reviews and will have been vetted for their quality.

7 What is the date of the review, and of the studies it reviews?

Systematic reviews are always more out of date than the studies they review. Some topics date worse than others.

8 Is there any evidence that the reviewers are disposed towards or against particular kinds of practices, practitioners or client groups?

Some reviews are openly propagandist for particular approaches, others may suffer from the unwitting bias of the reviewers. It is worth looking for evidence of the reviewers' affiliations. Was the review funded by a drug company? Was a review with a conclusion favouring a social work practice written by a social worker committed to this practice?

9 Does the review address a clearly focused issue, or a set of clearly focused issues? Ideally the review should concentrate on studies asking similar questions about similar interventions, measured according to similar outcomes for similar kinds of people.

The possibility for reviewers to focus a review depends on what research is available for review. For example, the review by Roberts et al. in this volume (Chapter 4) deals with the effects of home visiting according to a wide variety of different kinds of injury occurring or not under a wide range of circumstances. That reflected the state of knowledge derived from RCTs at the time but it made for considerable difficulties in drawing general conclusions.

10 How widely and where has the reviewer looked for relevant studies to review?

Many systematic reviews are restricted to a single language, perhaps missing important papers in other languages. However, it is important to consider whether topics are culturally or institutionally bounded (see **3** above). Outcome measures such as 're-admitted to hospital' will not equate between societies where the structure of health services is different. There is a *publication bias* towards publishing studies which reach definite and positive conclusions. Good systematic reviews look for unpublished studies as well.

11 Did the reviewer ask authors to provide information missing from published accounts of their studies? Was this successful?

There are acute publishing constraints on how much information can be published. Sometimes it is not until a systematic review is conducted that it is clear what information is relevant.

12 What criteria did the reviewer use to decide which studies to include in the review. Are they appropriate criteria?

There will be two bases for such critieria. One is that they produce a group of studies where like can be compared with like. The other basis is that the criteria exclude poorly conducted studies. The latter criteria are similar to satisfactory answers to 'Questions to Ask about Experiments'.

13 Did the inclusion criteria exclude some studies which might have been interesting to you?

Many self-styled systematic reviews exclude all non-experimental research, and many all but RCTs. But other kinds of research can be relevant to practice (see Parts 2 and 3 of this volume).

14 Did the reviewer evaluate each study included so that less convincing studies count less towards the overall conclusion than more convincing ones?

Simply treating each study as equally convincing runs the risk of poorly conducted studies crowding out the better ones. The evaluation questions which should be asked by the reviewer will probably be similar to 'Questions to Ask about Experiments'. In Chapter 4 Prendiville's criteria are explained and used to weight studies.

15 Were the reviewer's judgements on the use of criteria evaluated for their reliability?

Asking several judges to apply the same criteria independently is the standard way of testing this: an inter-rater reliability test (see Chapter 6, section 6).

16 If the results of studies are combined in a meta-analysis, was it reasonable to do this?

Meta-analysis may be problematic if the numerical data have been produced using different instruments in different studies and because there is a risk that a large and poorly conducted trial will overwhelm the results of smaller but better ones (see Table 1 in Chapter 4). Data transformations are often necessary (Chapter 6, section 4; Chapter 7, section 6). In addition, meta-analysis presumes a high degree of similarity in all the studies combined in terms of people involved, context of practice, clientele, outcomes measured and so on. (For interpreting a meta-analysis, see Chapter 7, section 5.)

17 Does the author suggest implications for practice? If so do these follow logically from the review?

This includes considering whether the review addressed all possible outcomes, benign and adverse which might arise from adopting a particular intervention. Numbers needed to treat (NNT) can be a useful statistic for practitioners but needs to be regarded with caution (see Chapter 7, section 10.5).

18 Does the review clearly identify gaps in knowledge which would benefit from further research?

One of the main purposes of systematic reviews is to review the state of knowledge and to identify priorities for future research.

QUESTIONS TO ASK ABOUT COST-EFFECTIVENESS STUDIES

Questions	Issues of internal validity You judge whether the findings were true for the research location	Issues of external validity or generalisability You judge whether the findings would be true/ could be/should be, made true elsewhere
1 Evidence of effects How was this derived and is it valid evidence?	The most convincing evidence about effectiveness comes from experimental research (Chapter 5). See 'Questions to Ask about Experiments'	Is achieving these effects a high priority for you? Note: that the smaller the difference shown in research in effectiveness and/or popularity between two interventions the less likely it is that the same differences will show elsewhere.
2 The range of costs and benefits considered: What costs and benefits, whose costs and whose benefits? Costs and benefits over what period of time? Monetary and non-monetary costs?	No study could hope to include *all* conceivable costs and benefits to everyone, but there should be a clear statement about what costs and benefits are being considered. For internal validity the study should be judged on how well the researcher has accounted for the costs and benefits s/he chose to focus on.	Is this the range of costs and benefits of interest to you? For example, does a study of hospital at home care fail to include social services costs? Is aiming for these benefits incompatible with aiming for something else desirable?
3 Costing	Is the methodology of costing fully described?	Would it be possible to find the same costing

Are the data on which costing is based:

- accurate?
- timely?

Was costing even-handed as between two alternative interventions?

data locally and substitute them for those in the study?

If not, how similar or dissimilar are the cost bases in the research location and the practice location? The more similar, the more applicable the study.

4 Sensitivity

Do the authors conduct sensitivity analyses (SA) to estimate the effect of varying important factors? If so, are the topics chosen for SA the factors which are both most likely to vary and most likely to affect the cost–benefit ratio?

Are there any reasons to assume that the cost basis is very different in the practice location?

How out-of-date are the costings? Don't bother about matters that can be updated by a simple inflation factor: consider costs which might have changed radically.

Do the authors' sensitivity analyses help to fit their study to your situation?

Do they provide enough data to allow you to conduct a sensitivity analysis of your own?

QUESTIONS TO ASK ABOUT SURVEYS, CASE FINDING (OR 'CLINICAL EPIDEMIOLOGICAL') STUDIES AND CASE CONTROL STUDIES

1 What kind of study is this?

- Is it a survey, with a sample taken to represent a wider population? If so start at **2** (count 'cohort studies' as surveys; see Chapter 10, Box 10.6).
- Is it a case finding (or 'clinical epidemiological') study with cases of something being looked for, and their frequency being expressed as a proportion/rate of the population in which they were looked for? If so start at **5** (for an example see the study by King et al., in Chapter 11, sections 1 and 2).
- Is it a case control study, with cases of something being looked for, and then matched with controls selected in a different way? If so start at **4** (for examples, see Chapter 10, section 9).

Questions [Surveys only]	Appraisal issues
2 The sample Of what population was the sample supposed to be representative?	Usually this will be a population of individuals, but sometimes it might be a population of agencies, areas, or time periods.
	Researchers should clearly state the population they are trying to represent since this is the starting point for selecting a sample and the basis for judging whether the sample was adequately representative.
At what level of detail was the sample supposed to be representative?	Samples may be of an adequate size to represent a population at one level of detail, but not of an adequate size to represent the same population at another level of detail (see chapter 10, sections 1, 6 and 7). Check that the researcher does not make claims about matters for which the sample was too small.

Was a sampling of individuals preceded by clustering to group respondents conveniently? See Chapter 10, Section 4

Many national surveys begin by sampling areas, and then sample individuals within them. Clustering may undermine the representativeness of the sample (see Chapter 10, section 4).

Was the sample stratified? See Chapter 10, section 3

Where comparisons between subgroups of different sizes are of interest separate samples may be chosen from each to avoid the sample for the smaller sub-groups being too small (see Chapter 10, section 3). If this is not done, check to see whether the researchers do not make comments about sub-groups for which the sample is too small (see Chapter 10, section 7).

What sampling frame (if any) was used? Was it a complete listing: were omissions likely to slant the sample away from representativeness?

Sampling frames may under-represent some groups of interest. Do the researchers' conclusions take this into consideration? (see Chapter 10: Sections 2 and 8)

What technique was used to select the sample and was this adequate for the purpose?

Various techniques of sampling are given in Box 10.1 of Chapter 10. Never accept any generalisation about frequencies in a population which are based on convenience samples, or self-recruited samples.

How large was the sample and was it large enough to represent at the level of detail aimed for?

Eyeball the data given in any tables. If *each* cell of the table is filled with a small number this is an indication that the sample was too small (see also Chapter 10, sections 6 and 7).

3 Non-response
What was the level of non-response?

Did the researchers have accurate data as to the characteristics of the population in order to judge representativeness?

See Chapter 11, section 2.

Were the characteristics of non-respondents checked against known characteristics of the population?

The size of the non-response is less important than the characteristics of non-respondents (see Chapter 10, section 8)

Were estimates made of the extent to which non-response might have skewed the sample away from representativeness?

See Chapter 10, section 8.

Were the results weighted to redress greater non-response by some section of the population? Was the process of weighting adequately explained?

See Chapter 10, section 8 and Chapter 11, section 1.

Now go to **6**

4 [Case control studies only]

How were the controls recruited, and matched to the cases found?

(If there was an attempt to make the controls representative of a particular population, go back to **2** and start there, but consider the questions only in relation to selecting controls – and don't forget the question about matching.)

Faulty matching will lead to confounding (see Chapter 10, section 9)

5 [Case control and case-finding (clinical epidemiological) studies]

How were the cases found and what means were taken to ensure:

- that the cases found were all of the same kind?
- that all the cases were found, or some estimate was made of the percentage not found?

Look out for unreliable categorisation (Chapter 6, section 5) and for ascertainment bias (Chapter 10, section 9)

6 Administration

How was the data collection instrument administered? (Postal questionnaire, telephone interview, face-to-face interview, data collected by clinical examination or assessment)

Is there any reason to believe that the way the research was done affected the results, overall or for sub-groups of respondents? Was it administered similarly for all respondents? Would the same situation have had different effects for different respondents?

What was the context in which the survey instrument was administered?

Is there any reason to believe that the context in which the survey was administered or the characteristics of the people administering the survey would have differential effects on different kinds of respondents: for example white interviewers with black respondents?

By whom was the survey instrument administered?

Were different interviewers trained to give a standardised performance/ follow a common protocol?

Were the results of the survey analysed interviewer by interviewer to investigate interviewer effects? For all above see Chapter 10, section 14.

In research that involved diagnosis or assessment by an expert were these judgements reached following a common protocol?

If expert judgement was involved was inter-rater reliability established? (see Chapter 6, section 6)

Instead of the questions in cells **7** to **11** you might prefer to use the questions in cell **22** of Questions to Ask about Experiments

7   Validation and piloting

Had the data collection instrument and procedures been piloted and amended in the light of this?

The re-use of tried and tested instruments has the dual advantage that the main problems will have been ironed out, and that the results of several pieces of research using the same instrument can be directly compared with each other (see Chapter 6, section 1).

8   Questionnaire or other instrument (for example, a self-completed diary or a diagnostic algorithm). Does the author give sufficient detail about the research instrument used?

Research that is reported without disclosing what instrument was used is virtually impossible to appraise; but for reasons of space details may be published elsewhere.

9   Questions (for each question)

Did the question ask people things they could reasonably be expected to know?

People are often willing to give answers to questions even if they don't know the answers, or to invent opinions on matters they have never considered before.

Was the question about something which happened some time in the past?

Answers to retrospective questions are often inaccurate about what really happened, though they may be accurate about what someone thinks happened.

Was the question asked in a concrete way: for example, 'How many times have you visited the doctor in the last seven days?' and not 'How often do you usually visit the doctor?'

People vary greatly in the way they generalise. One person's 'usually' may be another's 'rarely'.

Was the question 'leading' in any way – suggestive that one answer might be favoured by the interviewer rather than another?

What is a leading question for one person, may not be a leading question for another.

Was the question offensive, over-intrusive or upsetting in some way?

People vary in what they find offensive or intrusive.

Was the question phrased in a straightforward and unambiguous way, for the people intended to answer it?

Including whether questions were asked in a language some people didn't understand, or people with limited reading skills were asked to read a questionnaire.

Did any question have a particularly low response rate?

This is usually an indication that this was not an effective question and the results should be interpreted accordingly.

10 Responses

Were responses forced?

For forced choice questions were all the possible responses provided? For rating scales was there a 'neutral' middle position, or were respondents forced to opt for a positive or a negative answer?

Were responses open?

After the survey, responses to open-ended questions have to be coded into categories. How was this done?

Were respondents allowed to make more than one response to each question?

This leads to great difficulty in analysis, since loquacious respondents contribute more to the survey results than the reticent.

11 Analysis

Were the results presented with confidence intervals/sampling errors?

See Chapter 10, sections 6 and 7

Were differences tested for statistical significance?

See Chapter 7, sections 1 and 2

Were correlations expressed as correlation co-efficients and were these tested for statistical significance?

See Chapter 10, section 10

Were the conclusions based on figures that were large enough to bear them?

This can be a difficult question to answer, but see Chapter 10, sections 6 and 7.

Were the statistical tests used appropriate for the kind of data collected?

See Chapter 7, section 6

Was the commentary on the statistics commensurate with the statistical analysis of the data?

For example, does the author conveniently forget the non-respondents? Does the author make much of differences/correlations which are not statistically significant?

If frequencies were expressed as population rates, did the researcher have accurate data about the population?

Under-estimating the number of people 'at risk' will over-estimate the rate (see Chapter 11, section 2)

Did analysis involve age standardisation?	See Chapter 11, sections 1 and 2
Did analysis involve the use of deprivation indices?	See Chapter 11, section 4
How successful was the analysis in terms of creating categories for comparison similar in all respects except for the variable of interest?	See Chapter 10, section 11 (see also Chapter 5, sections 1 and 3)

12 Presentation of results

Did displays of data include all the data relevant to the conclusions drawn (for example 'don't knows' as well as those who gave answers)?	
If the survey involved non-proportional sampling (Box 10.1 in Chapter 10) is it made clear whether the results presented have been re-weighted to proportionality?	See Chapter 10, section 8 and Chapter 11, section 1
If results are presented in terms of a reference or standard population, is the standardisation fully explained?	See Chapter 11, section 1

13 Only if authors draw causal conclusions

Was this a contemporaneous/snap shot study or a longitudinal/prospective/cohort study?	Causal statements based on correlations found in contemporaneous surveys may well pose direction of effect problems which cannot be resolved from the survey or case control data (see Chapter 10, sections 11 and 12).

14 Other research

Does the author place conclusions in the context of wider literature? Does this strengthen or weaken the conclusions?	Usually more and better evidence is required to support findings that run counter to the weight of published research.

15 Conclusions

Do the authors' conclusions follow logically from the analysis of the evidence presented?	The authors' conclusions may simply be a generalisation from the sample to the population from which it was drawn. But an author may draw more speculative conclusions about other populations, about causal linkages (**13** above) or about the success or failure of policies and programmes. Generalisations about frequencies in populations should not be

drawn from case control studies (see Chapter 10, section 9).

16 Practice usefulness

Are the results presented in ways that allow for extrapolation of the results to a practice area?

A local practice area is most unlikely to show the same patterns as a national survey or a local survey elsewhere. Age standardisation, the use of deprivation index scores or presentation of results in terms of a reference population make it easier to extrapolate from a survey to practice (see Chapter 11)

Insofar as you find the conclusions convincing, is there any practical use to which you might put them?

For example:

- Providing a model for planning local surveys.
- Providing a tested questionnaire which you might re-use (see Chapter 6).
- Evaluating the impact/effectiveness of a policy/programme elsewhere in deciding whether to implement it locally.
- Bench-marking local performance on performance elsewhere (see Chapter 11).
- Identifying targets and 'at-risk' groups for intervention/prioritisation.

QUESTIONS TO ASK ABOUT QUALITATIVE RESEARCH

Questions

1 Is there a clear statement as to the aims of the research?

2 What kind of phenomena does the researcher think s/he is studying?

3 Does the author announce or imply a value position?

Appraisal issues

Qualitative research may not have a 'Research Question' as such, except 'What's going on around here and why?' This is a legitimate research question.

It makes a great deal of difference as to whether, for example, researchers think they are studying utterances as evidence of how people experience things/what they mean to them (see Chapters 12 and 13), or utterances as ways people do things with language at the time they speak (see Chapter 14). Assumptions about the phenomena being studied determine the appropriate way of collecting data and analysing them (see Chapter 16, sections 5 and 6, though the examples there by no means exhaust all the possibilities).

Qualitative research is sometimes 'value-led' with researchers wanting to draw attention to injustices, or to 'give a voice' to voiceless people. Given the great leeway there is for qualitative researchers to shape their data, out of sight of their readers, readers should beware of findings that exactly support the value position of the researcher. None of this is to say that allegedly 'value-free' research does not suffer from researcher bias (see Chapter 16, section 7).

4 Was this collaborative/participatory research (the researcher teaming with the subjects of the study to produce research together)?

What kinds of commitments might there have been between researcher and co-participants which might have shaped the way the findings were made public? (see Chapter 16, section 7)

5 Was this research an observation of events happening under natural circumstances, for example, a participant observation study of a clinic? If yes, go to **6**
Or
Was this research an interview/focus group study? If yes, go to **11**

6 The research location
Was the reason for the choice of research location explained?
Was the location suitable for the research undertaken?
How typical is the research location?

7 Time sampling
Does the author state how long was spent in the research location(s)? Was this long enough? For example, are claims made about the outcomes of what was observed which happened after the period of observation?

Which time periods were sampled, and which were not?

8 Activity/event sampling
Were there activities/events important to the topic of the research which were not observed?
Were the activities/events observed typical of this class of activities? Were observations of atypical activities/events used to illuminate typical ones? (deviant case analysis: Chapter 16, section 4)

9 Personnel sampling
Who were the people observed? Were those observed a representative selection of the people of interest in the research location? Representative might mean representative in the statistical sense, or representing important theoretical categories (see 'theoretical sampling' in Chapter 16, section 4).

In principle there is no reason why qualitative research should not be conducted anywhere at any time, in relation to any activities, or any people. But the questions opposite relate to the generalisability of the findings and the researcher's aspirations about making generalisations. For example, if generalisations are made from a study of a particular clinic, it is important that the clinic is representative of others in some ways, though not necessarily in the statistical sense of the term 'representative': note the difference between statistical and theoretical sampling in Chapter 16, section 4.

General claims about what happens in the research location covering times not observed should be treated with suspicion, as should general claims about activities when those observed may be atypical, and similarly general claims about types of people when only some of the type present in the research location have been observed.

Were the activities of idiosyncratic people used to illuminate those of people behaving more usually in this context? (deviant case analysis: Chapter 16, section 4)

10 Researcher's role and identity in the setting

How did other people understand what the researcher was doing?
How might this have affected what was said or done by them in the researcher's presence?
How might the role adopted have disbarred the researcher from certain settings, affected the way s/he was communicated with and so on?
Now go to **13**

The danger, of course, is that what the researcher sees is what happens when researchers are around, rather than what happens when they are not. In addition other people are often most anxious to make researchers see things in particular ways and not in others.

11 Sampling

How were the interviewees/focus group members selected?
Was this an appropriate way of selecting respondents for the topic of the research?
How many in total were there?

The importance of answers here depends on the researcher's aspirations about making generalisations. If generalisations are made on the basis of those who were respondents, applying to people who were not, then respondents need to be representative of the latter in some way. Representativeness does not have to mean statistically representative. It can mean representative of a range of theoretically interesting categories irrespective of their commonality or rarity. See the distinction between statistical and theoretical sampling in Chapter 16, section 4.

12 The interview/focus group situation

How were respondents briefed about the purpose of the research?
Does the author provide information as to what happened during the interviews/focus group which might have shaped the data produced?
Does the author provide information about the communicative behaviour of the researcher as well as about that of the respondents?

The ideal information comes from full transcriptions of interchanges between researchers and researched, but it is rarely practicable for authors to provide all that is necessary. None the less, there should be some data provided about the context in which the data were elicited so that readers can judge whether the 'findings' are an artefact of the context in which the data were gathered and/or of the communicative style of the interviewer.

Where interview respondents reported on what they did or said elsewhere, was there any means of verifying this, and were these means used?

(You might also like to look at cell **6** in 'Questions to Ask about Surveys')

There may be little relationship between what people themselves say they do, and what they can be observed to do.

13   Data recording

How (and when) did the researcher record the data? How did the researcher decide what to record?

The act of recording data can be intrusive and disruptive in observation research, but relying on memory and writing it up afterwards may suffer from selective remembering. Whether in observation or in interviews, handwritten notes about what people said are much less convincing than transcripts of tape/video recordings. Where records are made by audio or video recording they are already structured by decisions as to where to site the equipment and when to switch it on, but these are matters which are easy to know about. By contrast, where a researcher writes field notes in retrospect these will be shaped by implicit and difficult-to-know-about analysis in the form of selective attention, selective forgetting, and editing in terms of ideas of importance and relevance. Strategies such as a grounded theory approach (Chapter 16, section 4) make more of this explicit and accountable.

14   The analysis of the data

Does the author explain and *demonstrate* how the data analysis was done: for example, is a specimen transcript provided with examples of codings? Are decision-rules for coding given?

Was the coding of the data checked for inter-rater reliability? (see Chapter 6, section 6)

Are frequency statements made about the commonality of particular responses/behaviours?

Qualitative researchers suffer from the weightiness of their data and it is not always possible for them to provide readers with all that is needed to make an informed judgement about the adequacy of the analysis. However, it is not reasonable to expect readers to take matters entirely on trust.

What data were excluded is an important question. It is all too easy to carve a story out of a large amount of

Is an explanation given for what data were included and what excluded from the analysis?

data simply by ignoring most of it. The question of frequency relates to this. 'Most' only has a meaning in relation to what is counted as 'all'.

15 Fallibility testing
Did the researcher submit the findings to the people researched for their opinion about their accuracy?

Fallibility testing is popular with some researchers, but it is certainly not an acid test of the accuracy of findings. People may accept findings because they like them, reject them because they don't and findings which are acceptable to some people may be objectionable to others.

16 Triangulation
Were data produced by various methods compared (for example from observations and interviews, or from interviews and clinical measurements)? Did all the data support the same conclusions?

Conclusions supported by data collected by more than one method are more convincing than those based on a single data-collecting strategy. However, sometimes triangulation by method will lead to incompatible conclusions.

17 Overall, do the data support the conclusions the author derives from them?

18 Other research
How does this research relate to other research in the same field?

All other things being equal, it requires more convincing evidence to undermine existing findings.

19 Generalisability
Is it possible to use/does the author use data from elsewhere to locate this study in a wider context?

For example, for Blaxter (Chapter 12) the Health and Lifestyle Survey findings provided a kind of map in terms of which those she interviewed could be located. They may not have been statistically representative, but at least it was clear where they fitted in the wider picture.

Does the author generate any useful analytic concepts?

Qualitative research has generated many useful general purpose concepts, such as stigma, career, total institution, deviancy amplification and so on.

Is there anything you have learned from this study which helps you to understand other people, or social or psychological or organisational processes better?

It is sometimes claimed that the main function of qualitative research is to produce vicarious experience, providing insight into the worlds of other people (see Chapter 16, section 8).

QUESTIONS TO ASK ABOUT ACTION RESEARCH

1 Was the research design 'experimental' in the sense that there was some attempt to compare the effects of an intervention with the effects of no intervention, or of some different intervention; was there some degree of control built into the research? (see Chapter 5, section 3)
If yes, use 'Questions to Ask about Experiments' and Chapters 5, 6 and 7
If no, go to **2**

2 What strategies were used to produce evidence?
If this involved telling the inside story, see also 'Questions to Ask about Qualitative Research', cells **6** to **10** and **13** to **16**, and Chapter 16
If this involved loosely structured interviews, see also 'Questions to Ask about Qualitative Research', cells **11** to **16**, and Chapter 16
If this involved questionnaire research, see also 'Questions to Ask about Surveys', cell **6**, and Chapter 10
If this involved other kinds of data collecting instruments, see also 'Questions to Ask about Data Collection Instruments' and Chapter 6

Questions	Issues
3 Does the study provide convincing evidence that the 'action' actually led to the effects claimed for it? How was the situation prior to the research investigated and characterised? How was the situation at the end of the research investigated and characterised?	For example, if it is claimed that the research was successful in improving the knowledge and competence of those involved, what measures were there of this prior to and at the end of the research? Or if it is claimed that at the end of the research there was a more cohesive community – what measures were used to indicate more and less cohesiveness? Or if the claims are about improving the quality of service, what criteria were used to judge service quality and how were these turned into measures of quality? If testimonial evidence is used, is it reasonable to assume that those who bear witness are:

- Reliable witnesses – know what they are talking about?
- Have not been specially selected by the author to give a clean bill of health to the project?
- Are representative of all those affected by the action research?

Were effects for all people involved reported?

Are real or possible adverse effects reported as well as 'success' stories?

4 Replicability
Is sufficient evidence provided for readers to be able to carry out the same intervention elsewhere? This includes information about:

- What was done.
- The characteristics of people who benefited, and of those who did not.
- About the practitioners involved; their skills and other relevant characteristics.
- About the resourcing of the project.
- About the organisational structure of practice and/or political context.

Most action research features 'complex' interventions (Chapter 5, sections 9 and 12), involving many activities, often customised to individuals and circumstances and carried out over a longish time period. They may be particularly difficult to specify, thus leading to difficulties of knowing which aspects of the intervention had which effects, if any at all, and what someone would have to do to produce the same results elsewhere. Better studies attempt to specify the conditions necessary for the same actions to have the same effects elsewhere.

5 'Experiment effects' (see Chapter 5, section 5)
Is it clear how much of what happened was because of the actions taken, and how much of what happened was due to the commitment and enthusiasm of those involved?

Effects produced by mobilising the enthusiasm of participants may be real enough, but may not be replicable by someone else adopting the same strategy elsewhere.

6 Biased reporting
How likely is it that the research report was written to give a favourable picture of the practitioners and clients involved, an agency, or a favoured way of working?

Publication bias ensures that most published action research consists of 'success' stories, and most is written by researchers with strong value commitments, or commitments to particular forms of practice. Much is collaborative or participatory, such that the final report will reflect a consensus among those involved. Considerations of image and reputation may influence what is published, and some action research is specifically designed to improve the public image of the participants.

7 What insights and understandings does the study provide which might improve the way another practitioner practices?

The answer to this depends partly on the answers to the earlier questions but this is also a question about 'naturalistic generalisation' as discussed in Chapter 16, section 8.

APPENDIX

FINDING PUBLISHED RESEARCH IN HEALTH AND SOCIAL CARE

Because this is such a rapidly changing field readers are urged to use the recommended Internet sources or contact the specialist organisations to identify the most up-to-date sources.

1 Printed Sources – Books, Journals and Reports

Books

This is a small selection from the many textbooks designed to help practitioners apply research to practice.

Evidence-Based Healthcare: How to Make Health Policy and Management Decisions
  Gray, J.A.M. (1997) Churchill Livingstone ISBN 0–443–05721–4
A practical guide for those who manage or purchase health services or make health policies, condensed from the practical experiences of many people and projects.

Evidence Based Healthcare: a Practical Guide for Therapists
  Bury, T.J. and Mead, J.M. (1998) Butterworth–Heinemann ISBN 0–750–63783–8
A guide to evidence based practice written particularly for radiographers, physiotherapists, occupational therapists, podiatrists, speech therapists and other professionals allied to medicine.

Evidence-Based Medicine: How to Practise and Teach EBM
  Sackett, D.L. et al. (1997) Churchill Livingstone ISBN 0–443–05686–2
An explanation of how to apply the key principles of evidence based practice in your everyday clinical work.

Evidence-Based Social Work Practice with Families: a Lifespan Approach
  Corcoran, J. (2000) Springer ISBN 0–826–11303–6

How to Read a Paper: the Basics of Evidence Based Medicine
  Greenhalgh, T. (1997) BMJ Publishing Group
This book aims to introduce non-experts to finding medical articles and assessing their value and has also been published as a 'How to read a paper' series in the *British Medical Journal*.

The ScHARR Guide to Evidence Based Practice (1997)
A bibliography and resource guide:
ScHARR Information Resources, University of Sheffield, Regent Court, 30 Regent Street, Sheffield S1 4DA
The guide can be downloaded from the main ScHARR Netting the Evidence site and is freely distributed within the University and NHS sectors.
http://www.shef.ac.uk/~scharr/ir/ebpfin.doc

Journals and newsletters

While relevant research articles may be found in the majority of professional and academic journals in health and social care, there are also journals which specialise in reviewing the results of research and its relevance for practice. These include the following.

Bandolier
NHS monthly newsletter on local and national initiatives and literature on the effectiveness of health care interventions.

Clinical Effectiveness in Nursing
Quarterly nursing journal focusing on the effectiveness of clinical interventions.

Clinical Evidence 99
A six monthly, updated compendium of evidence on the effects of common clinical interventions. (BMJ Publishing Group)

Educational Action Research
Despite the title, this is a major source of published action research in health and social care as well as in education. The 'Educational' in the title reflects the notion that a major purpose of action research is that those involved as researchers or subjects should learn from doing it.

Effective Health Care Bulletins
Bi-monthly bulletin from the Centre for Reviews and Dissemination which examines the effectiveness of a variety of health care interventions, summarises results and makes clear recommendations for practice. (Distributed free within the NHS)

Effectiveness Matters
Annual updates on the effectiveness of important health interventions for practitioners and decision makers in the NHS. (Distributed free within the NHS)

Evidence-Based Health Care
Bi-monthly aiming to provide managers with the best evidence available about the financing, organisation and delivery of health care.

Evidence-Based Medicine
Bi-monthly to alert clinicians to important advances in all areas of medicine. Also available on CD-ROM Best Evidence (see below).

Evidence-Based Mental Health
Quarterly journal containing clinically useful and accurate selected articles on clinically relevant advances in treatment and the organisation of care, diagnosis, aetiology, prognosis/outcome research, quality improvement, continuing education and economic evaluation.

Evidence-Based Nursing
A quarterly journal which identifies and appraises high quality, clinically relevant research.

Evidence-Based Social Care Newsletter
The newsletter published three-times a year by the Centre for Evidence Based Social Services (CEBSS).

Health Evidence Bulletins, Wales
Signposts to the best current evidence across a broad range of evidence types and subject areas.

Health Expectations
Quarterly journal aiming to promote critical thinking and informed debate about all aspects of public participation in health care and health policy.

Journal of Clinical Effectiveness
Quarterly journal focusing on evidence based practice, clinical effectiveness, guidelines and clinical audit.

Journal of Evaluation in Clinical Practice
Quarterly journal containing articles and systematic reviews of research on clinical effectiveness and the implementation of evidence based care.

Journal of Health and Social Policy
This journal covers many health and health-related professions and focuses on all aspects of policy – its development, formulation, implementation, evaluation, review and revision.

Journal of Social Service Research
A publication exclusively devoted to empirical research and its application to the design, delivery and management of the new social services.

Reports

Reports may provide in-depth coverage of a piece of primary research or an overview and review of a number of primary research studies. In fields that have a large number of relevant research studies, they can provide an invaluable way of assessing the literature. They may be published by government departments, professional bodies or voluntary organisations.

CRD (NHS Centre for Reviews and Dissemination) Reports
CRD Reports discuss the results of a systematic review of research in more depth than an Effective Health Care Bulletin (see above). Press releases, executive summaries and some reports in full text are available on their website.
   http://www.york.ac.uk/inst/crd/crdrep.htm

Department of Health Reports
The Department of Health produces many reports which review the research evidence. These publications may be traced using the POINT search engine available at
   http://www.doh.gov.uk/pointh.htm
Details are also available from Health Literature line: Tel 0800 555 777.
Reports may be published as White and Green Papers but often as other Department of Health series, e.g. the guidance on commissioning cancer series which summarise the research evidence on questions relating to improving outcomes for cancer treatments, or the Confidential Enquiry reports into areas such as maternal and infant deaths.

Development and Evaluation Committee Reports
The Development and Evaluation service aims to provide commissioners in the South West and South East Regions with reliable, timely information about the cost-effectiveness of health care technologies. Reports contain information on the quality of evidence for both proposed and current treatments, and a measure of effect size and costs.
   http://www.hta.nhsweb.nhs.uk/rapidhta/

Health Technology Assessment Reports
Results of the NHS Health Technology Assessment Programme into the costs, effectiveness and broader impacts of health technologies are published as reports, many available in full text.
   http://www.hta.nhsweb.nhs.uk/

Joseph Rowntree Foundation Reports
This organisation's programme of R&D projects in housing, social care and social policy are published in various formats. Details are available on their website.
   http://www.jrf.org.uk/

University of York Social Policy Research Unit Reports
This Unit produces a series of publications including SPRU papers (short reports providing up-to-the-minute commentary as well as a reflective and critical presentation of research and research findings), and Social Policy Reports (covering research findings, comments on methodology, and discussion of policy and practice).
   http://www.york.ac.uk/inst/spru

2 Electronic Sources – On-line Databases and Internet Resources

Databases

This section lists a selection of databases which can be used to search for evidence based practice information. Some or all of these should be available in specialist health care/social care or academic libraries.

AgeInfo
CD-ROM database on age and ageing from the Centre for Policy on Ageing.

AMED (Allied and Alternative Medicine)
Offers access to resources in non-traditional medicine and covering reference articles from 350 journals, many not indexed elsewhere.

Best Evidence
A CD-ROM database of abstracts from *ACP Journal Club* (1991–) and *Evidence-Based Medicine* (1995–) which cover reviews from more than 90 journals world-wide.

British Nursing Index (BNI)
A database of articles from over 220 nursing journals. Available in printed form, on CD-ROM and on the Internet.

CANCERLIT
The treatment of cancer and information on epidemiology, pathogenesis and immunology.

CAREDATA
Contains abstracts of books, research papers and journal articles from social work and social care publications. Available on CD-ROM and the Internet.

CINAHL
The nursing and allied health database covers all aspects of nursing and allied health disciplines such as health education, occupational therapy, emergency services, social services in health care.

The Cochrane Library
This is the premier source of information on the effectiveness of health care interventions. It is produced by the Cochrane Collaboration, an international network of individuals committed to 'preparing, maintaining, and disseminating systematic, up-to-date reviews of the effects of health care'. It contains the following databases:

(i) **Cochrane Database of Systematic Reviews (CDSR)**, a rapidly growing collection of regularly updated, systematic reviews of the effects of health care.

(ii) **Database of Abstracts of Reviews of Effectiveness (DARE)**, includes structured abstracts of systematic reviews from around the world. Also available through the CRD.

(iii) **The Cochrane Controlled Trials Register (CCTR)**, a bibliography of controlled trials as part of an international effort to hand search the world's journals and create an unbiased source of data for systematic reviews.

(iv) **The Cochrane Review Methodology Database (CRMD)**, a bibliography of articles on the science of research synthesis and on practical aspects of preparing systematic reviews.

(v) **ACP Journal Club abstracts**, available on CD-ROM and the Internet.

EMBASE
European equivalent of MEDLINE, the Excerpta Medica database focuses on drugs and pharmacology. Other aspects of human medicine covered include health policy, drug and alcohol dependence, psychiatry, forensic science and pollution control.

ENB Healthcare Database
References and abstracts from more than 80 UK journals, 1985 onwards, produced by the English National Board for Nursing, Midwifery and Health Visiting.

HEALTH-CD
A database launched in 1997 of many publications and documents from the Department of Health and the Stationery Office.

HealthSTAR
Covers literature on the non-clinical aspects of health care delivery such as administration and planning of health care facilities and evaluation of patient outcomes. Available as CD-ROM, on Internet or as hard disk. International (published in US).

Health Technology Assessment (HTA) Database
Contains abstracts produced by INAHTA (International Network of Agencies for Health Technology Assessment) and other health care technology agencies.

HMIC
The Health Management Information Consortium database consists of the combined catalogues of the Department of Health, the King's Fund and the Nuffield Institute for Health whose main subject focus is health care management in the UK. Available as CD-ROM.

MEDLINE
The US National Library of Medicine's bibliographic database covering all aspects of medicine and health care.

National Research Register (NRR)
Contains 42,000 project records recording ongoing research primarily funded by the NHS.

NHS Economic Evaluation Database (NEED)
This database is produced by the CRD and contains abstracts of economic evaluations of health technologies (coverage: 1990 to date).

Outcomes Activities Database
Contains details of recently completed activities connected with health outcomes work in all settings within the health service.

PsycLIT / PsycInfo
Contains abstracts of the world's journal literature in psychology and related disciplines and is compiled from the *PsycInfo* database. Available on CD-ROM.

SIGLE
The System for Information on Grey Literature in Europe, best defined as literature which is difficult to identify or obtain. Available as CD or hard disk.

Internet resources

The Internet is an excellent resource for evidence based practice information. There are a number of sites which act as gateways to the huge range of information available:

Core List for Evidence Based Practice
A list of books, reports, and journals suggested as a starting point for a UK library or clinical audit/effectiveness unit.
    http://www.shef.ac.uk/uni/academic/R-Z/scharr/ir/corelist.html

CTI Centre for Human Services – Social Work
A gateway to sites with information on education, research and training for social work teaching and practice.
    http://www.soton.ac.uk/~chst/

DrsDesk
The Doctors Desk is an integrated desktop information and communications system that a GP needs for evidence based practice.
    http://drsdesk.sghms.ac.uk

Evidence based health electronic discussion list
For teachers and practitioners in health-related fields; to announce meetings and courses, stimulate discussion, air controversies and aid the implementation of EBH. To subscribe e-mail: mailbase@mailbase.ac.uk
    http://www.ncl.ac.uk/ucs/email/mailbase.html
Other discussion lists of interest can be browsed through, and subscribed to, via the Mailbase website at the University of Newcastle.

Evidence Based Healthcare – a resource pack
Reading and key references concerning the background and current thinking on evidence based health care and details of the groups and organisations involved in this movement.
   http://drsdesk.sghms.ac.uk/Starnet/pack.htm

McMaster University EBM
A Canadian site which contains a huge amount of evidence based health care information, and links to other useful resources.
   http://www-hsl.mcmaster.ca/ebm/

Nursing and Health Care Resources on the Net
Helps you find the Internet source that meets most closely your interest.
   http://www.shef.ac.uk/~nhcon/

OMNI–Organising Medical Networked Information
A gateway to Internet resources in medicine, biomedicine, allied health, health management and related topics.
   http://omni.ac.uk/

ScHARR (Sheffield School of Health and Related Research) Lock's Guide to the Evidence
A guide to printed sources of evidence, focusing on grey literature from UK academic and quasi-governmental sources.
   http://www.shef.ac.uk/uni/academic/R-Z/scharr/ir/scebm.html

ScHARR (Sheffield School of Health and Related Research) Netting the Evidence
Online guide to journal articles, contact organisations, Internet discussion groups and definitions in all areas of evidence based practice.
   e-mail: a.booth@sheffield.ac.uk
   http://www.shef.ac.uk/~scharr/ir/netting.html

SOSIG (Social Science Information Gateway)
Internet resources gateway covering sociology, psychology and social welfare.
   http://www.sosig.ac.uk/

3   Projects, Initiatives and Organisations

Action Research Network Health Care Group
A network of practitioner–researchers interested in action research in health care contexts.
   Contact: Dr Ralph Nichols, Dementia Care Services, Shackleton, 57 Pellhurst Road, Ryde, Isle of Wight, PO33 3GT

Aggressive Research Intelligence Facility (ARIF)
A specialist unit at the University of Birmingham set up to help health care workers access and interpret research evidence in response to particular problems.
   Tel/Fax/Answering System: 0121 414 7878
   http://www.hsrc.org.uk/links/arif/arifhome.htm

Centre for Evidence-Based Child Health
Aims to increase the provision of effective and efficient child health care through an educational programme for health professionals.
  Tel: 0207 905 2606
  Fax: 0207 813 8233
  e-mail: rgilbert@ich.ucl.ac.uk
  http://www.ich.bpmf.ac.uk/ebm/ebm.htm

Centre for Evidence Based Medicine
Aims to promote evidence based health care and provide support and resources to anyone working or interested in the field. The CEBM website contains links to other bodies and organisations.
  Tel: 01865 221321
  http://cebm.jr2.ox.ac.uk/

Centre for Evidence Based Mental Health
Resources for promoting and supporting the teaching and practice of evidence based mental health care, including the journal *Evidence Based Mental Health*, the Royal College of Psychiatrists guidelines in full-text and OXAMWEB (a mental health evidence links site).
  Tel: 01865 226476
  Fax: 01865 793101
  e-mail: cebmh.enquiries@psychiatry.ox.ac.uk
  http://www.psychiatry.ox.ac.uk/cebmh/

Centre for Evidence Based Nursing
Identifies evidence based practice through primary research and systematic reviews and promotes the uptake of evidence into practice through education and implementation activities.
  Tel: 01904 435222/435137
  Fax: 01904 435225
  e-mail: health.matters@pulse.york.ac.uk
  http://www.york.ac.uk/depts/hstd/centres/evidence/ev-intro.htm

Centre for Evidence Based Pharmacotherapy (CEBP)
Researches the methodology of medicines assessment, pharmacoepidemiology and pharmacoeconomics.
  Aston University, Aston Triangle, Birmingham B4 7ET
  Tel: 0121 359 3611
  http://www.aston.ac.uk/pharmacy/cebp/

Centre for Evidence Based Social Services
Aims to improve the knowledge base of social work education and practice and to facilitate the implementation of research findings.
  University of Exeter, Amory Building, Rennes Drive, Exeter, EX4 4RJ
  Tel: 01392 263323
  e-mail: S.E.Bosley@exeter.ac.uk
  http://www.ex.ac.uk/cebss/

Centre for Health Information Quality
Working to support the development of patient information that is clearly communicated, evidence based and involves patients.
  Tel: 01962 863511 ext. 200
  Fax: 01962 849079
  e-mail: enquiries@centreforhiq.demon.co.uk
  http://www.centreforhiq.demon.co.uk/

CRD (NHS Centre for Reviews and Dissemination)
Funded by the NHS as part of their Research and Development Strategy, the CRD aims to review the effectiveness of health care interventions and to disseminate the findings to key decision makers in the NHS and to consumers of health care services.
  Tel:
  01904 433634 (general enquiries)
  01904 433707 (information service)
  http://www.york.ac.uk/inst/crd/welcome.htm

Dynamic Quality Improvement Network (DQI Network)
Part of the RCN's DQI Programme which undertakes a range of activities relating to clinical effectiveness, clinical guidelines, clinical audit and quality improvement.
  http://www.rcn.org.uk/services/promote/quality/quality.htm#dqi

FACTS (Framework for Appropriate Care Throughout Sheffield) Project
A project developing methods to help GPs tackle effectiveness in their practice.
  Tel: 0114 275 5658
  e-mail: Facts@Sheffield.ac.uk
  http://www.shef.ac.uk/uni/projects/facts/

King's Fund
An independent health policy organisation. The King's Fund library is concerned with health care management and organisational development and has a range of 'grey literature'.
  Tel: 0207 307 2400
  Fax: 0207 307 2801
  http:www.kingsfund.org.uk/default.htm

MIDIRS (The Midwives Information and Resource Service)
A charity providing information to health professionals involved in maternity care through a variety of sources.
  Tel: 0800 581009
  e-mail: midirs@dial.pipex.com
  http://www.midirs.org/

National Centre for Clinical Audit (NCCA)
Aims to improve the quality of clinical audit activities within the NHS. Also holds databases. The website and functions of this Centre are being absorbed and incorporated into the National Institute for Clinical Excellence (NICE) (see below).

National Co-ordinating Centre for Health Technology Assessment (NCCHTA)
Funded by the Department of Health, this initiative between the Wessex Institute for Health Research and Development at Southampton University and the University of York aims to support and develop the NHS Health Technology Assessment programme.

The Centre for Health Economics, University of York, York, YO10 5DD
Tel: 01904 433718
e-mail: CHEweb@york.ac.uk
http://www.york.ac.uk/inst/che/2314.htm

National Electronic Library for Health (NELH)
The aims of the NELH are to provide easy access to best current knowledge and to improve health and health care, clinical practice and patient choice. Details of the developing Library and its Virtual Branch Libraries can be found via the website.

http://www.nelh.nhs.uk/
or from

Robert Ward, NHS Information Authority, Room 1 N35C Quarry House, Quarry Hill, Leeds LS2 7UE
Tel: 0113 254 6245
e-mail robward@doh.gov.uk

National Institute for Clinical Excellence (NICE)
A national NHS initiative launched in April 1999. The Institute has been set up to appraise health interventions and will offer clinicians and managers guidance on the best treatments for patients. It will act as a centre of guidance for health professionals in the NHS, as well as patients and the general public. The Institute has also absorbed the functions of the National Centre for Clinical Audit (NCCA).

90 Long Acre, Covent Garden, London WC2E 9RZ
Tel: 0207 849 3444
Fax: 0207 849 3162
e-mail: ncca@ncca.org.uk
http://www.nice.org.uk/

National Institute for Social Work (NISW)
NISW is one of the groups looking after professionals working in the social care and social welfare fields. It provides professional development opportunities and information for both practitioners and users of social care services in the UK. It is involved with the latest initiatives to set up a new National Electronic Library for Social Care, and produces the Caredata abstracts database, now available free to people in Scotland.

http://www.nisw.org.uk/

National Primary Care Research and Development Centre (NPCRDC)
A multi-disciplinary centre aiming to improve primary and community health care in the NHS through the generation, dissemination and application of

knowledge and ideas relevant to the funding, organisation and delivery of health services.

   Tel: 0161 2757633

   Fax: 0161 2757600

   e-mail: maria.cairney@man.ac.uk

   http://www.cpcr.man.ac.uk

PACE (Promoting Action on Clinical Effectiveness)

A three-year programme seeking to investigate whether a co-ordinated approach to implementation can secure changes in clinical behaviour. The PACE Network provides links and a series of publications are available.

   http://www.kingsfund.org.uk/pace/evidence.htm

UK Cochrane Centre

The UK headquarters of the international Cochrane Collaboration. Aims to facilitate, maintain and disseminate systematic, up-to-date reviews of randomised controlled trials of health care.

   Tel: 01865 516300

   Fax: 01865 516311

   e-mail: general@cochrane.co.uk

   http://www.update-software.com/ccweb/default.html

Wisdom Project

A pilot project to create an on-line environment, using the Internet to train primary care professionals in informatics with evidence based practice a focus of the group.

   The WISDOM Centre, Institute of General Practice and Primary Care, Community Sciences Centre, Northern General Hospital, Sheffield S5 7AU.

   Tel: 0114 271 5095

   e-mail: n.j.fox@Sheffield.ac.uk

   http://www.shef.ac.uk/uni/projects/wrp/index.html

INDEX